Textbook of Physiotherapy in Surgical Conditions

AF541827

Textbook of Physiotherapy in Surgical Conditions

Pushpal K Mitra

BSc (Physiotherapy) MIAP SRP (UK) MCSP (UK)
Senior Faculty
National Institute for Orthopaedically Handicapped
Kolkata, West Bengal, India

Examiner and Paper Setter
West Bengal University of Health Sciences, Kolkata, West Bengal, India
Utkal University, Bhubaneshwar, Odisha, India
Patna University, Patna, Bihar, India
Guru Nanak Dev University, Amritsar, Punjab, India
Delhi University, New Delhi, India
Nagpur University, Nagpur, Maharashtra, India

Foreword

SS Rau

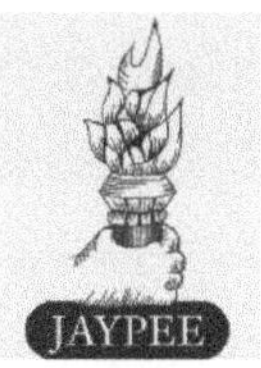

JAYPEE BROTHERS MEDICAL PUBLISHERS
The Health Sciences Publisher
New Delhi | London

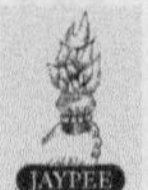

Jaypee Brothers Medical Publishers (P) Ltd.

Headquarters
EMCA House
23/23-B, Ansari Road, Daryaganj
New Delhi 110 002, India
Landline: +91-11-23272143,
+91-11-23272703
+91-11-23282021, +91-11-23245672
E-mail: jaypee@jaypeebrothers.com

Overseas Office

JP Medical Ltd.
83, Victoria Street, London
SW1H 0HW (UK)
Phone: +44-20 3170 8910
E-mail: info@jpmedpub.com

Corporate Office
Jaypee Brothers Medical Publishers (P) Ltd.
4838/24, Ansari Road, Daryaganj
New Delhi 110 002, India
Phone: +91-11-43574357
Fax: +91-11-43574314
E-mail: jaypee@jaypeebrothers.com

EU GPSR Authorised Representative
Logos Europe, 9 rue Nicolas Poussin
17000, La Rochelle, France
Phone: +33 (0) 6 67 93 73 78
E-mail: Contact@logoseurope.eu

Website: www.jaypeebrothers.com
Website: www.jaypeedigital.com

© 2013, Jaypee Brothers Medical Publishers

All rights reserved. No part of this book may be reproduced in any form or by any means without the prior permission of the publisher.

Inquiries for bulk sales may be solicited at: jaypee@jaypeebrothers.com

This book has been published in good faith that the contents provided by the author contained herein are original, and is intended for educational purposes only. While every effort is made to ensure a accuracy of information, the publisher and the author specifically disclaim any damage, liability, or loss incurred, directly or indirectly, from the use or application of any of the contents of this work. If not specifically stated, all figures and tables are courtesy of the author. Where appropriate, the readers should consult with a specialist or contact the manufacturer of the drug or device.

Textbook of Physiotherapy in Surgical Conditions

First Edition: **2013, Reprint: 2025**

ISBN 978-93-5090-206-6

Printed in India

Foreword

The *Textbook of Physiotherapy in Surgical Conditions* written by my colleague Pushpal K Mitra, will be useful for students, practitioners and teaching physiotherapists alike.

The topics covered in this textbook have been explained in a lucid and simple manner, which makes it easy-to-comprehend for the beginners in the profession.

Dr Mitra has used his vast clinical experience in explaining each topic in adequate detail, which enhances the appeal and style of the book.

Each topic is self-explanatory, adorned with ample illustrations and tables, and therefore appropriate for the practitioners and students of physiotherapy.

Practitioners and students of allied disciplines like occupational therapy and even nursing may also find the volume useful for their purpose.

As far as I know, no Indian author has till now written a book on the therapeutic management of surgical conditions, and I appreciate the labor and dedication put in by the author in writing this textbook.

In my opinion, this volume will definitely live up to its promise in helping the new generation of professionals in physiotherapy and allied disciplines.

SS Rau DPT BPT MPT
Professor and Head
Department of Physiotherapy
and Incharge Academics
National Institute for the Orthopaedically Handicapped
Kolkata, West Bengal, India

Foreword

The *Textbook of Pharmacology* [illegible] by my colleague [illegible] will be useful for students, practitioners and teaching physicians [illegible].

The topics covered in this textbook have been explained in a simple and lucid manner, which makes it easy to comprehend for the beginners [illegible].

[illegible] has used his vast clinical experience in explaining each topic in a manner [illegible] which [illegible] style of the book.

Every topic is self-explanatory [illegible] illustrations, [illegible] tables, and mnemonics appropriate for the [illegible] students [illegible] pharmacology.

The students and [illegible] of allied disciplines [illegible] may also find the volume useful for their purpose.

As [illegible] has [illegible] of [illegible] and I [illegible] the author [illegible] for writing the textbook.

In my opinion, this volume will definitely [illegible] in the new generation of [illegible] and allied disciplines.

[illegible]

Professor and Head

[illegible]

National Institute for the Orthopaedically Handicapped [illegible]

[illegible]

Preface

Surgery is an invasion of the living body. It is a veritable blow to the closed environs of the body, upsetting many self-regulating physiological functions, causing anatomical derangement and disfigurement, as well as causing anxiety and depression in the patient.

The adverse outcome of surgery in the short-term are acute pain, hemorrhage, respiratory and circulatory failure, infections, muscle weakness and general debility. In the long-term, it may give rise to complications such as chronic pain, cardiovascular deconditioning, respiratory incompetence, non-healing wounds, incisional hernia, scarring, contractures, deformities and disability.

Preoperative care of the patient focuses on identifying and treating pre-existing disorders that can create problems after the surgery and for preparing the patient's body and mind for the rigors of surgery, so that the postoperative complications can be minimized.

Recovering from a surgery begins from the day after. It is a process that can be both physically and emotionally challenging. The postoperative care focuses on minimizing complications after the surgery, so that the patient can resume normal life at the earliest.

Apart from inputs from the doctor incharge of the case, successful preoperative and postoperative care involves the inputs from nurses, physical therapists and occupational therapists, working as a part of the surgical team.

It has been my experience, that barring one or two exceptions, comprehensive textbooks on role, scope and techniques of therapeutic interventions in general surgery do not exist.

This volume is designed to provide the students and practitioners of nursing, physical therapy and occupational therapy with an insight into various aspects of common abdominal surgery, cardiothoracic surgery, breast surgery, burns and plastic surgery, obstetrics and gynecology.

Information in adequate detail, tailored to meet the needs of the therapists and nurses, has been provided about the indications and contraindications of surgery, outline of surgical procedures adopted and fundamentals of preoperative and postoperative care. It has been my conscious effort to keep the language as simple as possible, drive home a point with the aid of copious illustrations, figures, tables and charts, frequent "Points to ponder" to summarize important issues and an annexure that holds important information in a nutshell. I shall consider my effort amply rewarded if this volume proves to be useful to the students and fellow professionals for whom it has been written.

Pushpal K Mitra

Preface

[illegible]

[illegible]

[illegible]

[illegible]

[illegible]

[illegible]

[illegible]

[illegible]

[illegible]

Acknowledgments

I humbly acknowledge the eager anticipation of my beloved students and encouragement of my colleagues at National Institute for the Orthopaedically Handicapped, Kolkata, West Bengal, India and elsewhere, for providing the motivation to present this volume on applied aspects of physiotherapy.

Acknowledgments

I humbly acknowledge the great inspiration of my beloved students and the encouragement of my colleagues at [illegible] Institute for their [illegible] for providing the opportunity to present this volume on [illegible]

Contents

Chapter

Role and Scope of Physical Rehabilitation after Surgery

Any surgical intervention on the human body is a traumatic event. Undergoing and then recovering from a surgical operation can be both physically and emotionally challenging for the patient. Restoring the patient's health after surgery is the job of the surgeon and the physician. But restoring the patient to gainful and enjoyable life is the task of the postoperative rehabilitation team.

This is achieved through preoperative evaluation to identify potential red flag areas that may lead to postoperative complications, followed by appropriate treatment measures to manage potential trouble before for the surgery.

As soon as the patient has stabilized after surgery, diligent post operative assessment is needed to identify short-term complications, as they develop, and long-term problems, even before they manifest.

It is the responsibility of the entire surgical team—acute care and rehab personnel, to work in tandem to get optimum outcome of the surgery.

Any efficient surgical team works like a symphony orchestra. The surgeon as the leader, like the conductor of an orchestra, guides the team consisting of a group of professionals, each having a specific jurisdiction and set of responsibilities, through the preoperative and postoperative stages of recovery.

Pre- and postoperative care combines the efforts of the nurse, the physical therapist and occupational therapist, apart from the medical and surgical inputs from respective specialists. Final rehabilitation, however may need inputs from medical social worker, clinical psychologist and vocational counselor.

Role and scope of various surgical team members in postoperative rehabilitation process.

ROLE OF NURSING CARE

The embodiment of care in human suffering is the nurse. Every individual patient is unique. So, too, are their needs, the extent and type of care required for them. Understanding physical and mental needs of the patient for optimal well-being is necessary for best care of the patient.

Specially trained nurses are an important part of the surgical team. Apart from assisting the surgeon in the operation theater, they closely monitor the condition of the patient and render care as advised by the surgeon immediately after the surgery and may continue to do so throughout the hospital stay.

On discharge after the surgery, the patient may have specific issues such as catheterization, nasal tube feeding, pressure sore or wound care, all that require follow-up care by a trained nurse. Therefore transitioning from a hospital back home can be difficult without the proper rehabilitation nursing services.

ROLE OF PHYSICAL THERAPY

Physical therapy is a health care profession, which views human movement as central to the health and well-being of an individual.

Physiotherapists treat a patient by stimulating natural healing mechanisms of the body without the use of drugs, to restore the patient to optimum functional ability.

Physiotherapists are expected to identify and maximize movement potential through health promotion, preventive health care, treatment and rehabilitation.

Physiotherapy is a holistic approach to health care, and plays a vital part in pain relief, healing of injured musculoskeletal tissue, improving cardiorespiratory fitness and functional rehabilitation in most surgical conditions.

Physiotherapy has its applications in all most all disciplines of modern surgery— Orthopedics, Neurology, Cardiothoracic, Oncology, Obstetrics and Gynecology, General Surgery, Plastic Surgery and Cosmetic Surgery, etc.

In pre- and postoperative situations, the physiotherapist are required to assess the nature of actual or potential postoperative complication, identify the site and actual cause of a problem and relate it to the complaints and clinical background of the patient before arriving at a working diagnosis.

Once a clinical decision has been made, the situation should be explained to the patient and then the most appropriate therapeutic treatment should be started with the concurrence of the surgeon. The response to the treatment should be reviewed at every treatment session and the therapy modified as required.

Physical therapy should attempt to prevent or treat the common postoperative complications such as postoperative atelectesis, DVT, pressure sores, etc. Physical therapy can also help in minimizing long-term disability in those patients who have lost, partially or totally, cardiopulmonary fitness due to prolonged bed rest or the use of a body part that has been damaged due to the adverse effect of surgery, thereby depriving the patient of functional independence. Physical therapy helps patients to regain fitness, improve muscle strength and postural balance, improve mobility and restore walking skills, and to cope better with the pain and trauma associated with surgery. The benefits of physical therapy are multiple, meaningful and mostly permanent, as each patient can receive help and guidance tailored specifically for his/her individual needs.

ROLE OF OCCUPATIONAL THERAPY

Occupational therapy provides therapeutic benefits through structured activities that are designed to help patients to achieve the best possible level of independence in their daily life. It focuses on training of self-care skills like independent eating and dressing, mobility skills like transferring from bed to wheelchair and wheelchair handling and grooming skills like toileting and bathing.

Occupational therapy intervention also aids in easing emotional stress and promotes social and vocational adjustment necessitated due to permanent loss of function following surgery. All this helps the patient to cope better with the aftermath of a surgery, with or without residual disability and helps early return to work.

ROLE OF PROSTHETICS AND ORTHOTICS

Postoperatively, particularly after trauma or orthopedic reconstruction or following amputation, a patient may become functionally deranged and need external support in the form of simple splints, straps, belts or advanced orthosis. If an Amputee, he will also need a replacement for lost extremity in the form of prosthesis. The prosthetics and orthotics specialist is kept aware of the needs of the patient and has to work closely with the surgical team to assess, take measurements, fabricate the device and prepare the patient before the fitment of the orthotic/prosthetic devices. After fitment of the device, the checkout is done by the physiotherapist in presence of the prosthetics and orthotics engineer to ensure comfortable fit and therefore better compliance in using of the aids and appliances provided.

ROLE OF FOLLOW-UP MEDICAL CARE

After surgery, some medical issues, sometimes pre-existing, may persist with the patient. These issues include long-term complications of surgery itself or pre-existing medical conditions such as diabetes, hypertension, ischemic heart disease, which may complicate the outcome of the surgery. During hospital stay the patient will be monitored on a day to day basis by the house physician. Follow-up with a family physician usually is sufficient once the patient goes home.

ROLE OF DIETETICS AND NUTRITION

After a major surgery, specifically involving the gastrointestinal (GI) tract, a patient may be unable to eat properly and thus become a victim of malnutrition. A qualified dietician is needed to guide the postoperative nutrition plan once the patient is allowed to take oral food. The diet plan will need to workout the Required Daily Intake (RDI) of various foods such as carbohydrates, proteins, fat, essential trace elements and vitamins for a well-balanced nutrition, thus ensuring rapid repair of the body after surgery.

ROLE OF CLINICAL PSYCHOLOGY, VOCATIONAL AND SOCIAL SERVICES

As mentioned earlier, surgery of any kind is a stressful event. This stress multiplies several times when the patient has serious issues such as multiple fractures, burn, cancer, etc. for which extensive surgery is needed. Depression and anxiety are a constant companion of such patient and since morale of the patient in such cases play a great role in the rate of recovery after the surgery, counseling by a qualified clinical psychologist plays a great role in the final outcome of the surgery. Ensuring social support and future economic well-being are within the purview of the social worker and the vocational counselor. Their task may begin well before the surgery and ends only when the patient has been gainfully integrated in the society.

How can Physiotherapy Help after Surgery?

The benefits of physical therapy after any kind of surgery are undisputed. Physiotherapy, a medically oriented therapeutic practice has been around since Ancient Greece. The overall goal of physiotherapy is for the patient to regain a proper degree of normalcy in all aspects of their life after any illness, including surgery.

The physiotherapist needs to interact closely with the surgeon to understand the preoperative needs of the patient, surgical approach planned for surgery, precautions needed, possible postoperative complications, etc. Only then the therapist should evaluate the options available for the rehabilitation process and make an informed decision on the available assessment data.

The principal reasons why someone would need the aid of a physical therapist after surgery are as follows:

1. to control and minimize postoperative pain
2. to promote rapid healing of surgical wounds
3. to reduce respiratory incompetence
4. to combat loss of cardiac conditioning due to prolonged bed rest
5. to strengthen and mobilize weakened and stiff muscles
6. to prevent worsening of pre-existing disorders, such as arthritis.

Each of the above and other similar conditions can benefit greatly from physical therapy.

Broadly postoperative physiotherapy involves the use of:

- Corrective positioning of the body and passive/assisted/active movements of the extremities
- Breathing exercises
- Electrotherapy modalities for pain management, muscle reconditioning, fluid mobilization and tissue healing
- Soft tissue massage to promote blood circulation and lymphatic drainage.

ROLE OF CORRECTIVE POSITIONING AND EXERCISES

Pain, weakness and stiffness arising from prolonged bed rest after surgical operations can greatly decrease the quality of life in an individual. Physical therapists prescribe and demonstrate to the primary caregiver procedures such as proper positioning on bed using rolls and pillows, two hourly turning of the patient from one side to the other and give passive/assistive/active exercises that will prevent contractures and help the patient regain normal use of the body, improve function, reduce pain, and restore mobility.

Individually tailored exercises are prescribed for increasing flexibility, strength, and rebalancing of muscle action, increasing coordination, improving breathing efficiency and restoring function. Progressive resistance exercise programs (PRE) are indicated for postoperative patients in the final stages of recovery. Main benefit of movement therapy concerns secondary joint pain arising from pre-existing disorders such as arthritis.

The therapist will assist the patient in performing exercises and procedures aimed at regaining optimum range of motion that the joint once enjoyed. Usually, joints become stiff due to lack of use because of the pain that patients do not wish to endure. Therefore, the patient should perform activities to loosen up joints that will restore movement and overall ease discomfort.

Abdominal surgeries, which may include removal of diseased gut, ovarian cysts, hernia repairs, hysterectomy, and numerous other techniques, may downgrade abdominal muscle power and efficiency of intra abdominal pressure, so essential for spinal stability, respiratory and circulatory functions. After abdominal surgery, patients tend to decrease their activities to avoid pain, thus allowing muscles of abdomen to weaken further. Weak abdominal muscles lead to poor posture, compromises venous return from lower extremities and reduces diaphragmatic excursion. Simple isometric exercises of the abdominal muscles in most cases can be given once the sutures have healed, if not otherwise forbidden by the surgeon.

A physical therapist will provide a thorough evaluation and help manage the debilitating effects of abdominal surgery. Physical treatment may include some of the following:

- Exercises to perform while in bed during recovery to maintain good blood flow and prevent stiffness.
- Movement techniques to lessen the stretch on the incision.
- Deep breathing and coughing techniques.
- Exercises and self-help techniques to help reduce postsurgical pain from abdominal gas.
- Relaxation training.
- Instructions in home exercises to help promote strengthening of the back, abdominal and pelvic muscles.
- Instructions in wound and skin care, including scar care after healing.
- Instructions in proper lifting and movement techniques to make daily activities safe and easier.

ROLE OF CHEST PHYSIOTHERAPY

Breathing exercises can be used to optimize gas exchange, promote lung expansion, minimize postoperative atelectasis, decrease dyspnea, and promote secretion removal. The postoperative and even preoperative regime of physiotherapy will focus on two major types of breathing exercises with different benefits:

1. Those used to promote lung expansion and minimize atelectasis in individuals with no pre-existing lung disease. These techniques include deep breathing, deep breathing with breath stacking, deep breathing with inspiratory hold, and incentive spirometry.
2. Those used to reduce dyspnea (shortness of breath—SOB), to promote lung expansion and to minimize atelectasis in individuals with moderate to severe chronic respiratory disease such as chronic obstructive pulmonary disease (COPD). These include all of the above techniques in addition to teaching breathing control, minimizing work of breathing, improving exercise tolerance and pursed lip-breathing techniques to cope with severe SOB.

ROLE OF ELECTROTHERAPY

Electrotherapy devices work in different ways, depending on what type of problem they are treating. Certain devices excel at treating pain, while others specialize in muscle rehabilitation and fluid movement.

Electrotherapy in Pain Management

Electrotherapy devices that help control both chronic and acute pain fall into one of three categories: Interferential, Microcurrent, or Transcutaneous Electrical Nerve Stimulation (TENS). Each type of device works in a slightly different way, but they all provide an effective, non-narcotic alternative or supplement to drug therapy.

Interferential Therapy

Interferential therapy devices use two separate electrical frequencies that work together to stimulate large impulse nerve fibers—ones that "close the spinal gate of pain". Their frequencies interfere with the transmission of pain messages at the spinal cord level, and help block their transmission to your brain. Obviously, the fewer pain messages that make it through, the less it hurts. Interferential therapy uses two independent frequencies that deeply penetrate muscles and stimulate parasympathetic nerve fibers for increased blood flow. Like hundreds of tiny rivers, these vessels and capillaries quickly flush out old waste and usher in new blood.

Microcurrent Therapy

Microcurrent therapy is thought to mimic the body's own electrical system. It uses subtle current to build upon naturally occurring impulses to decrease pain. Microcurrent devices take what the patients already have and make it stronger, amplifying the ability to heal oneself, otherwise known as bio-feedback.

Transcutaneous Electrical Nerve Stimulation (TENS)

Transcutaneous electrical nerve stimulation (TENS) devices use a two-pronged approach to pain relief. First, they target sensory nerves, stimulating them to block pain signals and prevent their transmission to the brain. Second, TENS also promotes production of endorphins, the body's natural pain reducing substances. Because of its effectiveness, TENS therapy is routinely used to treat back and cervical muscular and disk syndromes, RSD, arthritis, shoulder syndromes, neuropathies and other painful conditions. It is also a very effective replacement for narcotic analgesics, often a habit forming drug used to control postoperative pain. However, to be effective in postoperative pain TENS may be needed to be applied continuously at the operation site, through surface electrodes fixed on either sides of the suture line and that the patient may not take any narcotic analgesic at all before or after surgery.

Electrotherapy in Muscle Rehabilitation

Neuromuscular Stimulation

It is a fact that exercise is good for you. Whether you are biking, walking or playing tennis, your movements are a carefully choreographed series of muscular contractions. Each contraction begins as an electrical impulse generated by your body. Only through repeated motion do your muscles stay strong and healthy.

When injury sets in, muscles become stationary. Fluid builds up between the cells and they begin to lose their strength. Electrotherapy has the ability to counter these effects through neuromuscular stimulation (NMS) and high or low voltage pulsed direct current therapy.

An injured muscle usually experiences little-if any-movement. NMS therapy remedies this by using low-voltages to stimulate motor nerves to cause involuntary muscular contractions. Neuromuscular therapy induces muscle contractions which pump fluid through both the venous and lymphatic systems. This helps to resolve the swelling or fluid build-up in the area. NMS devices have the ability to increase or decrease the strength of each muscular contraction.

Like exercise, NMS helps to strengthen the injured area and has been found to effectively treat a variety of musculoskeletal and vascular conditions. Common candidates for NMS therapy are patients recovering from orthopedic surgery, muscle strains or tears, or athletes who have undergone cartilage or tendon repair.

High or Low Voltage Pulsed Direct Current Therapy

Injured tissues are often surrounded by an excess of fluid, which prevents nutrient- and oxygen-rich blood from reaching them. Pulsed direct current devices remove excess fluid and increase blood flow to the injured site to encourage return to normal function. Fluid (swelling) is primarily composed of negatively-charged proteins. Placing a positive electrode over the injured site within the first 24–48 hours helps prevent the build-up of excess fluid. A negative electrode placed over the injured site after the first day or two causes the fluid to disperse from the site of the inflammation. This treatment reduces swelling, allowing new blood to move in and speeding up the recovery process. High voltage pulsed direct current therapy utilizes two oppositely charged electrodes to move the plasma proteins, which comprise excess fluid and leak into spaces between cells. Initially, the stimulus prevents fluid build-up. Later, using a different protocol, it repels fluid that has built-up.

Electrotherapy in Fluid Movement

Excessive fluid build-up, known as edema, is detrimental to any healing process. Not only does it cause swelling around the injured area, but it also prevents removal of waste products and hinders circulation. Electrotherapy uses Interferential, NMS, and high or low voltage pulsed direct current devices or faradism under pressure to move excess fluid from injured areas back to the circulation.

Interferential Therapy

Interferential therapy uses two independent frequencies that deeply penetrate muscles and stimulate parasympathetic nerve fibers for increased blood flow. Like hundreds of tiny rivers, these vessels and capillaries quickly flush out old waste and usher in new blood.

High or low voltage Pulsed Direct Current Therapy

High voltage pulsed direct current therapy utilizes two oppositely charged electrodes to move the plasma porteins, which comprise excess fluid and leak into spaces between cells. Initially, the stimulus prevents fluid build-up. Later, using a different protocol, it repels fluid that has built-up.

Neuromuscullar Stimulation

Neuromuscullar therapy induces muscle contractions which pump fluid through both the venous and lymphatic systems. This helps to resolve the swelling or fluid build-up in the area. NMS devices have the ability to increase or decrease the strenth of each muscullar contraction.

ROLE OF MANUAL THERAPY, MASSAGE STRAPPING AND ACUPUNCTURE

1. Manual therapy and massage also called Hands on Treatment which includes passive mobilizing of joints, manipulation of joints, mobilization with movement, soft tissue techniques and manual traction with or without aids. A massage given by a physical therapist can help in any number of ways. For overall health, the benefits of the professional massage can reduce stress by unknotting muscles and causing the body to relax. Massages will even improve blood circulation, lymphatic drainage, range of motion and increase flexibility (Fig. 1.1).

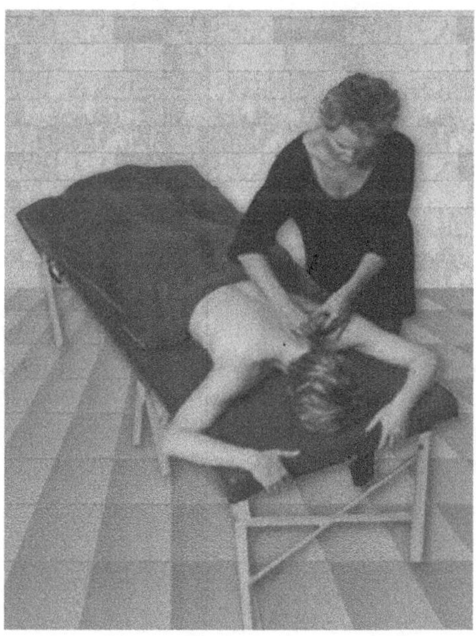

Fig. 1.1: Massage

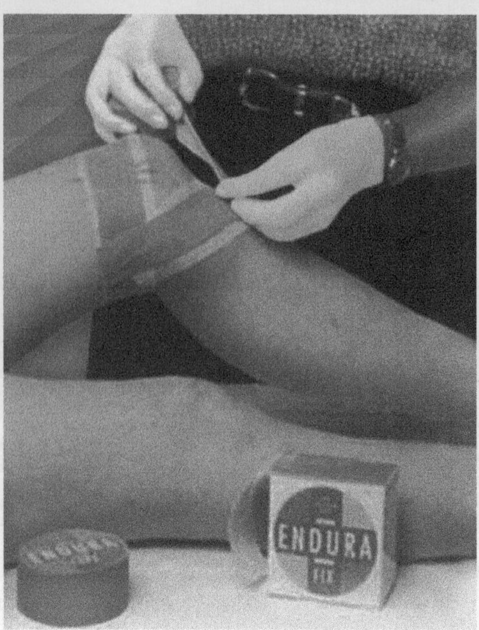

Fig. 1.2: Taping of the knee joint

2. Strapping techniques are a component of manual therapy which is very useful to rest painful tissues, if required. Sports taping techniques and manual therapy taping techniques, e.g. mulligan taping are commonly used following soft tissue release and repair surgeries (Fig. 1.2).
3. Soft tissue compression techniques such as Crepe bandage, Jones compression bandage, Jobst compression garments and intermittent pressure therapy help in preventing edema, minimizing scar formation and hypertrophy of scar along with controlling edema.

Acupuncture in Postoperative Care

Modern acupuncture with research back-up is practiced widely in physiotherapy as an effective modality for pain management. Acupuncture in postoperative cases is mainly sought for pain relief. Auriculotherapy or ear acupuncture is gaining wide acceptance in physiotherapy techniques used in surgical and traumatic conditions. Cold laser or low frequency TENS is often used to stimulate the acupuncture points as it is a sterile and safe procedure.

Chapter 2

Principles of Pre- and Postoperative Physiotherapy

An operation is like an athletic event. Before participating in any competitive event an athlete has to undergo extensive preparation under the close supervision of the trainer or coach. All athletes have some degree of natural talent and aptitude for the sport of his/her choice. The job of the trainer or the coach is to fine-tune this natural talent, detect the weaknesses in the athlete's skill, level of fitness, ability to avoid injuries and suggest ways and means to remedy these weaknesses for achieving success in the competition.

Similarly, when a patient is planned for surgery, a detailed preoperative evaluation, planning and training is mandatory to ensure succeess. Preoperative assessment is done primarily to evaluate the patient's general condition and level of cardiorespiratory fitness to undergo anesthesia. During these checkups one has to also look for potential risk factors such as pre-existing systemic disorders such as hypertension, chronic obstructive pulmonary disease (COPD) and diabetes; pre-existing reginal disorders such as arthritis, soft tissue tightness, contracture or deformities; history of smoking or alcoholism, obesity and bleeding disorders, any or all of which may adversely affect the outcome of the surgery. Preoperative asessment is mainly done by the anesthetist and in some cases by the physiotherapist as well. Preoperative screening of the patient by the physiotherapist primarily looks at patients musculoskeletal movement, cardiopulmonary fitness, including the extent of deconditioning because of being bedridden due to the actual disease process and must also include inputs regarding pre-existing co-morbidities such as COPD, arthritis, rheumatism, vascular disorders, etc. which may result in serious postoperative complications.

During preoperative physiotherapy assessment the therapist should specifically look for the following:

- *Respiratory issues* such as impaired air entry, inability to cough and clear secretions from the airway effectively.
- *Lifestyle issues* such as sedentary habits, obesity, smoking and alcohol abuse.
- *Cardiovascular issues* such as reduced exercise tolerance due to deconditioning, chest pain, varicosity, risk for developing deep vein thrombosis and persistent edemas of the feet or hands.

- *Musculoskeletal issues* such as arthritis, contractures, tightness and deformity and muscular weakness or incompetence, specifically related to the site of the operation and the extremities affected directly after the operation.

The outcome of this assessment must be recorded in the preoperative checkup report so that the entire surgical team, in particular the therapists in the team, will be aware of potential complications that may develop after surgery and take appropriate preventive measures before the operation to minimize the adverse effects of such pre-existing dysfunctions.

The idea behind preoperative assessment and management is to prepare the patient to the best possible level of physical competence to undergo the planned surgery and come out with best possible outcome. Therefore spending time and effort for preoperative therapy in the long run is extremely valuable for getting excellent outcome of an operation.

However, in case of surgical emergencies, such meticulous preoperative preparation is not feasible because there is simple no time available to perform this preoperative regimen. Under such circumstances the therapist has to anticepate, detect and tackle each complication as and when they develop, as early as possible, to the best of his/her skill, ability and resources available.

Respiratory Issues Needing Specific Attention of the Therapist

The deterioration of respiratory muscle function after spinal, brain, thoracic and abdominal surgeries contribute significantly to poor pulmonary function and this leads to the incidence of postoperative respiratory complications, increasing rate of morbidity and mortality in all types of surgical cases.

The onset and severity of postoperative pulmonary complications depend as much on the type of anesthesia as on the nature of the surgical procedure itself. The incidence of postoperative pulmonary complications is most common after general anesthesia and is more frequent after upper abdominal and thoracic surgeries. Among the important pathophysiological changes created by general anesthesia are hypoventilation, suppression of cough reflex and depression of cilliary activity, which contribute to retention of secretions in the lungs and CO_2 in the blood. Inhibition of chest expansion due to stretch pain of the sugrical wound and reduced respiratory muscular activity contribute significantly to development of common postoperative pulmonary complications such as reductions in pulmonary flows and volumes, leading to atelectasis, reduced cough efficiency, increased work of breathing.

Active smokers have an increased risk of postoperative pulmonary complications. They present a higher incidence of expectoration and a greater occurrence of pulmonary complications in the postoperative phase.

In general one of the primary preoperative requirements is cessation of the smoking habit.

Aims and Objectives of Preoperative Exercise Training of Respiratory Muscles

The programs of preoperative respiratory muscular training aims at preventing postoperative dysfunction in respiratory muscles, mostly through strengthening exercises. These are programmed activities that increase the load imposed on a respiratory muscle pump, through increments in frequency, duration and intensity of muscular contraction and, as in training of any skeletal muscle, obey physiological principles of muscular training.

The specific training of respiratory muscles can be obtained through breathing exercises with and without additional load, which increases muscular work, requiring greater effort. The breathing exercises can be done either by use of selected and controlled free breathing exercises or with breathing done through different apparatuses. In load-free breathing exercises done under voluntary control, it is possible to obtain adequate contraction of the muscles of inspiration, as well as expiration, that modify the rate, volume and depth of respiration.

The oscillation of pressure gradients and the modifications in chest-wall conformation, by pressure applied manually or through elastic strap, facilitate a selective distribution of airflow in the lungs, depending on the muscular groups activated and with the posture adopted by the patient.

In exercises done with apparatuses, the additional load is offered through systems with linear or nonlinear loads, against which the patient produces respiratory efforts. The utilization of additional loads permits better control of work intensity, since it is possible to adjust the load according to individual differences, contrary to respiratory exercises without additional load. Preoperative muscular training with apparatuses has been employed with the proposition of increasing respiratory muscular strength.[1]

The time of preoperative preparation described by different authors varies according to the program. Orientation programs are usually brief and can be done moments before the surgical procedures or a few days before surgery. However, the training programs prescribed before two weeks or more can significantly improve pulmonary function before surgery. Among other factors, the urgency of surgical procedure, the necessity or not of previous hospitalization and the viability of costs, also influence the time of preoperative preparation.[1,2] Respiratory exercises applied preoperatively for respiratory muscle training are useful in the prevention of pulmonary complications; however, its effect may vary in individuals with specific risk factors for developing postoperative pulmonary complications such as tobacco smoking.

Essential Preoperative Pulmonary Evaluation

The evaluation of pulmonary function is done through Spirometry and specifically through measurement of maximum inspiratory and expiratory pressures (PI max and PE max).

The Spirometry may done with the patient seated, using a portable spirometer to evaluate forced vital capacity in liters (FVC), forced expiratory volume in the first second in liters (FEV_1), inspiratory and expiratory peak flow in liters/sec (IPF and EPF) and maximum voluntary ventilation in L/min (MVV, L/min).

Protocol of Exercises to Improve Ventilation

i. *Diaphragmatic re-education*—Slow nasal inspiration and oral expiration aiming for an increased excursion of the diaphragm, observed through elevation of the abdomen and lateral expansion of the thorax. Repeat 15 times in one sitting.

ii. *Deep inspiration exercises*—Deep nasal inspiration until reaching the TLC followed by one oral expiration after a short pause of breath holding. During inspiration the arms are elevated. Repeat 15 times in one sitting.

iii. *Inspiratory hiccups*—Short and successive inspirations through nose, without holding breath, until reaching TLC, followed by a smooth expiration through open mouth, until resting state is reached, with the patient seated supporting the thorax laterally with the palms of the hands, creating a light pressure during expiration. Repeat 15 times in one sitting.

iv. *Resistive inspiration with linear pressure load*—Incentive spirometer may be used. The load utilized may vary from 30 to 50 percent of the value of PI max. Three series of 15 repetitions in one sitting with intervals for rest.

Specific Preoperative Preparation Needed for a Patient With COPD Needing General Anesthetic

History-taking and Assessing

During history taking, following information will be required concerning the disease:

- The length of time the person has suffered from COPD and how his/her condition is being treated, paying particular attention to the drugs that are being used coupled with the procedure/s for monitoring responses to these drugs and how stable, or unstable, the person's condition is or has been.
- To what extent the person understands his/her condition and is able to cooperate with the aims of treatment. An enquiry should be made concerning any previous experience involving anesthesia and surgical

procedures, paying attention to any difficulties that they have been experienced.

- Questioning can be tiring for someone who is breathless. Therefore keeping questions brief and to the point and asking only close ended questions whenever possible will lessen the degree of effort that has to be made.

While gathering information, an assessment will be taking place concerning the person's mental state. Hypoxia, if present, can impede mental performance. The degree of alertness and how well-orientated the person is, and the degree of knowledge and understanding they have concerning their proposed operation, are important observations to make.

Lifestyle Issues Needing Specific Attention of the Therapist

People who are classed as severely obese run a greater risk of developing complications while undergoing surgery. It is seen that the risk of a cardiac arrest before or during surgery is higher in obese patients. In addition, severely overweight individuals are in greater danger of developing noncardiac complications after operations and prolonged hospital stays than nonobese patients.[3]

Cardiac Issues Needing Specific Attention of the Therapist

- *Myocardial ischemia or infarction*—This is the leading cause of perioperative death.
- *Arrhythmias*—Can be caused by underlying heart disease or imbalance of electrolytes (particularly potassium), as well as due to acid-base abnormalities. The management of such arrhythmia is to correct the underlying cause.

Cardiac complications pose one of the most significant risks to patients undergoing major noncardiac surgery, mainly due to physiological factors such as blood loss, increased myocardial oxygen demand arising from raised heart rate and blood pressure due to stress from surgery, and an increase in postoperative platelet fragility.[1,2]

Three elements must be assessed to determine the risk of cardiac events:

- Patient specific clinical variables
- Exercise tolerance
- Surgery specific risk.

Patient specific clinical variables: A detailed history inquiring about previous ischemia, congestive heart failure, aortic stenosis, severe hypertension, and peripheral vascular disease, anxiety disorders, if any, is essential for effective risk assessment.

Exercise tolerance: An assessment of cardiac functional status may be performed. Patients with good functional status usually have a lower risk of complications. This measurement can be done easily by the therapist and expressed in metabolic equivalent (MET) levels. Risk of cardiac arrest during surgery is increased in patients unable to meet a 4MET demand during most normal daily activities.[3]

Indicators of cardiac competence related to functional status include the following:

- Can take care of self, such as eat, dress or use the toilet (1 MET)
- Can walk up a flight of steps or a hill (4 METS)
- Can do heavy work around the house such as scrubbing floors or lifting or moving heavy furniture (between 4 and 10 METS)
- Can participate in strenuous sports such as swimming, singles tennis, football, basketball, and skiing (>10 METS).

An important limitation to assessment of functional capacity as related to cardiac function is that, patients with vascular diseases often cannot complete exercise because of cramps in calf.

Predicting Risk of Cardiac Complications Before Surgery

Patients having two or more vascular risk factors often face a significant possibility of suffering a major cardiovascular complication and should be kept in a surgical ICU and monitored for at least 48 hours, taking serial readings of cardiac markers such as troponin. Myocardial infarction is the most common major cardiovascular complication, with most of those patients showing little or no sign of classical angina.

Surgery specific risk: The type and timing of surgery significantly affects the patient's risk of cardiac complications during surgery. Death due to cardiac arrest and nonfatal MI rate is greater than five percent, particularly in the elderly patients undergoing emergency major operations. Patients undergoing vascular surgery are likely fall into a high-risk category.[3]

Intermediate risk is generally less than five percent in patients undergoing surgical procedures such as carotid endoarterectomy, head and neck surgery, intraperitoneal and intrathoracic surgery, orthopedic surgery and prostate surgery.

Low risk is generally less than one percent in patients undergoing the surgical procedures such as endoscopy procedures and cataract removal (See also Annexure 2.1).

Vascular Issues Needing Specific Attention of the Therapist

Any surgical intervention in the thorax, abdomen or in the long bones of the extremities can upset the efficiency of venous return from the distal most points of the body to the central circulation. This happens because of multiple postoperative factors such as inhibition of the autonomic reflexes controlling vascular tone, increased viscosity of blood, increased bleeding time, reduced clotting time and increased platelet count and clotting factors in blood. All or some of these factors may lead to stasis or pooling of blood in the calf that may lead to formation of a deep vein thrombosis (DVT). Additional risk factors for developing DVT are diabetes, smoking, hyperlipidemia, and the principle causes are prolonged bed rest or injury to the inner lining of the veins due to pressure on the calf on the edge of the operating table while under anesthesia during the surgery or indirect traumas causing injury to the intima of the calf veins. A clot may develop gradually within the lumen of deep veins without any overt symptoms. Such clot may break off at its tip to form an embolus that is carried by the bloodstream to cause an embolic stroke in the heart or the brain. This is a silent condition that is very difficult to detect till it has been well-established and even more difficult to treat. Hence, prevention is always better than cure in case of DVT. In the preoperative stage the therapist must advise the patient to do ankle-foot pumping exercise five times every hour as long as he is awake. In patients who are confined to bed may be advised to put on pressure stocking to facilitate venous return. Active exercises in conscious patients or passive movements to the lower extremities in case of unconscious or paralyzed patients, done throughout the full ROM are the best possible prophylaxis for DVT. The therapist in course of his daily rounds should dorsiflex the foot of the postoperative or bed ridden patient to detect presence of any pain in the calf. Pain in the calf with forceful dorsiflexion is called the Homan's sign. In case Homan's sign is positive, i.e. a DVT is suspected, all therapeutic exercises must cease immediately and the physician informed. Primary management of DVT includes administration of anticoagulants such as intravenous heparin. This in itself is a dangerous modality in immediate postoperative stage due to risk of triggering hemorrhage. The physician has to weigh the risk and benefit and take the most appropriate course of action.

Musculoskeletal Issues in the Postoperative Stage Needing Specific Attention of the Therapist

Pre-existing musculoskeletal disorders such as periarthritis of the shoulder or degenerative joint disorders of the spine and lower limb joints may worsen after surgery.

- In specific surgical conditions such as mastectomy or thoracotomies, a pre-existing shoulder pain and stiffness can get worse due to postoperative immobilization of the shoulder on the affected side, as usually seen in case of radical mastectomy.
- Pain inhibition may be another cause of stiffness of shoulder and secondary scoliosis of spine on the operated side in case of high level thoracotomies. The cervical spine may also be similarly affected in such cases.

- Muscles controlling the shoulder girdle may be divided during the mastectomy or thoracotomies, resulting in weakness and therefore inefficiency of function of the entire shoulder girdle.
- Incision of the abdominal wall invariably weakens the core muscles, resulting in increased lumbar lordosis and sometimes scoliosis. Such derangement of spinal alignment may give rise to or worsen pre-existing chronic low back pain.

The therapist is expected to anticipate such problems before they develop and take preventive measures in the form of posture toning exercises to maximize the functional efficiency of the spine.

Objective Preoperative Assessment

This includes:

- Recording the temperature, pulse, blood pressure and respiratory rate (baseline clinical recordings)
- Testing and charting a specimen of urine
- Measuring the person's weight
- Assessing the person's skin condition (particularly important if the person's mobility is restricted, and also if the person's skin is compromised, e.g. as a result of taking steroids)
- Peak flow recordings (pre- and postnebulizer/inhaler/s)
- Recording of oxygen saturation levels
- Sputum culture and sensitivity tests may be required, particularly if the person has a productive cough
- The anesthetist may need pulmonary function studies, which will be equally useful for the therapist.

Planning Postoperative Care

A care plan will need to be developed which addresses the potential trouble spots uncovered during the assessment process and also to incorporate specifics such as whether a conventional general anesthesia or a spinal or epidural procedure is to be performed. Opinion may be taken from the physiotherapist, the respiratory nurse specialist, and the theater nurse who is to be responsible for the person's postoperative care regarding the pro and the con of the type of anesthesia in the individual concerned. These members of the care team will need to visit the patient before the operation, introduce themselves and discuss the part each of them will play during the preoperative and postoperative periods.

Implementing

Preoperative information and education contributes greatly to the reduction of stress and anxiety of the patients, common in hospital admission for whatever reason and even more so when scheduled for surgery.

For someone who has underlying respiratory disease, the degree of insecurity and anxiety experienced while waiting for surgery can be quite intense. Information needs to be given to the patient regarding procedures that will be performed and the difficulties to be expected in the postoperative period. If the patient is aware what physical discomforts and limitations to expect just after the surgery and in the days thereafter, he/she is likely to be better prepared mentally and will have less stress and anxiety.

Chest physiotherapy, along with maintenance exercises that need to be carried out postoperatively, must be taught to the patient early in the preoperative stage and the importance of these exercises in uneventful recovery must be stressed by the therapist repeatedly during each training session.

Additional Points to Consider

People with asthma, chronic bronchitis and emphysema tend to have irritable airways. Endotracheal intubations during general anesthesia and nasogastric tubes may injure the upper respiratory passage and provoke coughing attacks as soon as the patient is concious. Inhaled oxygen and anesthetic gases used in general anesthesia dries the mucus membrane and can also act as irritants to the bronchial mucosa triggering hypersecretion of mucus. Adequate humidification of the inhaled gasses during anesthesia can reduce this adverse effect of general anesthesia.

General Postoperative Complications and its Care

All patients having an operation under general anesthesia (GA) are in a potentially unstable cardiorespiratory state. Close monitoring of the cardiopulmonary system is therefore essential in the immidiate post operative stage. Patients usually need inhaled oxygen guided by O_2 saturation levels, IV fluid support, monitoring and correction of the fluid-electrolyte balance.

The acute care of the postoperative patient does not end when the patient's eyes open after anesthesia. It is a continuous process, starting 24 hours before surgery and continues into the early recovery period, when most complications are expected to occur and when adequate analgesia is of utmost importance. The postoperative recovery room should be a warm, well lit area close to the operating theaters, where patients are allowed to calmly reorient themselves and are monitored after coming out of anesthesia. Nursing staff monitor vital signs, such as heart rate and rhythm, blood pressure, respiratory rate, oxygen saturations, temperature, fluid input, urine output and level of consciousness. They also assess the level of patient's pain and gives analgesics as advised to keep the pain at bare minimum level. Adequate analgesia is one of the main pre-conditions for rapid improvement in patients condition after surgery. Once the anesthetist is satisfied that the patient is hemodynamically stable, following the criteria

Table 2.1: Criteria that a patient should meet before transfer to the ward
• Independendly maintains a secure airway with intact airway reflexes (cough) • Spontaneously breathing with adequate oxygen saturations • Hemodynamically stable (a patient whose cardiac output and rate is stable) • Awake, not febrile and pain free (often with sufficient analgesia)

Table 2.2: Signs of airway obstruction
• Stridor—Audible statorous breathing • Tachypnea (rapid respiration rate), sometimes with tachycardia (rapid pulse rate) • Tracheal tug (downward displacement of trachea during inspiration) • Use of accessory muscle during inspiration • Caving in of the intercostals and supraclavicular muscles during inspiration • Persistent reduced oxygen saturation (SaO_2) and later on hypoxemia (PaO_2)

laid down in Table 2.1 as a guide, plans are made for transfer the patient to the ward.

Most of the postoperative patients may experience some or other complications immidiately after the surgery. Postoperative recovery rooms, with adequate infrastructure in terms of staff, equipment and medication are essential in tackling such complications rapidly.

Although problems are usually minor, like nausea or vomiting, in some cases, airway obstruction, cardiorespiratory distress or hemorrhage may appear and such issues may require immediate expert attention and specialized care, which is easily imparted in a postoperative recovery room.

Common Respiratory Complications

Airways obstruction: It may be caused by many factors, including laryngospasm, soft tissue swelling around the pharynx (often in children), foreign bodies (loose teeth), hypotonia of pharyngeal muscles from the residual effect of anesthetic, and viscous fluids blood in the airway, especially from maxillofacial surgery. The signs of an obstruction to the airway are given in (Table 2.2). In all patients developing airways obstruction, a patent airway must be achieved immediately with a head tilt chin lift positioning, and using airways adjuncts like oropharyngeal tubes and suction, or if required endotracheal intubations.

Hypoventilation: The reduction in the ventilatory capacity of the lungs can be caused either by a depressed respiratory drive or by mechanical obstruction in breathing. Common causes of a reduced respiratory drive include the effect of anesthetics, opioid pain killing drugs, hypothermia and a metabolic alkalosis secondary to intermittent positive pressure ventilation. Impaired chest expansion can result from lung disease such as COPD due to smoking; (Table 2.3), muscle weakness arising from electrolyte imbalance, inhibition of diaphragm movement due to incission pain

Table 2.3: Postoperative complications in patients with pre-existing lung disease
• Develop severe pneumonias after general anesthesia • Need prolonged ventilatory support • Have greater mortality rate • Smoker need care in high dependence surgical recovery area for longer duration • Asthmatics may have exacerbations from histamine releasing anesthetic gasses

or obesity and the residual effect of paralyzing muscle relaxants on the chest wall musculature.

Hypoxemia: The PaO_2 may be lower than that expected in a postoperative patient. Thoracic and abdominal surgery can have huge effects on the expansibility of the chest, leading to a substantial drop in the oxygen saturations of blood. The principal causes of postoperative hypoxemia include:

1. A reduced inspired oxygen fraction was more common when nitrous oxide was frequently used in anesthesia, whereby the speed of air entry into the alveolar spaces was far quicker than the speed at which nitrogen could diffuse out. A so-called "diffusion hypoxia" occurred from the relative dilution of the surrounding oxygen fraction.
2. Hypoventilation (described above)
3. Ventilation or perfusion mismatch (for example, lung collapse or atelectasis, bronchospasm, pulmonary edema, pneumothorax, and pulmonary embolism).

Hypovolemia

Changes in blood pressure are common postoperative complications. Loss of fluid from the intravascular space due to bleeding and extra vascular space due to vomiting, diarrhea, and sweating leading to generalized dehydration can contribute to a hypovolemic state (Table 2.4). Patients in the postoperative period may often be profoundly dehydrated because of their general ill health and catabolic state, as well as being "nil by mouth" before surgery. Dilatation of blood vessels through relaxation of smooth muscle in the vessel wall also contributes to a reduced blood pressure; the residual effect of general anesthetic agents can cause this postoperatively. Finally, leaky blood vessels and the subsequent seepage of intravascular fluid may occur due to sepsis and anaphylaxis. These patients are often very ill and aggressive fluid management in addition to other measures are needed to restore their hemodynamic stability.

The prescription of fluid treatment should always be given in light of following clinical signs (Table 2.5).

- Loss of skin turgidity.
- The tongue dry and furry.

Table 2.4: Causes of extraordinary fluid loss in postoperative patients: in addition to normal fluid loss

Kidney	*Gastrointestinal tract*	*Physiological and emotional*	*Vascular*
Drug induced Impaired renal Tubular function increasing clearance of fluid and reducing reabsorption of fluid and electrolytes	Reduced oral intake of fluid; in patients under "nil by mouth" instruction before and after operation	Hyperventilation due to pain and anxiety	Hemorrhage
Diabetes insipidus	Increased fluid and electrolyte loss due to vomiting, nasogastric aspiration, fistula and diarrhea Acid-base imbalance; hypoacidity in pyloric stenosis, hyper-alkalinity in pancreatic fistula Hidden causes; intestinal obstruction	Fever and sweating	

Table 2.5: Ordinary fluid input and output over 24 hours in a healthy 70 kg adult

In	Food—1000 ml, Drink—1200 ml, Metabolic oxidation—300 ml
Out	Urine—1500 ml, Feces—100 ml, Insensible (respiration and sweating)—900 ml
Total	In and out—2500 ml

- The patient peripherally shut down with cold and clammy skin and a prolonged capillary refill time (press on the nail bed and note the time taken for the blanching to diminish).
- Abnormal sweating and tachycardia.
- A persistently low urine output (< 0.5 ml/kg/hour) may be an indication of inadequate fluid replacement, and this needs prompt treatment to avoid renal compromise (known as prerenal failure).

Intravenous fluid replacement and a urinary catheter are often used as simple, first line measures in the management of hypovolemia.

Oliguria

Urine retention due to obstruction of the urinary catheter is the common cause of oliguria. In the postoperative period, low limit of urine output is about 35 ml/hour in a 70 kg adult. Always flush the catheter with 10 ml normal saline as a first step. Acute tubular necrosis due to acute ischemia following prolonged hypoperfusion of the renal parenchyma due to

Table 2.6: Clinical assessment of hypovolemia in a 70 kg patient

Blood loss (ml)	≤ 750	750–1500	1500–2000	≥ 2000
Blood loss (% of blood volume)	≤ 15	15–30	30–40	≥ 40
Heart rate (beats/min)	< 100	> 100	> 1–20	≥ 140
Blood pressure	Normal	Normal	Reduced	Reduced
Pulse pressure	Normal	Reduced	Reduced	Reduced
Capillary return	Normal (< 2s)	Prolonged	Prolonged	Prolonged
Respiratory rate (breaths/min)	14–20	20–30	30–40 ≥ 35	
Urine output (ml/hour)	> 30	20–30	5–15	Negligible
Mental status	Normal	Anxious	Confused	Drowsy

hypovolemia (prerenal failure) may also cause oliguria. It can also be caused by toxic injury; antibiotics, such as gentamicin, and nonsteroidal anti-inflammatory drugs are common culprits. So, one should always review the drug chart to look for clues.

Thirst as an Important Early Warning Sign

Extracellular dehydration, which occurs commonly in the postoperative period, is detected by cardiovascular receptors, such as the pressure receptors in the aortic arch and carotid sinus, and volume receptors in the atria and large veins of the thorax. A patient is often asymptomatic until the circulating volume of blood has decreased by at least 10 percent—only then may the patient become thirsty. Remember that a patient complaining of thirst may be giving you an early warning of ensuing shock. All other vital signs are still within normal range at this stage (Table 2.6).

Pathophysiology of Hypovolemic Shock

Vasoconstriction squeezes blood from the capacitance vessels, mostly leg veins, back into the heart to maintain cardiac filling and the resultant output. Subsequently, the vasculature of certain noncritical organs like the gastrointestinal system and skin is shut down through controlled vasoconstriction in favor of perfusing the critical organs like the brain and heart. Simultaneously, fluid from the extravascular space is moved back into the circulation to maintain a filling pressure.

Once the circulating intravascular volume is critically reduced, the perfusion of distal tissues becomes compromised and tissue ischemia occurs. Hypoperfusion of the brain causes nonspecific neurological symptoms, such as confusion. Remember that elderly people tend to decompensate much earlier than young people, partly because of the inability of smooth muscle in the blood vessel wall to contract efficiently. In addition, the dilatation of blood vessels secondary to the effects of general anesthetic agents may precipitate cardiovascular collapse in elderly patients with volume depletion; extra caution is always needed.

Fluid Replacement Therapy

I have described above the complications that result from hypovolemia. Conversely, however, excessive fluid loading, particularly in patients with renal failure can induce congestive heart failure due to fluid overload.

A formula given below is used to estimate the quantity of fluid needed for replacement is:

Replacement fluid = Resuscitation + Maintenance + Losses (including hidden, third space).

Requirements of maintenance fluid are 1.5–2 ml/kg/hour, i.e. between 2.5 and 3.5 liters in 24 hours for a 70 kg adult, irrespective of the type of surgical procedure a patient is undergoing. Daily maintenance of sodium is 1–2 mmol/kg/day (140 mmol a day) and potassium 1 mmol/kg/day (70 mmol a day). If blood has been lost, the volume of normal (0.9%) saline replacement needed is three times that of the estimated blood loss (only a third of the volume remains intravascular). If a considerable amount of blood is lost, replacement with whole blood is optimal. An example of a maintenance fluid regimen is one bag of saline (1 liter contains about 150 mmol sodium) and two bags of 5 percent dextrose; 20 mmol potassium can be added to each of the three bags.

To calculate losses, you need the weight of the patient and the suspected percentage loss in blood volume (Table 2.6). For example, consider a 70 kg patient with an estimated 10 percent circulation volume loss. Since 60 percent of body weight is water (70 × 0.6 = 42 liters) 10 percent circulatory volume loss equates to 42 × 0.1 = 4.2 liters. This needs to be replaced, in addition to the maintenance requirements of about 3 liters per day.

A fluid challenge in the form of an intravenous bolus of a fixed volume of crystalloid or colloid is often used both to assess and treat volume depletion, particularly in acutely ill patients. Monitoring the central venous pressure during this is often helpful for guiding further administration of fluid. For example, if the central venous pressure rises and then falls after a fluid challenge, more fluid is needed.

Which Fluid?

- Crystalloids are electrolytes dissolved in water. One example, normal (0.9%) saline, tends to disperse into the extracellular spaces after its intravascular administration because of the sodium content. Five percent dextrose is essentially water (the sugar is metabolized very quickly) and this disperses throughout the intracellular and extracellular compartments; it has little use as a resuscitative fluid.
- Colloids contain high molecular weight molecules and can be natural (albumin) or synthetic (gelofusin); they remain in the intravascular space for longer and are, therefore, used when maintaining sufficient blood pressure is the priority.

- With substantial bleeding however replacement with whole blood is optimal. A blood sample is needed for the transfusion department to make the correct cross-matched units of blood for infusion, and this takes about an hour. If the patient needs immediate resuscitation with blood, then one can give type O negative.

Hypertonic saline is becoming increasingly popular in recent times since it has the ability to move fluid from the body's own extravascular space, drawing fluid into the circulation across a sodium gradient.

Neurological Complications after Anesthesia

Delayed Emergence from Anesthesia

Delayed emergence can be caused by:

- Perioperative opiate analgesia and anxiolytics. These cause respiratory depression and hypoxia, resulting in a confused and disorientated patient. Reversal agents can be used to correct this (naloxone for opiates, flumazenil for benzodiazepines)
- Metabolic disturbances (electrolyte or acid-base) also contribute to a prolonged state of unconsciousness
- Comorbidity in the patient, especially relating to the hepato-renal system, affects the clearance of many drugs
- Stroke can be masked by sedation. Strokes are often seen in patients undergoing neurosurgical and vascular interventions (particularly in the arterial pathologies with cardiovascular risk factors such as hypertension).

Temperature Change

The artificial and physiologically hostile environment to which the patient is exposed during surgery can lead to marked changes in the body's temperature. Hypothermia is caused by heat loss from the exposed skin and viscera during prolonged open abdominal procedures, leading to confusion as well as dangerous coagulation disorders. Hyperthermia may result after overzealous rewarming techniques but can also be the sign of an underlying sepsis.

Postoperative Pain

Pain is unpleasant and associated with worse physical outcomes. Basic postoperative analgesia consists of opioids (morphine, tramadol), nonsteroidal anti-inflammatory drugs (diclofenac), and paracetamol. Epidural and regional blocks can be invaluable as supplemental analgesia after a procedure. In addition, local infiltration of the incision site, usually with a long-acting local anesthetic at the time of wound closure gives good pain control in the immediate postoperative period.

This can be followed by patient controlled analgesia. The patient presses a button to infuse a bolus, often of morphine, when the pain is bad. This is good in the first few days postoperatively but only with the aim of switching to oral alternatives, which give continuous analgesia so that the patient is always pain-free.

A combination of opiates, nonsteroidal inflammatory medicines, and paracetamol-based preparations are usually prescribed on the drug chart preoperatively by the surgical team house officer. Postoperatively, these can be titrated depending on the patient's response.

Transcutaneous electrical nerve stimulation (TENS) is an effective pain reliever in acute postoperative stage. However it is most effective only when the patient has had no or very little opiates in the immediate post of stage.

Postoperative Nausea and Vomiting

Postoperative nausea and vomiting are less common now because of reduction in the use of nitrous oxide and the introduction of propofol as an induction agent. Postoperative nausea and vomiting can be managed by various drugs. Serotonin (5-HT_3) antagonists are effective but expensive. Cyclizine is a cheap antihistamine commonly prescribed whenever opiate analgesia is given because opioids cause nausea. Alternatives include dopamine antagonists, such as metoclopramide. Steroids also work but are not as commonly used as antiemetics because of the many body systems that can be adversely affected. It should also be pointed out that the actual cause of nausea and vomiting should be detected; other than the surgery itself. The patient may also have a source of infection that needs tracing, a deep venous thrombosis and pulmonary embolism, or perhaps may be feeling sick from electrolyte imbalance.

The Postoperative Ward Round

After surgery, the consultant surgeon will want to know a few important points. The patient's temperature and vital signs are a good start. Most patients feel washed out after a surgical procedure and are often drowsy afterwards. Adequate analgesia is important and the switch from patient controlled analgesia to oral analgesia is often tried. Recovery of the patient's appetite is important. Patients are often started on sips of water followed by free fluids and then a light diet. In patients who have had bowel surgery, a steady approach to nutrition needs to be taken to make sure the bowel is adequately prepared for digestion. It is important to ask whether patients have opened their bowels since the operation—this process is often not immediate. Passing urine freely without difficulty is also important. Drains need inspection in terms of the color and volume of their content. And the wound site also needs inspection for any signs of infection. Also one shoud not forget general examination of the patient to assess hydration, to check for developing chest infections, and to examine for any evidence of a deep vein thrombosis. Postoperative blood tests, such as a full blood count, urea, creatinine, and electrolytes as well as C-reactive protein are also often asked for.

CONCLUSION

In the postoperative state, the patient continues to remain vulnerable not only because of the pathological changes caused by disease but also to the physiological variations induced by the surgery. The level of care given after the operation should be in no way less than that given during the procedure.

Although the surgeon is in charge of manipulating the patient's anatomical structures, it is the surgical team's responsibility to maintain the patient's physiological integrity and to negotiate the transition from intraoperative care through recovery and return to normal life.

REFERENCES

1. Wong T, Detsky A. Preoperative cardiac risk assessment for patients having peripheral vascular surgery. Ann Intern Med 1992;116:743.
2. Paul S, Eagle K. Assessing the cardiac risk of noncardiac surgery. Contemp Intern Med 1994;6:47.
3. Eagle K, Brundage B, Chaitman B, et al. Guidelines for perioperative cardiovascular evaluation for noncardiac surgery: Report of the American College of Cardiology/American Heart Association Task Force on Practice Guidelines (Committee on Perioperative Cardiovascular Evaluation for Noncardiac Surgery). J Am Coll Cardiol 1996;27:910.

ANNEXURE 2.1

A study by Lee et al aimed to devise an index to help physicians predict risk in patients undergoing noncardiac surgery. Looking at 4,315 patients undergoing noncardiac surgery, they discovered six independent predictors that replace the nine predictors of Goldman's original cardiac risk index for noncardiac surgery:

- History of ischemic heart disease defined as a history of myocardial infarction, positive exercise test, current complaint of ischemic chest pain, nitrate use, or ECG with pathological Q waves (patients with prior coronary bypass surgery or angioplasty are only counted if they still meet other criteria for ischemic heart disease)
- History of congestive heart failure defined as a history of heart failure, pulmonary edema or paroxysmal nocturnal dyspnea; S_3 gallop or bilateral rales on physical examination; or a chest radiograph showing pulmonary vascular resistance
- History of cerebrovascular disease (i.e. stroke or transient ischemic attack)

- High-risk type of surgery—intraperitoneal, intrathoracic or suprainguinal vascular surgery
- Diabetes mellitus requiring treatment with insulin
- Preoperative serum creatinine > 175 μmol/L

Box 2.1

Number of risk	*Risk of perioperative cardiac death, nonfatal MI, or nonfatal cardiac arrest (Ref. 1)*
0	0.4 %
1	1.0 %
2	2.4 %
3 or more	5.4 %

- Box 2.1 shows the risk of patients suffering a major perioperative cardiac event based on their number of risk factors
- Analysis of this Lee Index (or Revised Goldman Risk Index) proved its superiority over other risk prediction indexes in identifying patients that are at a higher risk for cardiac complications when undergoing major noncardiac surgery.

Chapter

3 Physiotherapy in Abdominal Surgeries

What is Abdominal Surgery?

Abdominal surgery involves a surgical repair, resection or reconstruction of organs inside the abdominal cavity (Fig. 3.1). This may include surgery on the stomach, gallbladder, small intestine, large intestine (colon), liver, pancreas, spleen, esophagus, and appendix, affected by infection, obstruction, cancerous growth, or inflammatory bowel disease.

Abdominal surgeries can be performed either by *open approach* or by *keyhole approach*. Traditionally, during open abdominal surgery, the surgeon operates through an incision given over the abdominal wall or laparotomy, which is subsequently closed with staples or sutures (Fig. 3.2).

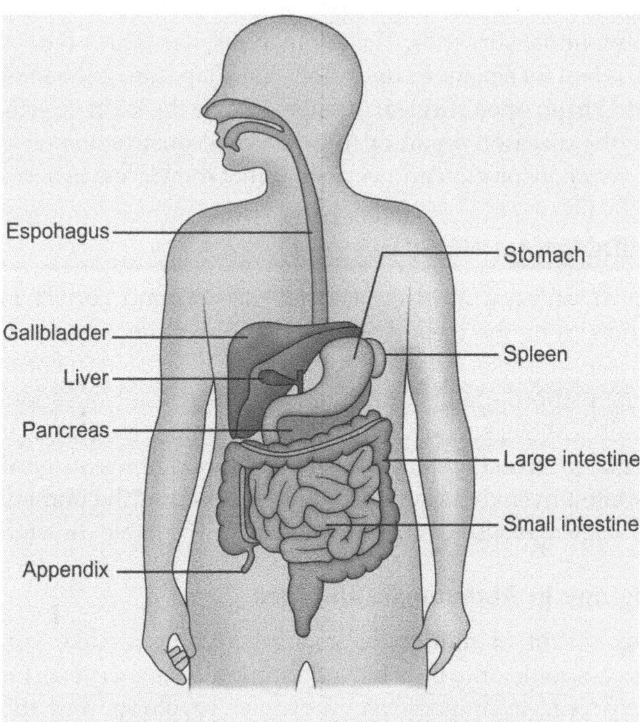

Fig. 3.1: Contents of the abdominal cavity

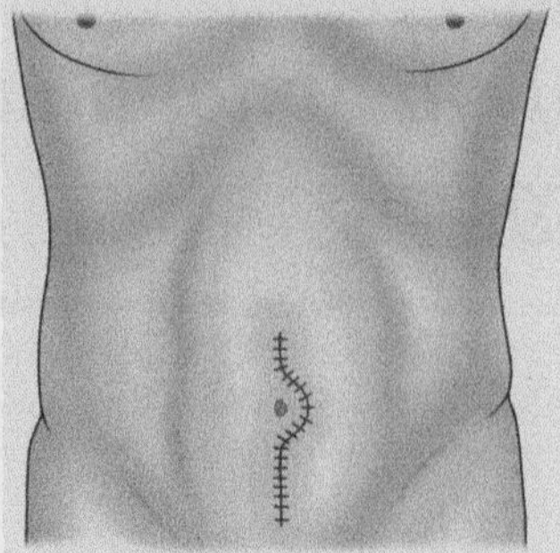
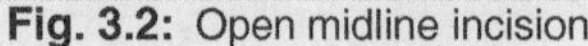

Fig. 3.2: Open midline incision

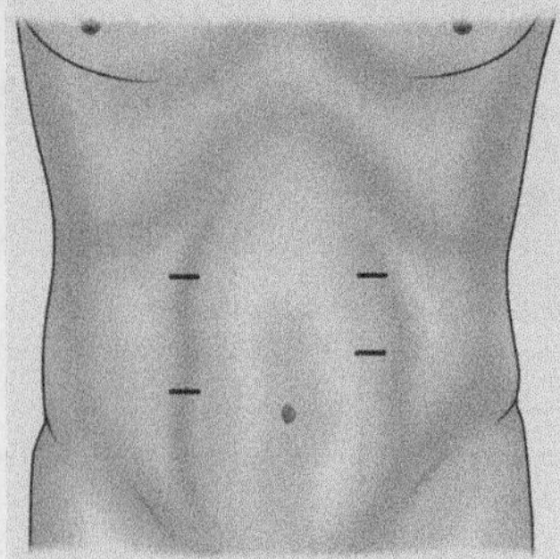

Fig. 3.3: Laparoscopic port sites

Nowadays most surgeons prefer to use the minimally invasive key-hole approach, otherwise known as laparoscopy, for most routine surgeries of the abdomen. During a laparoscopic abdominal surgery, the surgeon operates through several tiny incisions on the abdominal wall, using instruments placed through long, hollow tubes attached to a television camera (Fig. 3.3). Such approach is preferred primarily because the surgeon can see the target organ without actually exposing it and thus causing minimal surgical trauma, very little blood loss and minimal scarring. As a result the patient recovers faster, with minimal complications and therefore has very short hospital stay. Laparoscopic approach is however not possible for all types of abdominal surgeries. The surgeon decides which type of surgical procedure is best for a planned operation. Some laparoscopic operations may be converted to an open surgical incision, in case the keyhole is inadequate to remove the diseased organ or to perform reconstruction or for greater degree of visual inspection and exploration of the viscera is necessary.

OPEN ABDOMINAL INCISIONS

In abdominal surgery, a wisely chosen incision and correct method of making and closing the wound are factors of great importance in the final outcome.[1] Any mistake, such as a badly placed incision, inept method of suturing, or inappropriate suture material, may result in serious postoperative complications such as hematoma formation, an ugly scar, an incisional hernia, or, worst of all, complete disruption of the surgical wound.[1] Inappropriate physiotherapy techniques adopted in the immediate postoperative stage may also contribute to such preventable disasters.

Physiotherapy in Abdominal Surgeries

Before the advent of minimally invasive techniques like laparoscopy, optimal access could only be achieved through open incisions. Endoscopic and laparoscopic technology has, however revolutionized these areas, facilitating patient friendly access to even the most remote of abdominal organs.[1] In an endoscopic approach, the surgeon looks into the lumen of the alimentary canal or any other tubular structure or organ cavity of the viscera, such as, within the airway (Bronchoscopy), within the uterus (Hysteroscopy), inside the colon (Colonoscopy), etc. whereas a laparoscopy involves looking into the abdominal cavity from outside the lumen of the alimentary canal.

It should be the aim of the surgeon to employ the type of incision considered to be the most suitable for that particular operation to be performed. In doing so, three essentials should be achieved:[1,2]

1. Accessibility
2. Extensibility
3. Security.

The incision must not only give ready and direct access to the organ to be investigated but also provide sufficient room for the operation to be performed.[1] The incision should be extensible in a direction that will allow for any probable enlargement of the scope of the incision, but it should interfere as little as possible with the functions of the abdominal wall. The surgical incision and the resultant wound usually cause most of the trouble after abdominal surgery.

PLANNING OF AN ABDOMINAL INCISION

In the planning of an abdominal incision, following factors must be taken into consideration:

a. Preoperative diagnosis.
b. The speed with which the operation needs to be performed, as in trauma or major hemorrhage.
c. The general condition of the patient.
d. Previous abdominal operation.

Ideally, an abdominal incision is made in the direction of the lines of cleavage in the skin so that a hairline scar is produced.[3] An incision is usually tailored to the patient's need, but is strongly influenced by the surgeon's preference. In general, re-entry into the abdominal cavity is best done through the previous laparotomy incision. This minimizes further loss of tensile strength of the abdominal wall by avoiding the creation of additional defects in the abdominal fascia.

Care is taken to avoid 'tramline' or 'acute angle' incisions (Figs 3.4A and B), which could lead to devascularization of tissues, causing delayed or weak healing, thereby leading to incisional hernia. This is particularly relevant for the physiotherapist, because after the operation it is the therapist who has to juggle intrathoracic and intra-abdominal pressures to achieve and maintain maximum air entry into and clearance of secretions from the lungs, without creating a rupture of the suture or an incisional hernia.

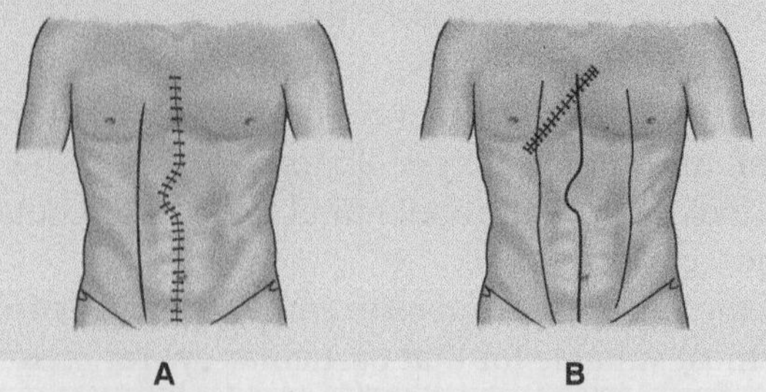

Figs 3.4A and B: (A) Tramline Incision, (B) Acute angle incision

Cosmetic end results of any incision in the body are most important from patients' point of view. Consideration is usually given wherever possible, to placing the incisions in natural skin creases or along Langer's lines. Much of the decision about the direction of the incision depends on the shape of the abdominal wall. In a short, stocky person needs a longer vertical incision and frequently gets better exposure if the incision is transverse. A tall, thin patient needs a short incision if it is made transversally, whereas a vertical incision affords optimal exposure.[2]

Certain operations are ideally done through a transverse or subcostal incision, for example cholecystectomy through a right Kocher's incision, right hemicolostomy through an infraumbilical transverse incision, and splenectomy through a left subcostal incision.

Certain incisions, popular in the past, have now been abandoned, and appropriately so. One example of this is the paramedian incision made at the lateral border of the rectus abdominis sheath. This incision was used until the mid 1940 primarily for the removal of the gallbladder, the spleen, and the left colon. It denervates the rectus abdominis muscle and produces an ideal environment for the development of postoperative abdominal wall hernia.[3]

CLASSIFICATION OF INCISIONS

The incisions used for exploring the abdominal cavity can be primarily classified as:

a. Vertical incision:
   1. Midline incision
   2. Paramedian incisions.
b. Transverse and oblique incisions:
   1. Kocher's subcostal incision
   2. Transverse muscle dividing incision
   3. McBurney's grid iron or muscle splitting incision
   4. Oblique muscle cutting incision
   5. Pfannenstiel incisions.
c. Thoracoabdominal spiral incisions.

Vertical Incisions

Vertical incisions include the midline incision, paramedian incision, and the Mayo-Robson extension of the paramedian incision.

Midline Incision (Fig. 3.5)

Almost all operations in the abdomen and retroperitoneum can be performed through this universally acceptable incision.[4]

Advantages

a. It is almost bloodless
b. No muscle fibers are divided
c. No nerves are injured
d. It affords goods access to the upper abdominal viscera
e. It is very quick to make as well as to close; it is unsurpassed when speed is essential
f. A midline epigastric incision also can be extended the full length of the abdomen curving around the umbilical scar.

Disadvantages

a. Due to poor vascularity of the incision site, healing is slow and usually of poor quality
b. In elderly obese persons, the anchorage of the suture is poor due to thin, largely fibrous nature of the abdominal wall. Tension sutures, catgut threaded through rubber tubing, is used to hold the thin abdominal wall together, without the suture cutting through the tissue

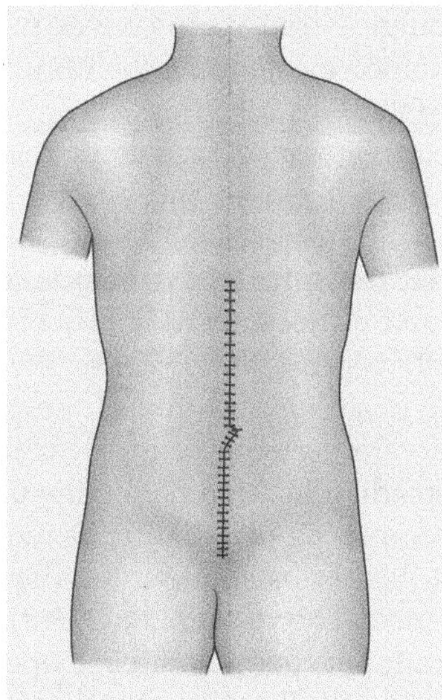

Fig. 3.5: Midline incision

c. Perfect site to develop an incisional hernia, therefore an abdominal binder may be needed immediately after and in some cases, ever after the surgery.

In the upper abdomen, this incision is made in the midline extending from the area of xiphoid and ending immediately above the umbilicus. Skin, fat, linea alba and peritoneum are divided in that order.

The infraumbilical midline incision also divides the linea alba. Because the linea alba is anatomically narrow at the inferior portion of the abdominal wall, the rectus sheath may be opened unintentionally, although this is of no consequence. In the lower abdomen, the peritoneum should be opened in the uppermost area to avoid possible injury to the bladder.

Paramedian Incision (Fig. 3.6)

The paramedian incision has two theoretical advantages:

1. The first is that it offsets the vertical incision to the right or left, providing access to the lateral structures such as the spleen or the kidney.
2. The second advantage is that closure is theoretically more secure because the rectus abdominis muscle which can act as a buttress between the reapproximated posterior and anterior fascia.[5]

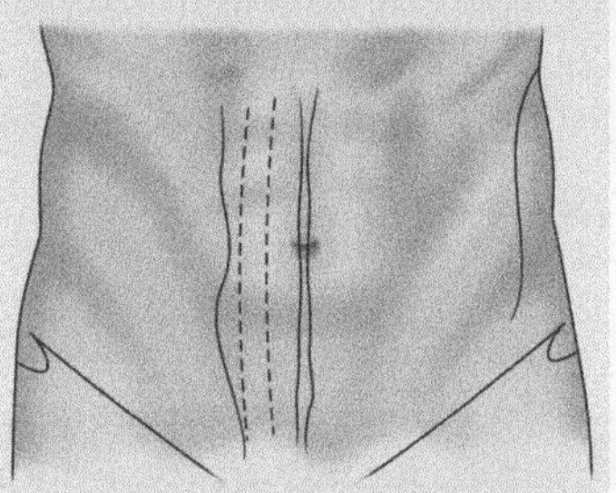

Fig. 3.6: Paramedian incisions

The skin incision is placed 2 to 5 cm lateral to the midline over the medial aspect of the bulging transverse convexity of the rectus muscle. Extra access can be obtained by slopping the upper extremity of the incision upwards to the xiphoid.

Skin and subcutaneous fat are divided along the length of the wound. The anterior rectus sheath is exposed and incised, and its medial edge is grasped and lifted up with hemostats. The medial portion of the rectus sheath then is dissected from the rectus muscle, to which the anterior sheath adheres. Once the rectus muscle is free of the anterior sheath it can be retracted laterally because the posterior sheath is not adherent to the rectus muscle. The posterior sheath and the peritoneum which are adherent to each other, are excised vertically in the same plane as the anterior fascia. A paramedian incision below the umbilicus is made in a similar manner. Some surgeons prefer to split the rectus muscle rather than dissect it free.[4] In this rectus-splitting technique, the muscle is split longitudinally near its medial border (medial 1/3rd), after which posterior layer of the rectus sheath and peritoneum are opened in the same line. This incision can be made and closed quickly and is particularly valuable in reopening the scar of a previous paramedian incision.

Disadvantages

1. It tends to weaken and strip off the muscles from its lateral vascular and nerve supply resulting in atrophy of the muscle medial to the incision.
2. The incision is laborious and difficult to extend superiorly as is limited by costal margin.
3. It does not give good access to contralateral structures.

The Mayo-Robson extension of the paramedian incision is accomplished by curving the skin incision towards the xiphoid process. Incision of the fascia is continued in the same direction to obtain a larger opening.[6]

Transverse Incisions (Fig. 3.7)

Transverse incisions include the *Kocher's subcostal incision, transverse muscle dividing, McBurney, Pfannenstiel,* and *Maylard incisions.*
A. Kocher's incision, B. Transverse incision, C. Rockey-Davis incision, D. Maylard incision, E. Pfannenstiel incision.

Kocher Subcostal Incision (Fig. 3.8)

Theodor Kocher originally described the subcostal incision; it affords excellent exposure to the gallbladder and common bile duct and can be made on the left side to afford access to the spleen.[7] It is of particular value in obese and muscular patients and most suitable in planned surgery.

The subcostal incision is started at the midline, 2 to 5 cm below the xiphoid and extends downwards, outwards and parallel to and about 2.5 cm below the costal margin. The rectus sheath is incised in the same direction as the skin incision, and the rectus muscle and the internal

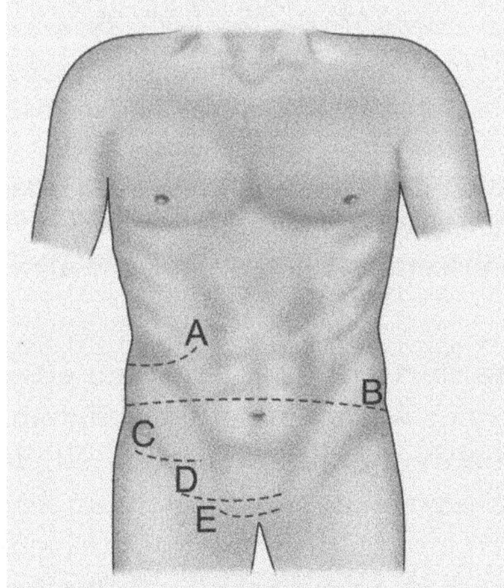

Fig. 3.7: Transverse and transverse-oblique incisions

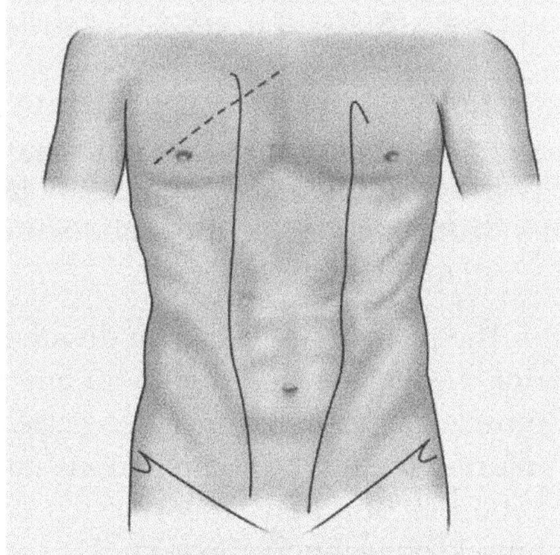
Fig. 3.8: Kocher's incision

oblique and transversus abdominis muscles are divided. Special attention is needed to control bleeding from branches of the superior epigastric vessels, which lie posterior to and under the lateral portion of the rectus muscle. The small eighth thoracic nerve will almost invariably be divided; the large ninth nerve must be seen and preserved to prevent weakening of the abdominal musculature.

In the recent years, many surgeons have advocated the use of a small 5–10 cm incision in the subcostal area for minilaparotomy cholecystectomy. This incision is similar to the Kocher's incision except that the length of the incision is much shorter.

The major advantages of this incision are:

a. Lesser postoperative pain
b. Early recovery from the surgery and return to work
c. Good cosmetic results.

But disadvantages are:

a. Poor exposure
b. Chances of injury to bile ducts or other structures.

a. ***Chevron incision (Fig. 3.9A):*** The Kocher's incision may be continued across the midline into a double Kocher incision or Gable or Chevron Incision (Fig. 3.9A), which provides excellent access to the upper abdomen. This is useful in carrying out total gastrectomy, operations for renovascular hypertension, total esophagectomy, liver transplantation, extensive hepatic resections, and bilateral adrenalectomy, etc.

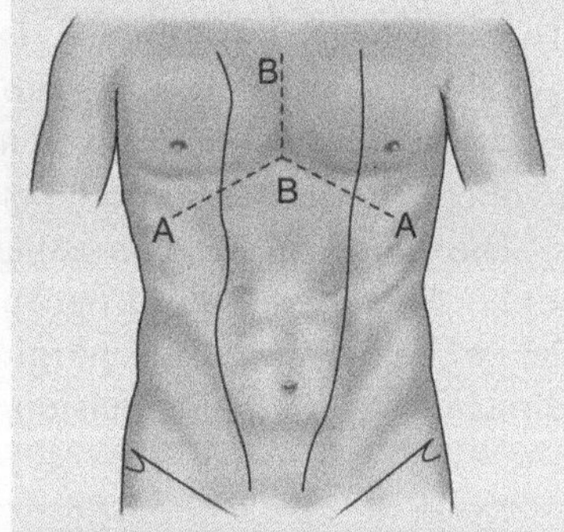

Figs 3.9A and B: A. Chevron incision; B. Mercedes Benz extension

b. ***The Mercedes Benz extension (Fig. 3.9B)*** consists of bilateral low Kocher's incision with an upper midline limb up to and through the xiphisternum.[8] Note the typical three pointed star logo of the famous car. This incision gives excellent access to the upper abdominal viscera and, in particular to all the diaphragmatic hiatuses.

The rectus muscle can be divided transversely. Its anterior and posterior sheaths are closed without any serious weakening of the abdominal muscle because the incision passes between adjacent nerves without injuring them. The rectus muscle has a segmental nerve supply, so there is no risk of a transverse incision depriving the distal part of the rectus muscle of its innervations.

Transverse Muscle-dividing Incision

The incision is similar to the Kocher incision. In newborns and infants, this incision is preferred, because more abdominal exposure is gained per length of the incision than with vertical exposure because the infant's abdomen has a longer transverse than vertical girth.[9] This is also true of short, obese adults, in whom transverse incision often affords a better exposure.

McBurney Grid Iron or Muscle-split Incision (Fig. 3.10)

The McBurney incision, first described in 1894 by Charles McBurney is the incision of choice for most appendicectomy.[10] Classically, the McBurney incision is made at the junction of the medial two thirds and the lateral one third of a line running from the umbilicus to the anterior superior iliac spine, the McBurney point. The level and the length of the incision will vary according to the thickness of the abdominal wall and the suspected position of the appendix. Good healing and cosmetic appearance are virtually always achieved with a negligible risk of wound disruption or herniation.

After the skin and subcutaneous tissue are divided, the external oblique aponeurosis is divided in the direction of its fibers; exposing the underlying internal oblique muscle. A small incision is then made in this muscle adjacent to the outer border of the rectus sheath. The opening is enlarged to permit introduction of two index fingers between the muscle fibers so that internal oblique and transversus can be retracted with a minimal amount of damage. The peritoneum is then grasped with a thumb forceps, elevated and opened.

The ilioinguinal and iliohypogastric nerves cross the incision for appendectomy and their accidental injury should be prevented which can

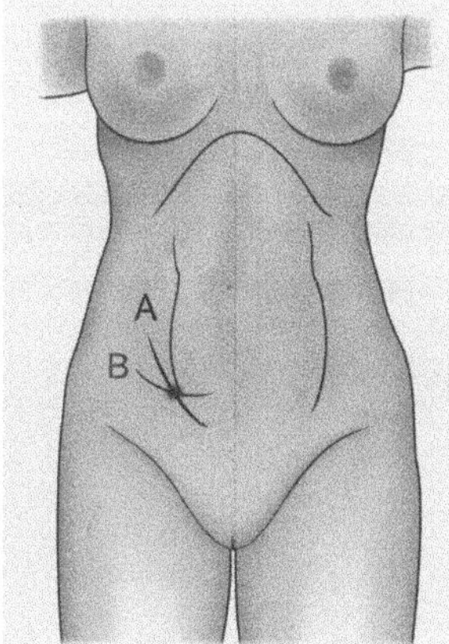

Fig. 3.10: McBurney grid iron or muscle-split incision A. The classic McBurney incision is obliquely placed; B. Most surgeons today use a more transverse skin-crease incision

predispose the patient to inguinal hernia formation in the postoperative period.

Pfannenstiel and Maylard Transverse Muscle Cutting Incision

The Pfannenstiel and Maylard incision is used frequently by gynecologists and urologists for access to the pelvis organs, bladder, prostate and for cesarean section.[11] The skin incision is usually 12 cm long and is made in a skinfold approximately 5 cm above symphysis pubis. The incision is deepened through fat and superficial fascia to expose both anterior rectus sheaths, which are divided along the entire length of the incision. The sheath is then separated widely, above and below from the underlying rectus muscle. It is necessary to separate the aponeurosis in an upward direction, almost to the umbilicus and downwards to the pubis. The rectus muscles are then retracted laterally and the peritoneum opened vertically in the midline, with care being taken not to injure the bladder at the lower end.

Thoracoabdominal Incision (Figs 3.11 and 3.12)

The thoracoabdominal incision, either right or left, converts the pleural and peritoneal cavities into one common cavity, thereby gives excellent exposure. Laparotomy incisions, whether upper midline, upper paramedian or upper oblique can be easily extended into either the right or left chest for better exposure.[3] The right incision may be particularly useful in elective and emergency hepatic resections. The left incision may be used effectively in resection of the lower end of the esophagus and proximal portion of the stomach. The patient is placed in the "corkscrew" position (Fig. 3.11). The abdomen is tilted about 45° from the horizontal by means of sand bags, and the thorax twisted into full side lying position. This position allows maximal access to both abdomen and the thoracic cavity. The abdomen is explored first through the abdominal incision to assess

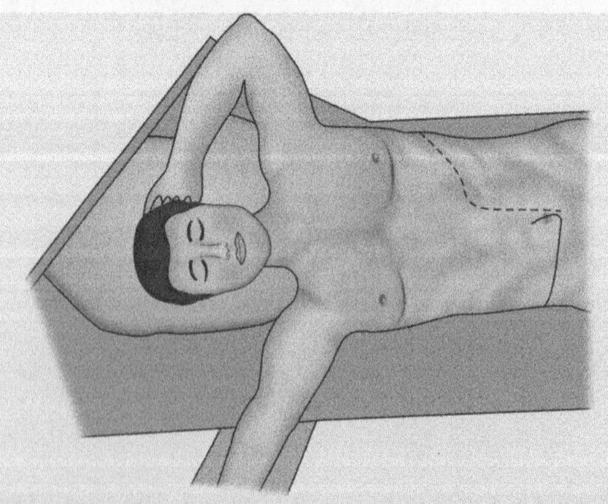

Fig. 3.11: "Corkscrew" position for thoracoabdominal incision

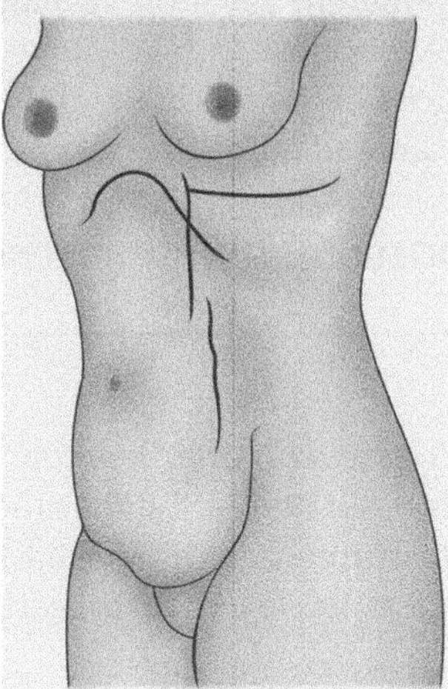

Fig. 3.12: Surface markings of the thoracoabdominal incision

for the operative exposure and necessity for thoracic extension. The incision is extended along the line of the eighth intercostals space immediately distal to the inferior angle of the scapula.

The thoracic incision is carried down through the subcutaneous fat and the latissimus dorsi, serratus anterior and external oblique muscles. The intercostals muscles are divided and pleural cavity is opened and lung allowed to collapse. The incision is continued across the costal margin, and the cartilage is divided in a V shape manner with a scalpel so that the two ends interdigitate and can be closed more securely. A chest retractor is inserted and opened to produce wide spreading of the intercostal space. After ligation of the phrenic vessels in the line of the incision, the diaphragm is divided radially.[12]

Why does a Physiotherapist Need to Know about Surgical Incisions?

Points to Ponder

- "Being forewarned is being forearmed"; this is the significance of the knowledge of surgical incisions to the therapist.
- Knowing which muscles are likely to be divided by a specific incision and thus become weak after surgery enables the therapist to undertake preoperative strengthening of these at risk muscles or muscle groups.
- Location of any incision near or across a key joint or a body segment can seriously compromise its movement. Any pre-existing movement loss, due to arthritis, etc. in that segment can worsen after the surgery. Knowing this enables the therapist to undertake preoperative mobilization of the segment/joint at-risk.

- Some incisions have inherent risks of developing hernias. Knowing about this enables the therapist to take preventive measures such as binders or braces which can be made ready before the operation and fitted onto the patient immediately after the surgery.

LAPAROSCOPY—ABDOMINAL SURGERY THROUGH KEYHOLE INCISION

Definition

Surgery performed through several tiny "keyhole incisions". A fiber-optic instrument is inserted through one of the incisions to view the inside of the abdomen. Surgical instruments are inserted through other incisions (Fig. 3.13). Laparoscopy can be used for a variety of procedures and operations.

Indications for Laparoscopy

Laparoscopy is done to examine, diagnose, and treat problems inside the abdomen and female reproductive system. The procedure is most often performed for the following reasons:

- Diagnose the cause of acute or chronic abdominal or pelvic pain
- Visualize and obtain a tissue specimen for biopsy, from a mass in the abdomen
- Evaluate the cause of female infertility
- Evaluate source of fluid accumulating in the abdomen
- Monitor the status of previously treated cancer
- Assist in determining the "stage" or spread of certain cancers.

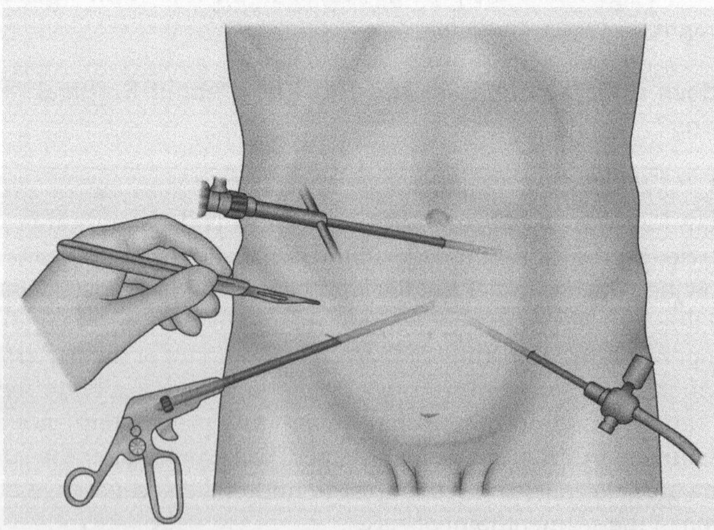

Fig. 3.13: Laparoscopic instruments being placed in the abdomen

Many types of surgery that have traditionally been performed with an open incision can now be performed laparoscopically, these include:

- Repair of inguinal or femoral hernia
- Taking biopsy sample of abdominal tissue
- Removal of appendix and gallbladder or gallbladder stones
- Ligation of the fallopian tube for family planning
- In ectopic pregnancy—removal of the fetus from within the fallopian tube
- Egg retrieval for artificial insemination in assisted reproductive technology (Test tube baby)
- Removal of tumors/cysts from the ovary, fibroids from the uterus or shaving inside the uterus in endometriosis and complete removal of whole uterus and/or ovary (hysterectomy/salpingectomy)
- Removal of parts of the liver, adrenal glands and spleen
- Removal of adhesions in the gut following diverticulum (twisted gut)
- Surgery of the urinary bladder as management of incontinence.

Risk factors for developing postoperative complications:

- Pre-existing heart or lung condition
- Previous abdominal surgery
- Obesity
- Diabetes.

Preoperative Protocol

Depending on the reason for the laparoscopy, the surgeon may do the following:

- Physical exam
- Review of medications
- Blood tests such as Hemogram and blood sugar, including pregnancy test, liver function, electrolyte status
- Urinalysis to rule out urinary tract infection or diabetes
- USG, CT and / or MRI of the abdomen.

Anesthesia

A laparoscopy may be done under local, spinal and general anesthesia, depending upon the surgeons preference.

Description of the Procedure

The surgeon cuts a small opening in the abdomen. The location of this incision varies depending on the procedure, either near the navel or in the lower abdomen for pelvic conditions. A needle is inserted and used to inject carbon dioxide gas into the abdomen. This gas causes the abdominal cavity to expand and makes it easier for the surgeon to see the internal structures. The surgeon then inserts a long, thin tubular instrument (laparoscope) that lights, magnifies, and projects an image of the internal organs onto a video screen. The internal organs are then inspected visually.

If necessary, several other tiny incisions may be made in the abdomen through which to insert instruments that can take biopsies or perform various types of surgery (such as repair or removal of an organ). After the laparoscope and any other tools are removed, the incisions are closed with stitches or clips and covered with a dressing. The procedure usually takes less than 1 hour, but this depends on the type of procedure being done.

After Procedure

A laboratory will examine the removed fluid or tissue samples for sign of infection or cancer.

Pain After Laparoscopy

Anesthesia prevents pain during the procedure. The patient may experience soreness for a couple of days during recovery, but can receive pain medication to relieve this discomfort. The patient may also feel bloated or have pain in shoulder girdle from the gas pumped in during the procedure. This can last up to three days.

Possible Complications

- Infection
- Gas embolism
- Excessive bleeding due to damage to blood vessels or organs, sometimes requiring immediate open surgery for repair
- Anesthesia-related problems
- Sometimes it becomes evident to the surgeon during laparoscopic visual inspection that the operation would be better carried out using a traditional, open incision. In such case, the usual complications after open abdominal surgeries may be encountered.

Average Hospital Stay

Most patients having a diagnostic laparoscopy go home the same day. Laparoscopic surgery may require a few days of hospital care, depending on the procedure.

Postoperative Care

The operative dressing can usually be removed the morning after surgery. The patient must—

- Avoid heavy lifting
- Do not drink carbonated beverages for two days
- Avoid constipation.

Outcome

Outcome of laparoscopy is usually uneventful. Depending on the procedure, the patient should be able to resume regular activities in about 1 week. If the laparoscopy was performed to help diagnose a condition, the surgeon will suggest further treatment options. Biopsy results may take 3 to 5 days. However the surgeon must be informed if any of the following occurs:

- Signs of infection, such as redness, swelling, increasing pain, excessive bleeding, or discharge from the incision site, including fever and chills
- Headache, muscle aches, feeling faint or dizzy
- Difficulty urinating
- Following general anesthesia: cough, shortness of breath, chest pain, or severe nausea or vomiting.

Preparing for Surgery

Use the following information as a general guide for yourself as well as your patient scheduled to undergo an operation.

The patient needs to make an appointment with the surgeon for a physical exam before surgery. One week before the surgery is the ideal time for the physical exam. However, physical exams up to one month before the surgery can be accepted.

The primary care physician/anesthetist will perform the initial clinical evaluation to make sure that the patient will be physically able to undergo surgery. He also informs the patient of any necessary lab testing or imaging (USG / CT / MRI) that may need before surgery.

What the Patient Needs to Know about Medications?

The patient must have a current list of medications and supplements he is taking and ask the surgeon/primary doctor if and when he should stop taking any of the routine medications. If taking any vitamins, herbal supplements, or over-the-counter medications, this must also be discussed with the surgeon and primary care doctor. Some of these medications may need to be stopped before surgery.

If taking blood-thinning medications such as aspirin, warfarin, clopidogrel, or nonsteroidal anti-inflammatory medications such as naproxen, or ibuprofen, the surgeon/primary doctor will tell the patient when to stop taking these medications before surgery.

If taking medications for diabetes such as metformin, glyburide, or glipizide or taking insulin for diabetes, the surgeon/primary doctor will advise the dosage and type of insulin, or whether NOT to take insulin, prior to the surgery.

Instructions to the Patient before Surgery

- Inform surgeon immediately about any changes in patient's health condition, such as a fever or cold, within 24 hours before the scheduled surgery.
- Be sure to inform surgeon if the patient is pregnant.
- If having colon or rectal surgery, the surgeon will give specific instructions for preoperative bowel preparation.
- *No food or drink allowed after midnight the day before surgery:* This includes water, coffee, and chewing gum unless otherwise indicated by the surgeon. If the patient accidentally had something to eat or drink, notify the surgeon.
- The patient must be strongly urged not to smoke or drink alcohol 24 hours before the surgery.
- The patient must leave all valuables at home or with relatives on the day of surgery and should not wear jewelry including rings and body piercing.
- Patient must take only the medications advised by the surgeon/ primary doctor or nurse—with a sip of water.
- The patient must arrive at the operation theater 2 hours before scheduled surgery. This time is required by the staff to help prepare the patient for surgery.

Planning Recovery

- After abdominal surgery, it is normal to feel weak and tired for several weeks after the patient returns home. Since each person is unique, the speed of recovery and ability to return to normal activities will vary.
- Pain from the incision is to be expected. It will vary from day to day and with activity level. Gradually, the pain should decrease over time. The surgeon usually prescribes pain medication at discharge from the hospital.
- The diet after abdominal surgery plays a crucial role in recovery and may vary significantly from the normal diet of the patient. The patient or the caregiver at home may get dietary inputs from the primary care physician/nutritionist and plan ahead to simplify meal preparation. If living alone, it is wise to do grocery shopping, prepare and freeze several meals before the patient comes to the hospital. Cooking utensils that are used frequently must also be placed within easy reach.
- Recreation during recovery plays a very important role in reliving postoperative anxiety and depression. A selection of reading material, music CDs and television should be kept ready for the patient to use during recovery period.
- The patient must check with the surgeon about how long one can expect to be off work because of surgery and arrange time off from work, so that he does not feel rushed during the recovery.

- Arranging for funds before the operation is crucial to a worry-free recovery. It is wise to have a cashless medical insurance policy, to take care of the hospital bills in case of eventualities even if one is obstinately healthy. Some petty cash should be left behind at home with the caregiver to look after immediate expenses.

COMMON ABDOMINAL SURGERIES AND THEIR POSTOPERATIVE PHYSIOTHERAPY MANAGEMENT

Operation of the Gallbladder

The gallbladder is located in the abdomen, on the upper right corner, underneath the liver. The gallbladder stores bile produced by the liver, and delivers it to the first part of the small intestine (duodenum), where it aids in the digestion of fat. The cystic and common bile ducts connect the gallbladder to the duodenum-bile passes through these ducts from the gallbladder to the duodenum.

Gallbladder surgery is done to treat gallbladder disease, which consists predominantly of the formation of gallstones in the gallbladder (cholelithosis).

Gallstones can cause:

- Obstruction of the cystic duct leading to severe abdominal pain (biliary colic)
- Infection or inflammation of the gallbladder (cholecystitis)
- Blockage of the biliary ducts leading to the duodenum (biliary obstruction).

In each of the above cases, removal of the gallbladder (cholecystectomy) is indicated.

Most gallbladder surgery today is done using laparoscopic surgical techniques. A laparoscopic camera is inserted into the abdomen near the umbilicus (navel). Instruments are inserted through two small puncture holes. The gallbladder is found, the supply blood vessels ligated and bile and cystic ducts cut, and the gallbladder removed.

If the gallbladder is extremely inflamed, infected, or has large gallstones, the abdominal approach (open cholecystectomy) is recommended. A small incision is made just below the margin of the rib cage on the right side of the abdomen. The liver is moved aside to expose the gallbladder. The cystic duct and artery leading to and from the gallbladder are cut and the gallbladder is removed. The common bile duct that drains the bile from the liver into the duodenum is examined for blockages or stones.

Most patients who undergo laparoscopic cholecystectomy can go home on the day of surgery or the next day, and resume a normal diet and activities within a week. Most patients who undergo open cholecystectomy require 5–7 days of hospitalization, are able to resume a normal diet after one week, and normal activities after 4–6 weeks.

Drainage Tubes

- A T-shaped drainage tube may be left in the common bile duct for several days to drain excess bile and exudates if there is inflammation or infection.
- This tube is located just below dome of the diaphragm under the right basal lobe of the lung. It impinges on the diaphragm during inspiration and the pain thus felt may inhibit the patient from taking a deep breath. In the long-term such inhibition may cause atelectasis of the right lung base.

Postoperative Care

After Open Cholecystectomy

Postoperative care for the patient who has had an open cholecystectomy, as with those who have had any major abdominal surgery, involves constant monitoring of:

- Blood pressure
- Pulse rate
- Rate of respiration
- Temperature.

Breathing tends to be shallow because of the effect of anesthesia, and the patient's reluctance to breathe deeply due to the pain caused by the proximity of the incision to the muscles used for respiration and location of the drainage tube just below the diaphragm.

The therapist must show the patient how to support the operative site when breathing deeply and coughing. The patient is also given pain medication as necessary. Fluid intake and output is measured, and the operative site is monitored for color and amount of wound drainage. Fluids are given intravenously for 24–48 hours, until the patient's diet is gradually advanced as bowel activity resumes. The patient is generally encouraged to walk eight hours after surgery and discharged from the hospital within three to five days. The sutures may be removed between 7 to 10 days after surgery. The patient is usually fit to return to work approximately four to six weeks after an open cholecystectomy procedure.

After Laparoscopic Cholecystectomy

Care needed immediately after laparoscopic cholecystectomy is similar to that of any patient undergoing surgery with general anesthesia. A unique postoperative pain may be experienced in the right shoulder related to pressure from entrapped carbon dioxide used in the laparoscopy to inflate the operative site for better visualization of the target organ. This pain may be relieved by lying down on the left side with right knee and thigh drawn up to the chest. Walking will also help increase the body's reabsorption of the gas. The patient is usually discharged the day after surgery and allowed to shower on the second postoperative day. The patient is advised to resume normal activities gradually over a three-day period, while avoiding heavy lifting for about 10 days after the surgery.

Repair of Inguinal Hernia

An inguinal hernia refers to a protrusion of the abdominal contents through a weakness in the connective tissue of the inguinal canal in the groin (Fig. 3.14).

Hernia and groin problems are common sports injuries, particularly in soccer where the pelvic region is subject to large torsion (twisting) loads. It is also common in elderly or over weight individuals with large visceral bulk and weak abdominal musculature.

Inguinal hernia surgery has been revolutionized over the past ten years. Most surgeons now perform hernia surgery under local anesthesia. Depending on the individual condition of the patient, considering their age, occupation, general health and the size and degree of the inguinal hernia, the surgical technique is chosen 'tailored' to the patient's need. Rehabilitation following inguinal hernia surgery is very rapid and exercises can begin the day after the hernia repair.

Common Signs and Symptoms of Inguinal Hernia

- Abdominal and groin pain that gets progressively worse, following sudden rise in intra-abdominal pressure, e.g. lifting of heavy weight, straining at stool, etc.

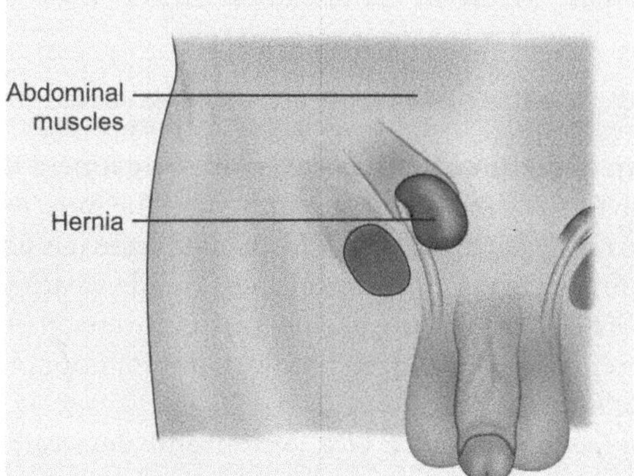

Fig. 3.14: Inguinal hernia

- Pain typically reproduced with coughing and sneezing.
- Groin pain when squeezing the legs together.

Pathomechanics of Inguinal Hernia

The inguinal canal is the region between the abdomen and inner thigh, through which the testes in male or the round ligament in female descend during childhood. The inguinal region is a weakpoint in the abdominal wall. The weakpoint results from the fact that the spermatic cord passes through this canal in men and the ligament of the uterus passes through it in women.

Prior to a true inguinal hernia, the abdominal muscle layers can become lax as a reaction to extreme strains in this region due to age, multiple pregnancies, obesity, repeated lifting without any external support and sports activities. The resultant pressure on the nerves passing through that region—particularly the genitofemoral nerve, can cause severe pain that can radiate to the upper thigh and the testes.

Diagnosis of Inguinal Hernia

- Any exertion that increases intra-abdominal pressure, such as coughing, sneezing or sporting activity can cause pain.
- In the early stages, the person may be able to continue ADL but the problem usually gets progressively worse.
- Typically, the day after a heavy strain, getting out of bed or a car will be uncomfortable.
- Pain in the groin and pelvis can be referred from a number of problems, including injuries to the lower back, the hip joint, the sacroiliac joint, the abdomen and the genitourinary system.
- Therefore, diagnosis of an inguinal hernia requires skilful differentiation.
- Because it requires an expert to diagnose an inguinal hernia it is not unusual for many weeks or months to pass before the correct diagnosis is made.
- A typical inguinal hernia can be confirmed with physical tests and an ultrasound scan.

Management of inguinal hernia conservative treatment through physiotherapy involves stabilizing and strengthening the muscles of the pelvic region, but this rarely cures the problem. In most cases it is usually possible to continue doing normal activities and sports while wearing compression girdle (Hernia Truss) or pressure garments (Compression Shorts) over the weak spot, to renifroce the abdominal wall, until an opportune time can be arranged for surgery.

Pressure biofeedback device is a very useful device that provides a visual indication of whether the patient is working the correct postural muscles, in the right manner, when performing specific exercises. Research has shown that this can relieve and prevent repeated herniation, back pain and neck pain. Size 19.5 × 10 × 10 cm (Fig. 3.15).

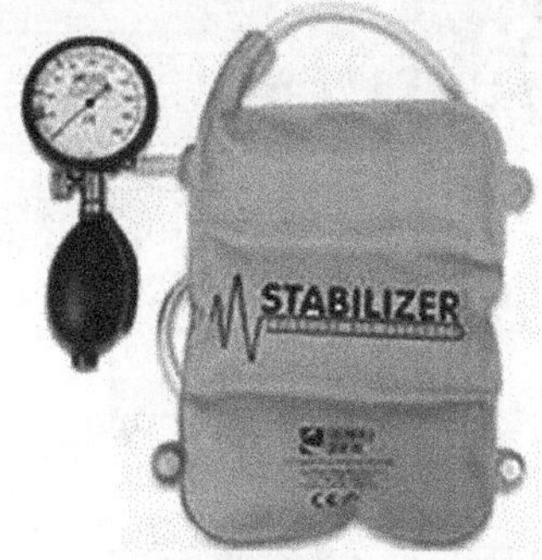

Fig. 3.15: Pressure biofeedback device

How Pressure Biofeedback Device Works?

The air bag is inflated using the hand pump. This is then placed against a specific part of the body, such as the lower abdomen.

The user then contracts the specific lower abdominal muscles which provide postural support to the affected region. The stabilizer helps by giving visual feedback that lets the user know whether they are using the correct technique.

With the correct technique the pressure reading on the dial changes, depending on the effort the person is exerting. The dial provides visual feedback and significantly improves the quality of the contraction of specific muscles (Fig. 3.16).

Compression Shorts

Compression shorts have a patented 'Core Activation System' for the treatment and prevention of hernia, osteitis pubis, pubalgia, gilmore's groin, hamstring, groin and thigh injuries. Compression shorts are specifically designed to stabilize the lower abdominal, pelvic and hip areas. The compression (20–30 mm Hg) provided by the criss-cross design helps to provide physical support and reassurance to the groin and pelvis, which improves stability and relieves symptoms of recurrent hernia (Fig. 3.17).

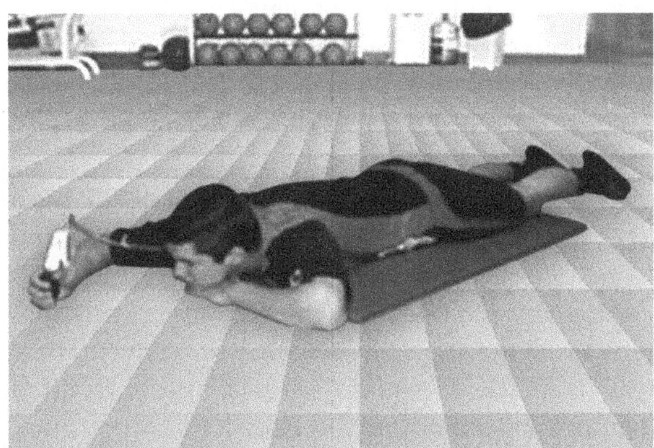

Fig. 3.16: Using a pressure biofeedback device

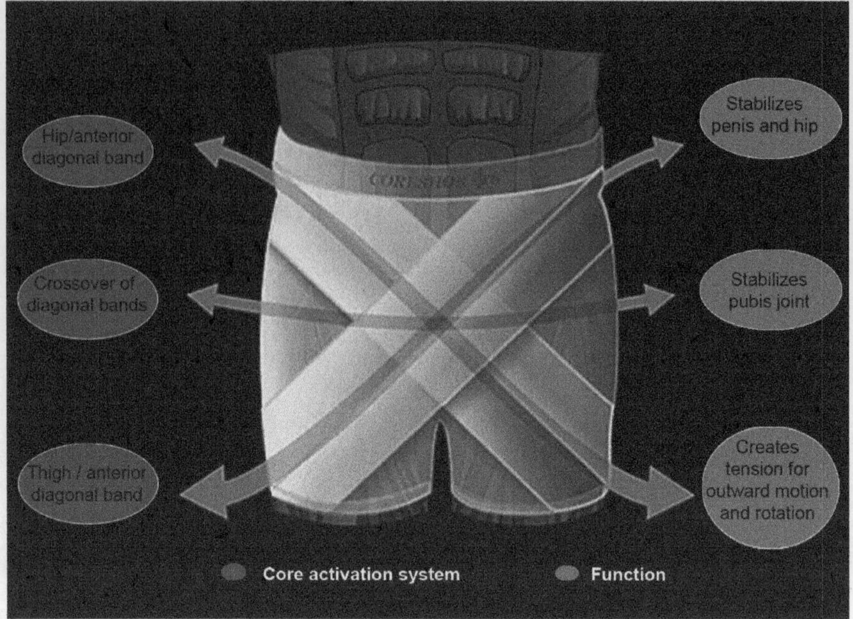

Fig. 3.17: Compression stockings

Surgical Repair of Inguinal Hernia

Eventually, there comes a time when the person can no longer continue to function normally using conservative methods and supportive devices. Then surgical repair and/or reconstruction of hernia is required to be done.

The surgical treatment of inguinal hernias has been revolutionized over the past ten years. The hernia surgeons now prefer to perform hernia surgery under local anesthetic. Depending on the individual circumstances of the patient, considering their age, occupation, general health and the size and degree of the inguinal hernia, the surgical technique is chosen which is 'tailor made' to the patient's need.

A minimal repair technique has been pioneered by Dr Ulrike Muschaweck, at the Hernia Center Munich. This tissue sparing technique does not use a surgical 'mesh' to repair the hernia and only the affected tissues are repaired. This is ideal repair for young persons or athletes who have a big defect in the fascia of the inguinal canal, while the muscle layers are still intact. Physical immobility is not required and the patient can begin physical activities a few days after surgery.

'Mesh' techniques have been developed for patients who have large defects in the wall of the inguinal canal or for older patients where the abdominal wall is weak. A square surgical mesh is stitched onto the muscle layers of the abdominal region in order to repair the hernia.

The principle of local anesthesia is pain elimination by blocking the nerves in the groin region with an injection. This is different from spinal anesthesia, such as an epidural injection. The advantages of a local anesthetic are that the patient is able to get up on their feet straight after the operation and there is no need for an overnight stay in hospital.

Patients can usually eat immediately after surgery, as they do not experience the side effects of a general anesthesia, such as nausea, vomiting, headaches and urinary retention.

Because these side effects are eliminated and the surgical repair is so unobtrusive, the rehabilitation process can begin immediately. Patients are encouraged to return to everyday activities and work the day after surgery. The patient can resume gentle exercise such as jogging or cycling. Elite athletes can begin sprinting after three or four days. Within five or six days there are no physical restrictions.

Prevention of Inguinal Hernia

Core strength and core stability exercises can improve muscle function across the trunk and pelvis. Core strength exercises on a mat and using a Gym Ball or Elastoplastic Straps (Theraband) are ideal, because the improved muscular strength and stability can help to counteract the large forces that are applied to the lower abdomen and pelvis. This can reduce the risk of developing a hernia.

Partial and Total Gastrectomy—Surgeries for Stomach Cancer

Worldwide, stomach cancer remains one of the most common forms of cancer, affecting approximately 800,000 new individuals annually. Stomach cancers are classified according to their tissue type. The most common type of stomach cancers are *gastric adenocarcinomas*, which arise from the glandular tissue lining the stomach.

Causes of Stomach Cancer

- *Diet* appears to play a major role in the development of stomach cancer. Nitroso compounds such as *nitrites* found in smoked meats or fish and *nitrates* used in food preservatives, and high salt intake, all are likely contribute to this disease, whereas fresh vegetables are protective. The question of whether green tea also has any protective effects remains debatable.
- *A bacterium called Helicobacter pylori*, believed to cause peptic ulcers, represents an additional risk factor for gastric cancer, particularly those cancers occurring in the distal portion of the stomach. This infection may lead to inflammation of the superficial layer of the stomach, inducing changes in the cells that line the stomach which eventually results in cancer. It should be stressed, however, that most patients with *H. pylori* infection do not develop gastric cancer.
- *Autoimmune gastritis*, associated with lack of hydrochloric acid secretion in the stomach and pernicious anemia, and adenomatous gastric

polyps, represent other precursors that increase a person's risk of developing stomach cancer.

- *Chronic GERD* (*gastroesophageal reflux disease*) can cause damage to the tissue lining the lower portion of the esophagus and proximal portion of the stomach resulting in the development of cancer at the GE junction.

Symptoms of Stomach Cancer

The symptoms of stomach cancer often mimic those of peptic ulcer disease, namely:

- A vague upper abdominal pain aggravated by food, heartburn, and indigestion. These symptoms are often initially treated with antacids and H-2 blockers.
- Loss of appetite and feeling full after eating only a small amount of food are other common symptoms.
- Large stomach cancers may result in partial blockage of the digestive tract and cause patients to vomit after meals.
- Stomach cancers may also bleed, resulting in the vomiting of blood or the appearance of black, tarry stools (melena).

Diagnosis of Stomach Cancers

Diagnosis is most frequently made by upper GI endoscopy, a procedure whereby a gastroenterologist can visualize the lining of the esophagus and stomach by insertion of a long flexible tube, with a fiber-optic cable inside, attached to a camera at the tip of the tube.

Tissue samples for Biopsy, of any suspicious lesions seen through the endoscope, can be taken during this procedure to confirm the diagnosis.

Further evaluation should include physical examination to look for enlarged lymph nodes particularly in the left supraclavicular region, enlarged liver, and ascites or fluid in the abdomen; routine blood and imaging tests such as—TC, DC, ESR and Hb; Cancer specific antigen study: chest X-ray; and an USG study and CT scan of the abdomen in all and specifically pelvis in females.

Staging of Stomach Cancers

Stomach cancer is staged by the TNM system.

- T refers to the depth of penetration of the tumor through the wall of the stomach and whether it invades into local structures;
- N refers to the presence or absence of lymph node involvement near the stomach;
- M refers to the presence or absence of metastatic spread of tumor to distant sites in the body.

This staging system is important in guiding treatment decisions and offering prognostic information to the patient. For example, early stage gastric cancers can be cured in more than 50 percent of the cases, whereas cancers which have metastasized to distant organs have a very slim chance (< 3%) of long-term survival.

Treatment of Stomach Cancers

From a treatment standpoint, the first question to address is whether the cancer is operable or not. This depends on a number of factors, including its location, how bulky the tumor is, whether it invades surrounding structures, the extent of lymph node involvement, and whether the individual is strong enough to undergo a major operation. Cancers arising in the lower portion of the stomach have better cure rates than those arising in the upper portion of the stomach. Cancers that have metastasized to distant organs cannot be surgically resected with the intention of a cure; however, in certain instances, e.g. if the tumor is causing severe obstruction or bleeding uncontrollably, it can be resected for palliative purposes. Bulky tumors in the upper portion of the stomach and the GE junction are sometimes treated first with chemotherapy and radiation, with the aim to shrink the tumor enough to permit a better chance of resecting the entire tumor.

The Operation

Partial and total gastrectomy are an important treatment for many stomach cancers. Cancers of the upper portion of the stomach are generally treated with a total gastrectomy, whereas patients with cancers of the lower portion of the stomach undergo partial gastrectomy. These surgeries are major undertakings and require reconstruction of the digestive tract, plus removal of surrounding lymph nodes. The results of surgery have improved in the last ten years, because nowadays the cancer is often found and treated earlier, and because better surgical methods have been developed. If the cancer is diagnosed at an early stage, a surgical operation may be all that is needed to cure it. This usually involves removing only a part of the stomach through a partial gastrectomy (Fig. 3.18).

If whole of the stomach is removed this is known as a total gastrectomy (Fig. 3.19).

Often, the lymph nodes close to the stomach are removed at the same time to see if the cancer cells have spread into them. Depending on the extent of the cancer, some other organs in the area of the stomach may be removed during the operation. These may include the lower part of the esophagus, the upper part of the small intestine (duodenum), the spleen or part of the pancreas. If the lower part of the esophagus has been

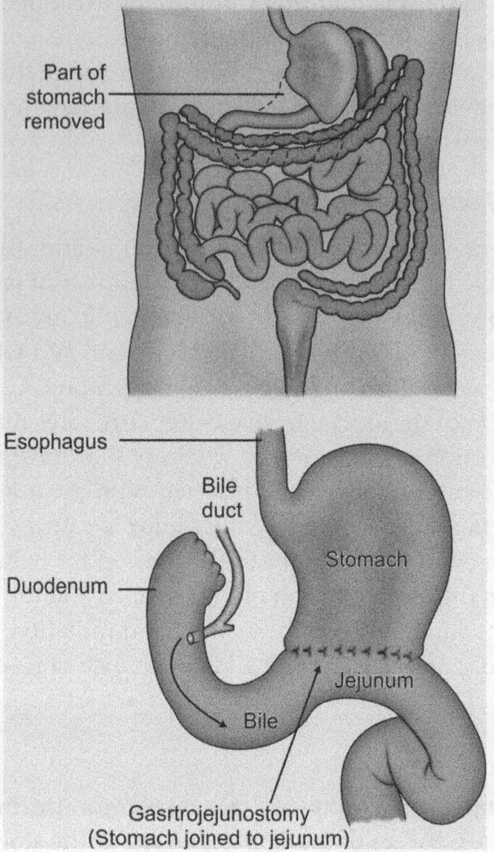

Fig. 3.18: Partial gastrectomy with gastrojejunostomy (Billroth II)

removed along with the stomach, the remaining portion of esophagus is reconnected directly to the small intestine.

Occasionally, before the surgeon decides to operate on the stomach, they may perform a laparoscopy. This is to help decide whether to remove whole or part of the stomach and any other organ that also needs removal during the procedure. This kind of laparoscopy is done under general anesthesia.

Following surgery, adjuncive treatment of conservative nature improves the final outcomes. This treatment typically consists of a combination of external-beam radiation and concurrent chemotherapy, most often a drug called 5-fluorouracil. An alternative strategy adopted for operable patients is to administer combination chemotherapy both before and after surgical resection.

For patients with metastatic disease at the time of diagnosis, the mainstay of treatment is chemotherapy. Aggressive combination chemotherapy regimens can produce an objective response in many patients.

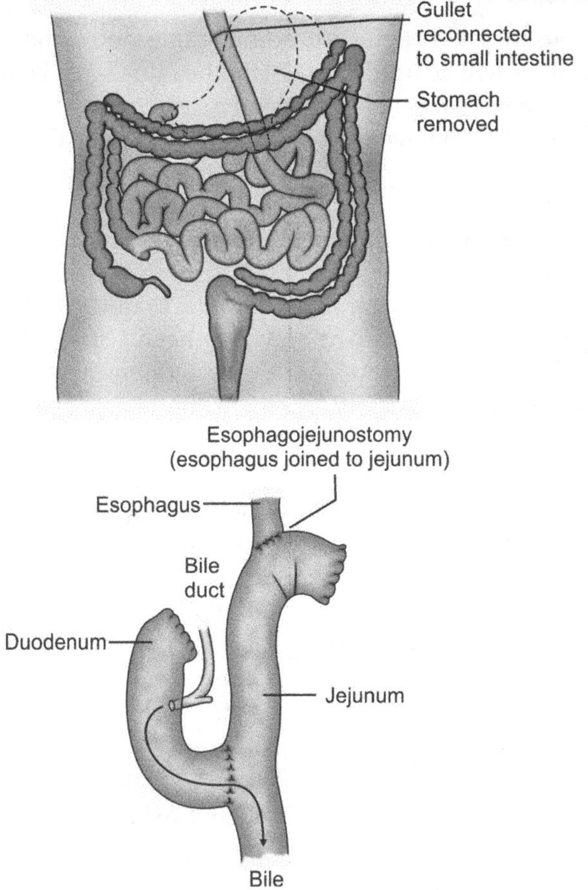

Fig. 3.19: Total gastrectomy—reconstruction with a Roux-en-Y procedure to prevent bile from entering esophagus

Bypass Surgery

Many patients may not be curable by an operation at their time of detection due to the advanced stage of their disease. However, those with bulky tumors that are causing pain, bleeding, or are impeding passage of food, can still be treated in a variety of manners to relieve their symptoms. These include a surgery to bypass the tumor; followed by an abbreviated course of radiation treatment; or placing a stent across the obstructed area to allow food to pass through more easily.

Immediately after this operation the patient should be encouraged to start moving about on the bed as soon as possible. This is an essential part of recovery. During initial 3–7 days bed rest the therapist must encourage the patient to do regular leg movements and deep breathing exercises.

Drips and Drains

An intravenous infusion of glucose, normal saline and some time blood or blood derivatives will be used to maintain the body's fluid and electrolyte balance until the patient is able to eat and drink again.

The patient will also have a nasogastric (Ryle's) tube in place. This is a thin tube that passes down nose into the stomach or small intestine and allows feeding of graduated quantity of liquid feed or excess gastric secretions to be removed so that the patient does not feel sick. It is usually taken out within 48 hours.

Sometimes a Foley's catheter is put into the bladder to drain the urine into a collecting bag. The patient may also have a drainage tube in the wound for a few days to make sure that postoperative exudates do not collect inside the operated cavity and the wound heals properly.

Drinking and Eating

After GA, the movement of the bowel slows down and vomiting is very common after partial gastrectomy. Hence it is important that the patient may only drink small amounts of liquid feed till the remaining portion of the stomach has dilated enough to accommodate food in sufficient quantity. After about 48 hours he will probably be ready to start taking small sips of water. This will be gradually increased after a couple of days until he is able to eat a soft, semisolid, light diet, usually four or five days after the operation.

In case of total removal of stomach the patient is nursed mainly on homogenized liquids in small and repeated feeds.

Pain

As is the case with other cancer types, patients with advanced stomach cancer may also require aggressive pain management with escalating doses of narcotics based painkilling drugs. These are usually very effective in controlling any pain.

Postoperative Complications

Removing part or all of the stomach can result in a number of problems postoperatively. These include:

- Patients may develop deficiency of certain vitamins and minerals that require the stomach/gastric acids for normal absorption, such as vitamin B_{12} and iron. These should be supplemented as needed.
- The dumping syndrome is common after surgery because food passes so quickly through the digestive system that there is little time for absorption. Symptoms of dumping syndrome include abdominal cramping, diarrhea, sweating, rapid heartbeat, nausea, and dizziness. These symptoms frequently get better with time. Eating several small meals throughout the day rather than three square large meals, and

eating foods lower in carbohydrate, can help. Input from a nutritionist is highly recommended.

- Symptoms of upset stomach may be related to alkaline backup, or reflux, of bile and intestinal secretions into the esophagus. These symptoms can be controlled with medicines, as well as, by simple measures such as sleeping with the head of the bed elevated and staying upright for at least an hour after eating.
- Occasionally, bacteria can grow in the loop of the duodenum bypassed by a connection of the stomach to the small intestine, producing what is called blind loop syndrome. These bacteria breaks down bile salts needed to properly digest fats, resulting in diarrhea and abdominal bloating. This condition can be treated with oral antibiotics.

Going Home

The patient will probably be ready to go home about two weeks after the operation, once the stitches have been removed. Some people take longer than others to recover from their operation depending on their general condition.

PRINCIPLES OF POSTOPERATIVE EXERCISES AFTER ABDOMINAL SURGERIES

Since surgical incisions divide or separate muscle fibers of the abdominal wall, any abdominal surgery can cause disruption of the normal biomechanics of the abdominal wall. The extent of such disruption depends up on age of the patient, the preoperative tone and power of abdominal muscles, length and location of the incision, extent of tissue dissection and secondary complications such as surgical wound infections, constipation, violent coughing, etc. The aim of the physiotherapist in such cases should be to build up the tone and power of key muscles of the trunk (core muscles) to the maximum possible limit, preferably before and definitely after the surgery. The principle behind such exercises is that if core muscles can be recruited or contracted, the trunk and pelvis will have much better support. This helps to counteract the shearing forces during activities such as lifting, coughing, and straining at stool, which can lead to abdominal laxity, increased lumbar curvature, low back pain and incision hernia.

Role of Core Muscles in Trunk Stability

In order to understand how these exercises are effective it is necessary to have a brief introduction to how the trunk is supported by muscles. The primary muscle we are concerned with is called *transversus abdominis*. This muscle arises from the midline of the abdominal wall and goes right around the trunk, attaching itself to the spine.

The transversus abdominis muscle acts as a natural corset and provides stability for the trunk and pelvis (Fig. 3.20).

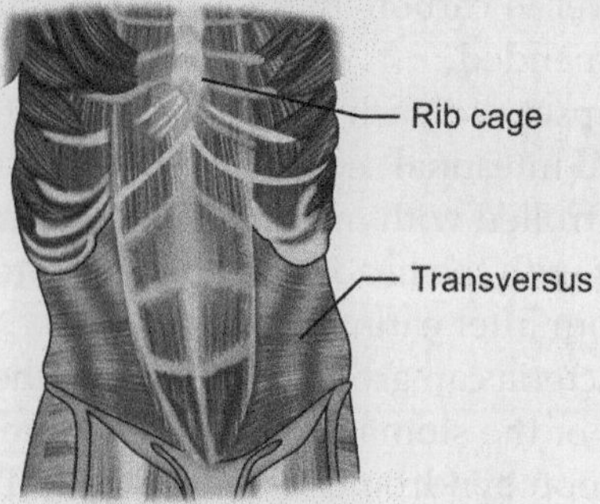

Fig. 3.20: Anterior core muscles

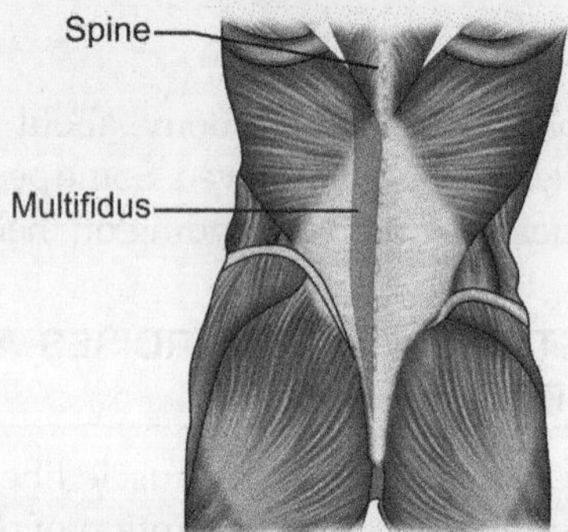

Fig. 3.21: Posterior core muscles

The second muscle involved in this exercise program is the *multifidus*. This muscle lies deep in the spine and attaches in between each vertebra. When it contracts it increases the stability of the spinal column (Fig. 3.21).

Usually, if one can contracts the transversus abdominis muscle, the multifidus muscle is also contracted automatically. This improves spinal stability and can relieve back pain.

What is the Core Strengthening Program?

The core strengthening program is an exercise program that aims to improve trunk stability and support to the spine. This is achieved by retraining specific trunk muscles, which may be under used.

Once these stabilizing muscles have been retrained the muscles of the arms and legs will have a more stable base to work from. This allows one to carry out lifting, arm and leg movements with more control and is thought to improve the quality of movement.

How will it Help During Postoperative Rehabilitation?

- It will provide more support for the back and may reduce the risk of back injuries.

- It will provide a more stable base for arm and leg movements, improving the control and quality of movements.
- It will improve muscular coordination during movement.
- As the stabilizing muscles gain more endurance a person will be able to perform movements without fatigue.
- Athlete's ability to hold off opponents in contact sports should improve.

Postoperative Rehabilitation Program

The program is broken down into stages and must be completed step by step. The patient should not progress to the next stage until he has mastered the exercises of the previous stage.

The stages are:

- ***Stage 1***
  Learn to contract the deep muscles which stabilize the spine. At first this takes quite a bit of concentration. Each individual will master this at their own pace. There is no set time, but perseverance is the key.
- ***Stage 2***
  Increase the endurance capacity of the deep stabilizing muscles of the spine, by practicing to contract them in different situations for as long as one can. This will become easier with practice.
- ***Stage 3***
  Begin arm and leg movements whilst contracting the deep stabilizing muscles of the spine.
- ***Stage 4***
  Progress to the core strengthening exercises, while contracting the deep stabilizing muscles.

There are two main deep stabilizing muscles that supports the lower back are:

- Multifidus muscle
- Transversus abdominis muscle.

In order to contract transversus and multifidus muscles simultaneously, it is easiest to get on all fours. Without moving the back, or pelvis, draw the stomach up gently-trying to draw the belly up towards the back. This is a very subtle movement so it is best to get the technique monitored by a physiotherapist.

Points to Ponder

- This movement should not be confused with breathing in—it is important to breathe normally while activating the stabilizing muscles.
- Do not use the muscles at the front of the stomach—using the 'six pack' is not the correct technique.

Another useful tool to aid the contraction of transversus and multifidus muscles is a pressure biofeedback device. This device is a bit like a modified blood pressure cuff and consists of an air bag and a readout dial, connected by a tube.

The easiest way to use this tool is to lie on a mat, with the airbag under the tummy. To contract the deep stabilizing muscles of the spine, gently pull in the tummy, until the needle on the dial drops by about 10 units.

- Once the contraction have been mastered, one should try to hold the contraction for four seconds, and repeat the exercise in sets of ten. Once this has been mastered, the patient is ready to move on to the stage 2.

To progress from stage 1, simply increase the duration of the contraction to ten seconds, then twenty, while continuing to practice in sets of ten. Then progress the contraction to as long as possible, aiming for five minutes, then longer.

At this point, one should progress to contracting the deep stabilizers in different positions such as sitting and standing. Practice this while doing everyday activities, such as sitting at the computer, watching TV or on an exercise bike. Once this has been mastered, the patient is ready to move on to the stage 3.

The whole point of the core strengthening program is to increase the support to the back and trunk in order to provide a more stable base for arm and leg movement. The best position to start these exercises is on all fours.

Commence by contracting the deep stabilizers (as described in Stage 1) and hold this contraction. Then raise the right arm straight out to the horizontal. Perform the movement slowly and in a controlled fashion—there should be no wobbling or unwanted movement of the trunk. Hold the arm up for four seconds and then slowly lower.

Next, while maintaining the same position, contract the deep stabilizers and then slowly lift the right leg up straight to the horizontal. Hold it there for four seconds and then slowly lower. The movement should be controlled and there should not be unwanted movement of the trunk or pelvis. Repeat for the left leg (Figs 3.22A to C).

Once these exercises have been mastered, maintaining a contraction of the deep stabilizer muscles, the patient can start doing the core strengthening gym exercises.

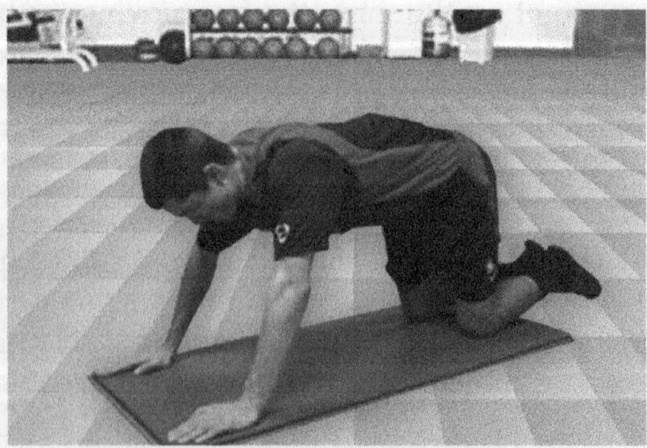

Fig. 3.22A: Prone kneeling

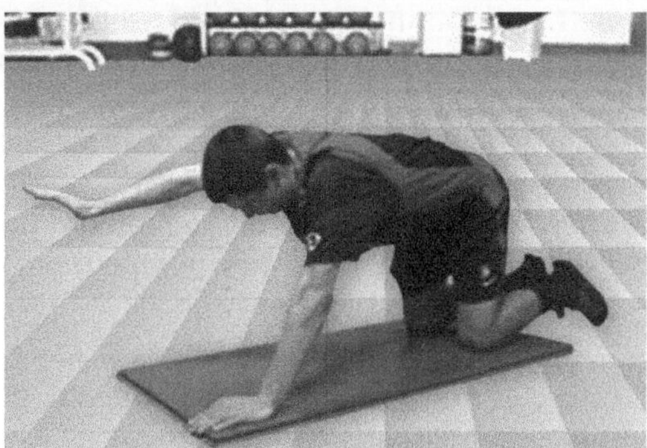

Fig. 3.22B: Single arm extension in prone kneeling

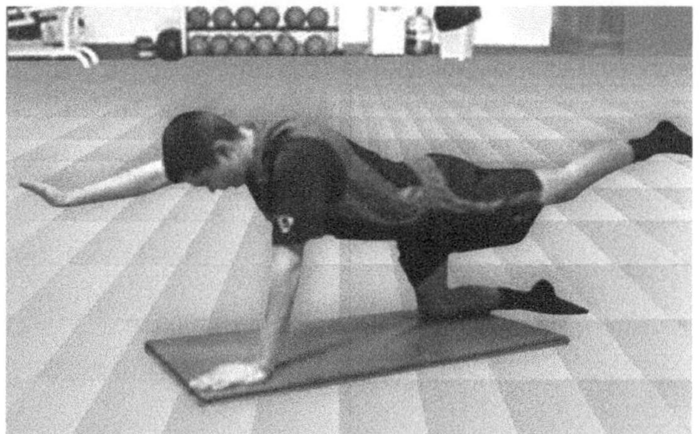

Fig. 3.22C: Crossed arm and leg extension in prone kneeling

The exercises of the core strengthening program are a progression from the previously described core stabilization exercises. It is very important to ensure that a controlled contraction of the core stabilizing muscles is maintained during all of these exercises.

Instruments Needed for Core Strengthening Exercises

Essential kits for core strengthening exercises are:

- Gym ball
- 6′ × 3′ exercise mat
- Medicine ball.

The following is an example day to day rehabilitation program designed to build-up the integrity of the abdominal wall for a professional footballer who has undergone surgical repair for 'Gilmore's Groin', a torn conjoined tendon and aponeuroses of the oblique abdominals.

Day 1

Check wound and start a daily change of dressing. The patient should be able to sit up on bed independently into an upright position, in order to promote scarring in functional position.

Start with isometric abdominal exercises: Lie supine with knees bent. Slide hands up thighs, then hold for four seconds at half way position (6 repetitions).

Then do knee rolls: Lying supine, roll both knees to the left, then to the right (6 repetitions).

Then flex one knee up to chest and straighten other knee out and keep it raised 10 cm off the bed. Repeat other side (6 repetitions).

Days 2–5

Carry out daily exercises as for day one (8 repetitions), three times each day. Initiate gentle cardiovascular work in straight lines using bike, stepper, cross trainer, etc. Discharge from hospital at discretion of surgeon.

From Day 6

Continue exercises as for days 2–5 (10 repetitions), three times each day. Continue cardiovascular work in straight lines with bike, stepper, cross trainer, etc. Initiate core strength exercises—2 sets of each exercise as detailed below.

Core Strength Exercises

1. *Side/holds with leg lift:* Lay on side, with the trunk straight, resting on the elbow. Raise the upper leg and hold for four seconds, then relax. Repeat 10 times (Fig. 3.23).
2. *Trunk twists (med ball between knees):* Balance on the trunk on a gym ball, with a medicine ball held between the knees. Hold another medicine ball in outstretched arms and twist slowly from left to right, then back again (Fig. 3.24).
3. *Lunges:* Lunge forward. Progress to lunging forward with a medicine ball in outstretched arms and then twist in alternate directions, right then left (Fig. 3.25).
4. *Ball rolls: shoulder, trunk and adductor exercise:* Place hands on the floor and feet balancing on the gym ball. Roll the gym ball first to the left then to the right. Repeat 10 times on either side (Fig. 3.26).

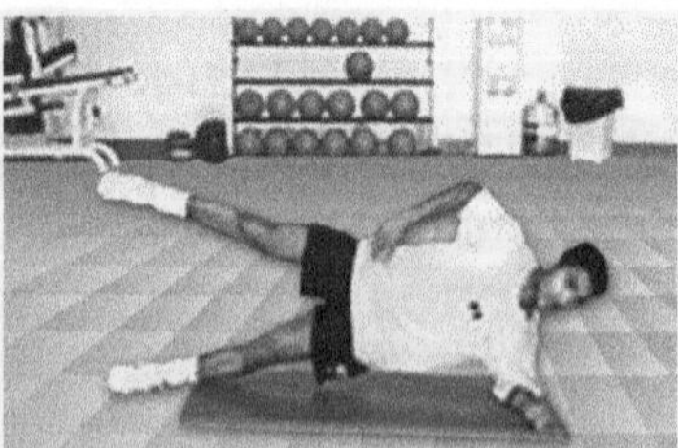

Fig. 3.23: Side/holds with leg lift in side lying on arm support

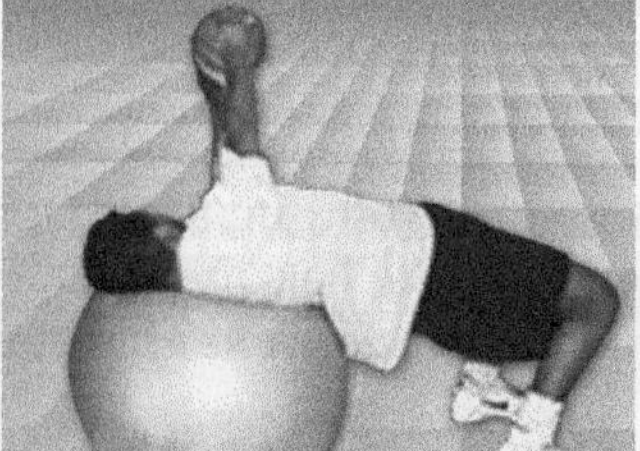

Fig. 3.24: Trunk twists back resting on gym ball

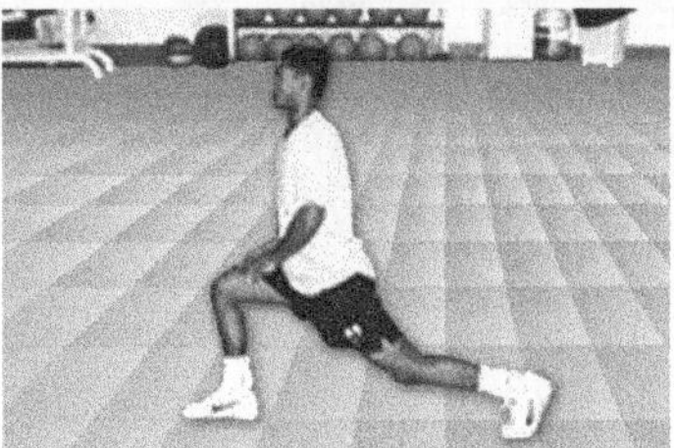

Fig. 3.25: Lunges—starting position

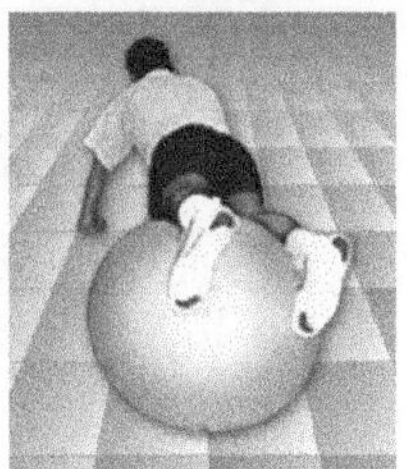

Fig. 3.26: Ball rolling exercises in arm support prone lying with legs resting on gym ball

5. *Adductor strengthening:* Lie on one side on an exercise mat. Bend the top leg as shown. Lift the underside leg off the floor and hold for a count of five. Repeat 5 times (Fig. 3.27).
6. *Hamstring exercises:* Lie on the back on the mat with heels on top of the gym ball. Dig the heels into the ball and lift the pelvis up. Hold for 4 seconds (Fig. 3.28).

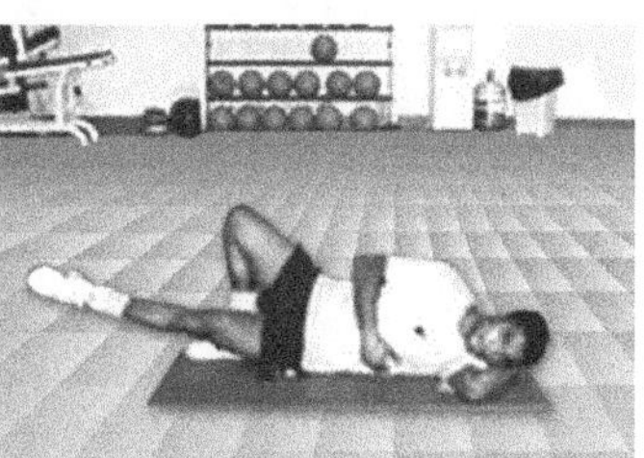

Fig. 3.27: Adductor strengthening exercises in side lying

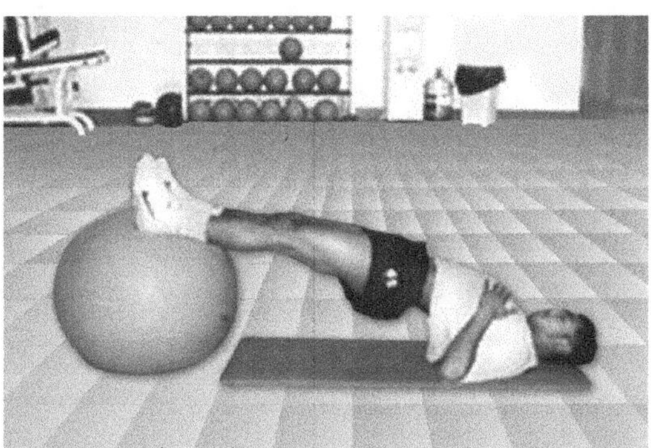

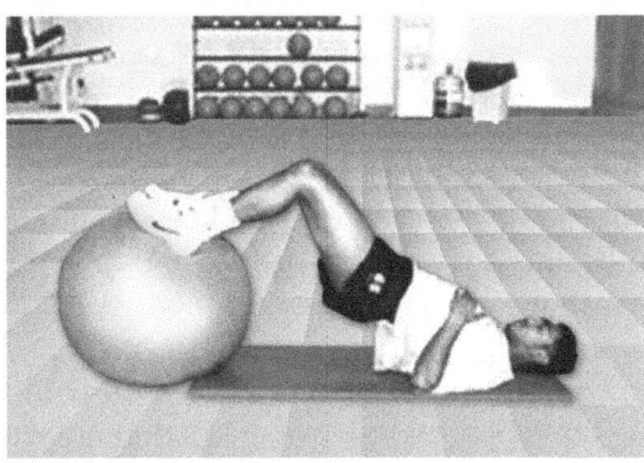

Fig. 3.28: Hamstring exercises—rolling a gym ball forward and back with feet

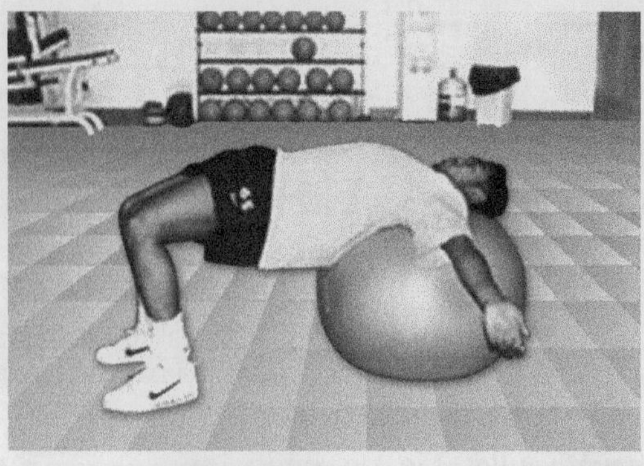

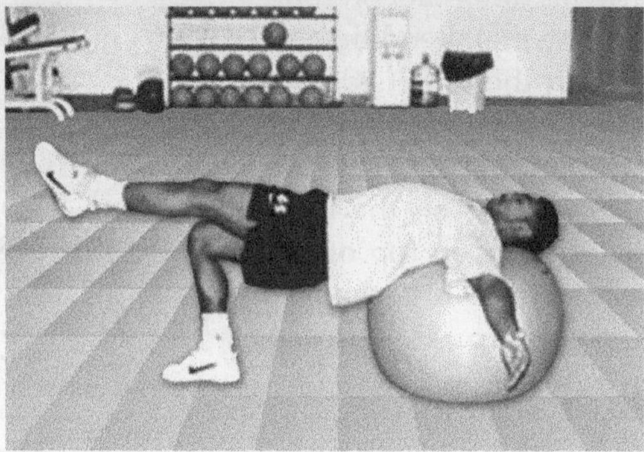

Fig. 3.29: Hamstring and gluteal exercises—trunk resting on a gym ball

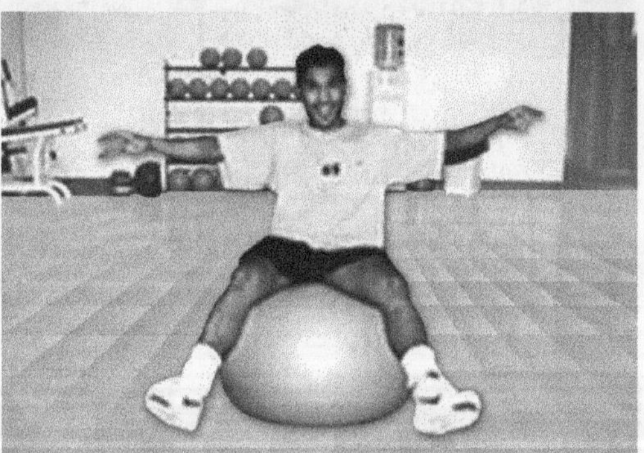

Fig. 3.30: Trunk exercises—sitting on a gym ball with feet off the ground

7. *Hamstring and gluteal exercise:* With the knees bent at 90° and ankles 15 cm apart, balance on the gym ball lying on the back. Tighten the bottom and push the pelvis up. Raise alternate legs to horizontal and hold for 4 seconds (Fig. 3.29).
8. *Trunk exercise*: Sit on the gym ball and balance with the feet off the ground. Note how long can one balance before touching the ground (Fig. 3.30).

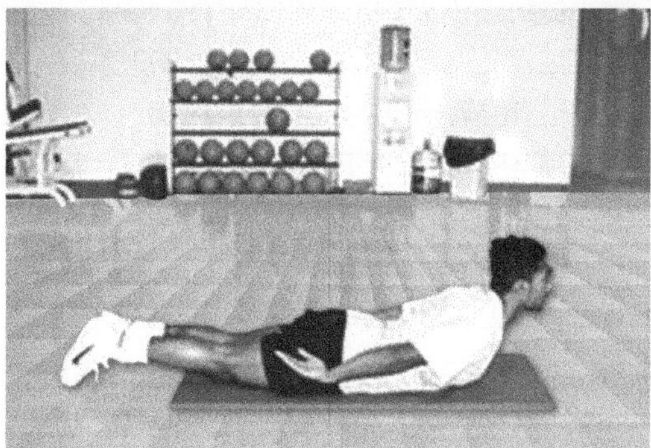

Fig. 3.31: Back extensor exercises—prone lying on a mat

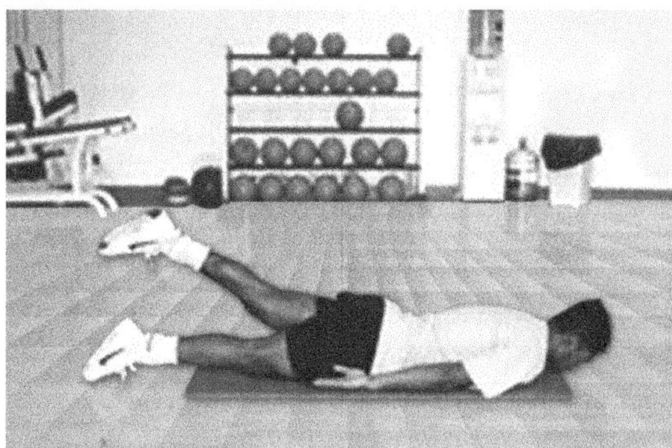

Fig. 3.32: Back extensor and gluteal exercise—prone lying on a mat, raising head and alternate legs simultaneously

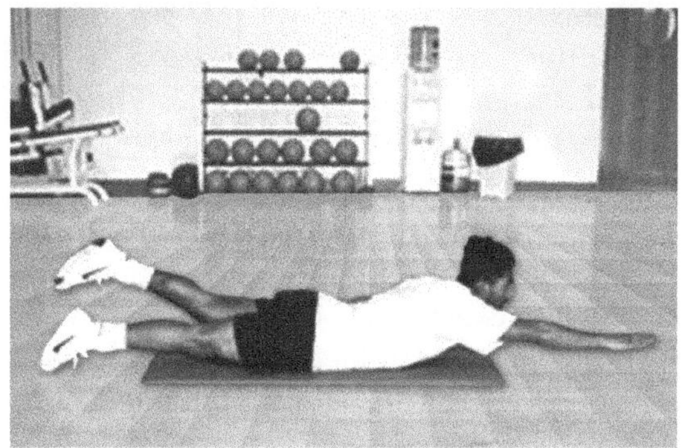

Fig. 3.33: Back extensor and gluteal exercise—prone lying on a mat, opposite arm and legs raised simultaneously

9. *Back extensor exercise*: Lying prone, slowly lift the head and shoulders up off the floor. Hold for 6 seconds (Fig. 3.31).
10. *Back extensor and gluteal exercise*: Lying supine, keep knee straight and slowly lift one leg up. Hold for 6 seconds then relax. Repeat with opposite leg (Fig. 3.32).
11. *Back extensor and gluteal exercise*: Lying supine, slowly lift opposite arm and leg. Hold for 6 seconds. Repeat on other side (Fig. 3.33).

From Day 7

- Discontinue mat exercises.
- Progress core strength exercises to 2 sets × 8 repetitions.
- Start bike, stepper, cross trainer progression.
- Once the wound is closed and stitches removed initiate hydrotherapy rehabilitation—aqua jogging in straight lines wearing buoyancy belt.

From Day 9

- Progress core strength exercises to 2 sets × 10 repetitions.
- Continue bike, stepper, cross trainer progression.
- Continue hydrotherapy progression.

From Day 12

- Progress core strength exercises to 3 sets × 8 repetitions.
- Continue bike, stepper, cross trainer progression.
- Continue hydrotherapy progression.

From Day 15

- Progress core strength exercises to 3 sets × 10 repetitions.
- Continue bike, stepper, cross trainer progression.
- Initiate straight line jogging (treadmill) at slow speed.
- Continue hydrotherapy progression.

From Day 18

- Progress core strength exercises to 3 sets × 12 repetitions.
- Continue bike, stepper, cross trainer progression.
- Progress speed of straight line running (treadmill).
- Continue hydrotherapy progression.
- Initiate single plane power exercises—squats, calf raises, clean and jerk.

From Day 21

- Progress core strength exercises to 4 sets × 10 repetitions.
- Continue bike, stepper, cross trainer progression.
- Progress speed of straight line running to three-fourth pace (treadmill).
- Continue hydrotherapy progression.
- Continue progression of single plane power exercises—squats, calf raises, clean and jerk.

From Day 24

- Progress core strength exercises to 4 sets × 10 repetitions.
- Continue bike, stepper, cross trainer progression.
- Progress speed straight line running to sprints. Introduce ball work to 75 percent straight runs.

- Continue core strength exercises to 4 sets × 12 repetitions as a preventive strategy.
- Continue bike, stepper, cross trainer progression.
- Continue straight line running sprints/ball work to 100 percent straight runs.
- Progress to full functional training.

REFERENCES

1. Patnaik VVG, Singla Rajan K, Bansal VK. "Surgical Incisions—Their Anatomical Basis Part IV-Abdomen" Journal of the Anatomical Society of India; 2001-07– 2001-12;Vol. 50(2).
2. Greenall MJ, Evans M, Pollock AV. Midline or transverse laparotomy ? A random controlled clinical trial. Part I: Influence on healing. British Journal of Surgery, 1980;67(3):188-90.
3. Nyhus LM, Baker RJ. Mastery of surgery. In : Abdominal Wall Incisions. 2nd edn. Little Brown & Co, Boston. 1992;444-52.
4. Guillou PJ, Hall TJ, Donaldson DR, et al. Vertical abdominal incisions—A choice? British Journal of Surgery 1980;67(6):395-9.
5. Cox PJ, Ausobsky JR, Ellis H, et al. Towards no incisional hernias: Lateral paramedian versus midline incisions. Journal of Royal Society of Medicine 1986; 79(12):711-2.
6. Pollock AV. Laparotomy. Journal of Social 1981;480-4.
7. Kocher T. Textbook of operative surgery, 2nd ed, Black London: England 1903.
8. Sato H, Sugawara Y, Yamasaki S, et al. Thoracoabdominal approaches versus inverted T incision for posterior segmentectomy in hepatocellular carcinoma. Hepatogastroenterology 2000;47(32):504-6.
9. Gauderer MWL. A rationale for the routine use of transverse abdominal incision in infants and children. Journal of Paediatric Surgery 1981;16 (Sup.1):583.
10. McBurney C. The incision made in the abdominal wall in cases of appendicitis, with a description of a new method of operating. Annals of Surgery 1894;20:38.
11. Ayers JW, Morley GW. Surgical incision for caesarean section. Obstetrics Gynaecology 1987;70(5):706-8.
12. Zinner MJ, Schwartz SI, Ellis H. Incisions, closures and management of the wound. In: Ellis H (Ed). Maingot's abdominal operation, landed. Prentice Hall International Inc. N Jersey 1997;395-426.

Chapter

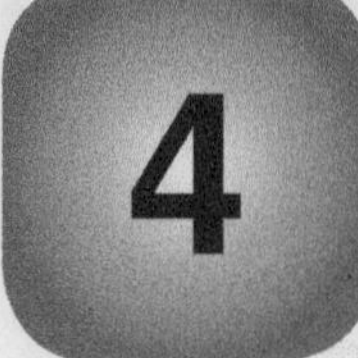

Physiotherapy in Cardiothoracic Surgeries

INTRODUCTION

The term "Thoracic" derives form the word "Thorax", which in ancient Latin and Greek stands for the chest. Anatomically, thorax refers to the area of the body that is located between the neck and the abdomen. It contains organs such as the heart, the great vessels, esophagus, lungs, trachea, bronchi, pleura, mediastinum, chest wall and diaphragm.

What is Cardiothoracic Suregry?

Cardiothoracic surgery is the use of surgical operation to treat diseases of the organs of the chest, specifically for removal of lung cancers and tumors contained in the chest cavity, correction of coronary artery and heart defects, heart or lung transplants, correction of abnormalities of the great vessels and heart valves. Though cardiothoracic surgery happens to be a specialty in surgery, in clinical practice thoracic and cardiac surgeons are two different super specialists who concern themselves with the lung and the heart respectively.

A thoracic surgeon specifically deals with patients with chest trauma, lung cancer, esophageal cancer, empyema and lung abscess, airway disorders like bronchiectasis, mediastinal tumors, diaphragmatic rupture or hiatus hernia and more.

A cardiac surgeon on the hand concentrates primarily with surgical correction of congenital or acquired defects of the heart; such as coronary artery bypass grafting, repair of septal defects, repair or replacement defective heart valve, heart transplantation, etc.

The Cardiothoracic Team

Any cardiothoracic unit works as a close nit team of highly trained professionals, who work under the leadership of the surgeon, but every member must have adequate exposure and experience about each others job to be able to manage in an emergency, till the surgeon can take control of the situation.

The cardiothoracic surgery team primarily consists of the surgeon, the anesthetist, the intervention cardiologist, the radiologist, the OT nurse, the perfusionist (heart-lung machine operator), the intensivist (ICU physician), the ICU nurse, the physiotherapist and the nutritionist.

Other support staffs include the oncologist, the pathologist, medical lab technicians, the clinical psychologist and the medical social worker. The procedures of cardiothoracic surgery include:

1. Noninvasive diagnostic/therapeutic techniques such as bronchoscopy (flexible or rigid)
2. Minimal invasive surgical techniques or keyhole surgery such as mediastinoscopy and thoracoscopy, also known as visually assisted thoracic surgeries or VATS and angiography/angioplasty.
3. Major Surgical techniques such as thoracotomy, sternotomy to conduct procedures like lobectomy, pneumonectomy, decortications, lung resection, thoracoplasty, mediastinal tumor excision, pericardial window and many more.

Indications for Cardiothoracic Surgery

The following are some of the common chest conditions treated through thoracic surgery.

- *Nontraumatic, noninfective chest disorders:* The most frequently encountered and curable condition in the young patients may be:
  - Mediastinal lymphadenopathy which require mediastinoscopy or thoracoscopy for diagnosis
  - Spontaneous pneumothorax, following rupture of a peripheral emphysematous bulla, which requires VATS bullectomy to seal off the air-leak into the pleural space.
  - Pleural effusion, which requires VATS biopsy to analyze the pleural membrane and fluid to rule out malignancy.
- *Chest trauma:* There is high prevalence of chest trauma in road traffic accidents or motor vehicle accidents. Increasing number of vehicles coupled with dangerous rash driving and lack of road safety awareness, result in large number of accidents every year. Many such patients, most often young persons, succumb to these injuries due to lack of appropriate care. Overall, thoracic injuries are directly responsible for up to 20–25 percent of all deaths after road accidents. Furthermore, chest trauma is implicated as a contributing cause of death in an additional 25 percent of patients who die from their injuries. Thoracic surgery, in all its variety, is frequently used to treat such injuries.
- *Infective disorders:* Such as pneumonia, empyema, bronchiectasis, drug resistant tuberculosis, aspergilloma and lung abscess are common clinical conditions seen in our country. It requires great deal of expertise on the part of the surgeon to understand the pathophysiology of the condition and to carryout appropriate surgical procedure suitable for the individual patient. Even simple procedures like chest drain insertion

and bronchoscopy clearance could save many lives that may otherwise suffer or succumb to these infections.

- *Malignancies:* In India, mainly due to growing tobacco smoking habit, numbers of lung cancer patients are increasing every year. We still continue to use asbestos in cement industries for manufacturing asbestos roofing sheet while it is banned in many countries. It is known to give rise to very serious lung problems; specifically to deadly cancer known as mesothelioma. At present, surgical resection of the diseased lung (lobectomy or pneumonectomy), followed up with radiation and chemotherapy, offers the only chance for cure for lung cancer. However, due to inadequate resources and small number of trained surgeons avaiable, such treatment can be offered only to very small proportion of patients in developing countries like India, compared to about 25–30 percent of patients diagnosed with lung cancer in developed countries.

Brief Outline of the Anatomy and Physiology of the Lungs

A quick refresher to the anatomy and physiology of the respiratory system is essential and appropriate before the reader begins to delve deeper into the surgical procedures done on the lungs. The respiratory system is made up of the organs involved in the interchanges of gases, and consists of:

- The upper respiratory tract includes the nose, nasal cavity, ethmoidal air cells and sinuses, larynx and trachea.
- The lower respiratory tract includes the lungs, bronchi, and alveoli.

The lungs take in oxygen, which cells need to live and carryout their normal functions. The lungs also get rid of carbon dioxide, a waste product of the body's cells. The lungs are a pair of cone-shaped organs made up of spongy, pinkish-gray tissue. They take up most of the space in the chest, or the thorax (the part of the body between the base of the neck and diaphragm).

The lungs are enveloped in a membrane called the pleura.

The lungs are separated from each other by the mediastinum. The mediastinum contains the heart and its large vessels, trachea, esophagus, thymus and lymph nodes.

The right lung has three sections, called lobes. The left lung has two lobes. When you breathe, the air enters the body through the nose or the mouth. It then travels down the throat through the larynx (voice box) and trachea (windpipe) and goes into the lungs through tubes called main-stem bronchi.

One mainstem bronchus leads to the right lung and one to the left lung. In the lungs, the mainstem bronchi divide into smaller bronchi and then into even smaller tubes called bronchioles. Bronchioles end in tiny air sacs called alveoli.

THORACOTOMY

Thoracotomy is the most common approach used in any lung and for closed heart surgery.

Definition

Thoracotomy is the process of making of an incision into the chest wall to gain access to the chest cavity. Reasons for the entry are varied. Thoracotomy allows for visual study (eyeballing) of the condition of the lungs; removal of whole or part of a lung; removal of a rib; and examination, treatment, or removal of any organs in the chest cavity. Thoracotomy also provides access to the heart, esophagus, diaphragm, and the portion of the aorta that passes through the chest cavity.

Types and Description

Thoracotomy incisions can of three types:

1. Standard or posterolateral axillary thoracotomy—commencing at the costovertebral margin, commonly passing through the 4th to 8th intercostal space, along the side of the rib cage upto the anterior axillary fold (Posterolateral Thoracotomy)
2. Anterolateral axillary thoracotomy—commencing from sternocostal margin passing under the breast upto the posterior axillary fold (Anterolateral thoracotomy)
3. Median sternotomy—on the front of the chest, vertically through the breastbone (median sternotomy).

The exact location of the incision depends on the level of the lung tissue to be removed. In most cases of lung surgeries and in case of closed heart operation, the incision may range from just under 5 inches (12.7 cm) to 10 inches (25 cm) long and is located at a level exactly opposite to the organ to be operated upon.

Median sternotomy splits the sternum vertically into two halves and is the incision of choice in case of open heart and mediastinal surgeries.

During thoracotomy, a tube is passed through the trachea up to the bronchial division, to keep the airway open for adequate gas exchange through the sound lung. The affected lung is deflated for examination and surgery, while the sound one is inflated with the assistance of a mechanical positive pressure ventilator.

Once the surgical procedure is completed, the chest wall is closed in layers. The layers of skin, muscle, and other tissues are closed with stitches or staples. If the sternum is divided vertically, as in the case of a median sternotomy, it is stitched back together with steel wire or staples.

Common Indications for Thoracotomy

- Thoracotomy is most frequently done to treat lung cancer. Tumors and metastatic growths localized in a small area of the lung can be removed through this incision by a procedure called segmental resection.
- A tissue sample from a lung tumor, can also be taken through this incision, and examined under a microscope for evidence of abnormal cells. This procedure is called a wedge resection. In case lung cancer is detected in the biopsy, the whole lobe (Lobectomy) or the whole lung (pneumonectomy) may be performed through similar incision.
- Thoracotomy is also indicated for removal of consolidated and fibrosed lung lobe following severe unresolved lobar pneumonia.
- Thoracotomy may also be used to resect a section of distorted airway along with its attendant lung segment in cases with severe bronchiectasis with persistent infection. This surgery is called sleeve resection.
- A resuscitative or emergency thoracotomy may sometimes be performed to resuscitate a patient who is near death as a result of a chest injury.

An emergency thoracotomy provides access to the chest cavity, to control stab-injury related bleeding from the heart, or to relieve pressure on the heart caused by cardiac tamponade—an accumulation of blood in the pericardial space, leaking through sutures on the heart wall after open heart surgery.

In the case of an emergency thoracotomy, the procedure performed depends on the type and extent of injury.

The heart may be exposed so that direct cardiac compressions can be performed manually to restart pumping; the surgeon may use one hand or both hands to manually pump blood through the heart. Internal paddles of a defibrillating machine may be applied directly to the heart, to restart the heart beat. Injuries to the heart wall causing the bleeding may be closed with either staples or stitches.

Preoperative Preparation

- Patients are told not to eat after midnight before surgery. This is important because vomiting during surgery, while under GA, can cause serious complications or death. For surgeries in which a general anesthesia is used, the gag reflex is often lost for several hours, making it much more likely that food particles will enter the lungs if vomiting occurs (Aspiration).
- Preanesthetic check should provide all information about all known allergies so that the safest anesthetics can be selected.
- Older patients must be evaluated for pre-existing heart ailments before surgery to assess the ability of their heart to cope with additional strain of surgical shock.

Preoperative Physiotherapy

- All candidates for cardiothoracic suregry and smokers in particular, need to be evaluated thoroughly regarding their pulmonary competence and respiratory reserve. This is usually done on an outpatient basis, much before the surgery by the physiotherapist attached to the cardiothoracic surgery team.
- Pre-existing COPD needs to treated and respiratory function optimized well before the operation through extensive respiratory physiotherapy.
- Any pre-existing disorder such as periarthritis of the shoulder on the side to operated needs to be addressed by the physiotherapist before the operation. After the operation the shoulder movements on the operated side is likely to be inhibited due to pain. Any pre-existing PA will most certainly worsened if not corrected before the operation.

Procedure

For a standerd thoracotomy, the patient lies on his or her side with one arm raised (A) an incision is marked into the skin of the ribcage, (B) skin and muscle layers are cut, and one or more ribs may be removed to gain access to the cavity, (C) retractors hold the ribs apart, exposing the lung, (D) after surgery, the periosteum of cut ribs are stiched back in place, and (E) new ribs will grow enetually from this periosteum. Layers of muscle and skin are stitched in layers to close the wound (F).

Aftercare

Opening the chest cavity means cutting through skin, muscle, nerves, and sometimes bone. It is a major procedure that often involves a hospital stay of five to seven days. The skin around the drainage tube to the thoracic cavity must be kept clean, and the tube must be kept unblocked.

The pressure differences that are set up in the thoracic cavity by the movement of the diaphragm make it possible for the lungs to expand and contract. If the pressure in the chest cavity changes abruptly, the lungs can collapse. Any air or fluid that collects in the pleural cavity puts a patient at risk for pleural effusion, or even collapse of the lung due to collection of air, called pneumothorax. Thus, any entry to the chest cavity requires that chest drainage tubes remain in place for several days to drain trapped air and exudate after the incision is closed.

The first two days after surgery may be spent in the intensive care unit (ICU) of the hospital. A variety of tubes, catheters, and monitors may be required after surgery.

Risks

The rich supply of blood vessels to the lungs makes hemorrhage a major risk in lung surgeries; a blood transfusion may become necessary during surgery. General anesthesia carries inherent risks such as nausea, vomiting, headache, unstable blood pressure, or allergic reaction. After a thoracotomy, there may be drainage from the incision. There is also the risk of infection; the patient must learn how to keep the incision clean and dry as it heals.

After the chest tube is removed, the patient is vulnerable to pneumothorax. Physicians strive to reduce the risk of collapse by timing the removal of the tube. Doing so at the end of inspiration (breathing in) or the end of expiration (breathing out) poses less risk. Deep breathing exercises and coughing should be emphasized as an important way that patients can improve healing and prevent pneumonia.

New Alternatives

Video-assisted thoracic surgery (VATS) is a less invasive alternative to thoracotomy. Also called thoracoscopy, VATS involves the insertion of a thoracoscope, a thin, lighted tube into a small incision through the chest wall. The surgeon can visualize the structures inside the chest cavity on a video screen. Such instruments as a stapler or grasper may inserted through other small incisions. Although initially used as a diagnostic tool to visualize the lungs or to remove a sample of lung tissue for further examination, VATS may be used to remove some lung tumors.

An alternative to emergency thoracotomy is a tube thoracostomy, a tube placed through chest wall to drain excess fluid. Over 80 percent of patients with a penetrating chest wound can be successfully managed with a thoracostomy.

Common Surgeries of the Lungs

A number of different procedures may be performed on the lungs through a thoracotomy incision (Fig. 4.1).

- A *lobectomy* removes an entire lobe of a lung, the right lung having three and the left lung two lobes. Lobectomy may be done to remove a small and localized cancer lesion that is contained by a lobe or a consolidated lobe following lobar pneumonia. When only the affected lobe of the lung is removed, the remaining healthy tissue is spared to maintain adequate lung function.
- A *segmentectomy* or *wedge resection,* removes a wedge-shaped piece of lung segment that is smaller than a lobe.
- Alternatively, the entire lung may be removed during a pneumonectomy.
- *Bullectomy:* After entring the thoracic cavity using one of the thoracotomy, the whole lung surface, particularly at the apex and the lung edges, are carefully searched for emphysematous bullae. Apical wedge resection or segmentectomy may be necessary to remove the diseased

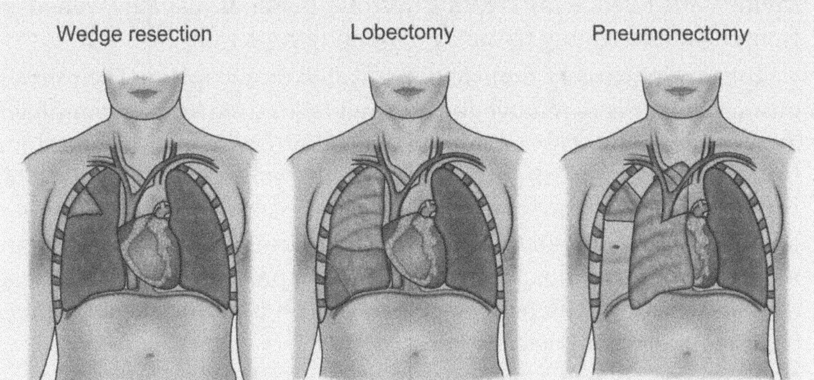

Fig. 4.1: Types of lung surgeries performed through thoracotomy incision

or damaged lung tissue. This is then followed by stapling or suturing to seal the affected area with fibrin sealant to reduce chance of postoperative leakage of air.

- *Pleurodesis:* After entering the thoracic cavity, mechanical abrasion of the pleural membrane is done to induce intrapleural inflammation that causes the parietal and the visceral pleura to stick togather, obliterating the pleural space. Without a space to become lodged, the problem of air entrapment in repeated pneumothorax is eliminated. Pleurodesis also can be done chemically, though less preferred to mechanical variety.
- *Pleurectomy (removal of the pleura):* The procedure may be done via a large thoracotomy or median sternotomy or by a small lateral incision in the fifth or sixth intercostal space. The procedure involves the complete removal of the pulmonary bullae and as complete as possible stripping of the parietal pleura.
- *Exploratory thoracotomy:* Opening of the chest wall for direct visualization of the lungs and other chest structures when there is evidence of an abnormality or disease that has not been verified by other diagnostic methods.

Common Causes for Lung Surgeries

Conditions of the lungs for which a lobecotomy may be performed include the following:

- *Tuberculosis (TB)*—it is a chronic bacterial infection that usually infects the lungs, although other organs may also be affected. TB is primarily an airborne disease that is spread by droplets from infected people when they cough or sneeze. In most cases TB is well controled by medication. In case of drug resistant bacteria, TB causes destruction of lung parenchyma resulting in formation of cavitites within the lungs. Such cavities are filled with creamy necrotic material, usually walled off from the remaing lung tissue by a tough fibrous wall.

The type of surgery done for TB is called thoracoplasty.The purpose of such sugery is to remove the infected lobe of the lung as completely as possible and create a limited collapse of cavities within the lung, through resection of ribs over the affected area, and allowing the chest wall to collapse inwards and adhere to the visceral pleura, eliminating the tubercular cavity in this process, eliminating oxygen supply to any residual TB bacterium that may have escaped resection and causes their destruction. The patient is then put on a multidrug antintubercular regime to complete the cure.

- *Lung abscess*—it is a localized collection of pus following any non-tubercular infection that may form in the lung. If the abscess does not resolve with antibiotic therapy, it may "wall off" within a fibrous tissue pocket within the lungs so that it does not infect the rest of the body. Such surgery is done to remove this pocket of infective material, with minimal collateral damage to healthy lung tissue.
- *Emphysema*—it is a chronic illness that results from the breakdown of the elastic fibers in the lungs, interfering with expansion and contraction of the lungs and formation of large cavities in the, called bullae, in the alveolar parenchyma of the lungs. Bullae may occasionally rupture, causing air to leak in to the pleural space, creating a spontaneous pneumothorax. Though Bullae may be removed by Bullectomy, Lobectomy may be needed sometimes to remove damaged lung lobe completely is the cavitation is wide spread and the loss of elastic recoil of the affected lobe is creating problems in the expansion and contraction of the remaining lung.
- *Benign tumor*—it is a a noncancerous mass, occupies space and causes compression of surrounding healthy lung issue, interefring with lung function. The type of surgery needed to remove this mass is either a segmental resection or a lobectomy, depending on the size of the tumor.
- *Lung cancer*—it is a group of cancers that may affect the bronchi, one or more lobes of the lungs, the pleural lining, and/or other lung tissue. In lung cancers, whenever operable, a lobe may be removed in very early stage of the disease and in later stages the entire lung needs to be removed in through Pneumonectomy. Aim of such sugery is to remove the affected lobe or the entire lung, along with all the lymph ducts and glands supplying the diseased lung, to prevent further spread of cancer.
- *Fungal infections*—fungi are a group of organisms that, although rare, may cause infections in various parts of the body, including the lungs. Fungal infections of lungs are diffuse, difficult to diagnose and treat. In few cases, badly involved lung segments in a lobe may need to be surgically removed through lobectomy.

Potential Complications of the Procedure

As with any surgical procedure, complications may occur following lung surgeries. Some possible complications include the following:

- Chest infection or generalized septicemia leading to shock.
- Tension pneumothorax—air becomes trapped in the pleural space, causing the lung to collapse.
- Hemorrhage.
- Bronchopleural fistula—an opening between the bronchus and pleural space causing leakage of air or fluid into the pleural space.
- Bronchopulmonary fistula—an opening between the stump of a bronchus and empty pulmonary space after pneumonectomy, causing siphoning of surgical exudates into the healthy lung.
- Hydrothorax—collection of fluid in the pleural space, causing the lung to collapse.
- Empyema—an accumulation of pus in the pleural cavity.

Postoperative Care after Lung Surgeries

After a minor procedure like thoracoscopy, most people can go home within 24 hours after the chest drains have been removed.

After a major procedure like thoracotomy, the patient may need to stay in the hospital for a week or more depending on the extent of surgical shock and secondary complications that may develop after the surgery.

After minor lung surgery, the patient will most likely go to a general care floor for one or two days, before being discharged. However after major thoracic surgery, a patient may need to be nursed in an intensive care unit until his condition is stable.

Pain Management

The patient will have pain near the incision and general soreness of the entire chest wall. Primary aim of postoperative nursing should be to make the patient feel as comfortable as possible. It is very important that the pain is managed aggressively well, so that the patient can cough, do deep breathing exercises, and move more easily in the bed. The medicine works better if started before the pain becomes too severe. Hence communication between the nurse and patient must be frequent and the patient feedback regrading intensity of pain must be given due importance.

During early recovery, an anesthesiologist may implement any of the following two pain control options.

- A patient controlled analgesia (PCA) pump is a pump that releases pain medicine into patient's veins. The patient will be able to control the amount of pain medicine he receives by pressing a button.
- An epidural catheter may be placed in the spine and delivers a constant amount of pain medicine.

- Once eating and drinking, the patient will be able to take pain killers by mouth.
- The physiotherapist may apply TENS along the suture line. This is very effective in controlling postoperative pain. The TENS can be started on a patient immediately after surgery. This however should be done in consultation with the surgeon or the intensivist in charge of the patient. Therapeutic measures such as breathing exercises and assisted coughing must be done only after adequate analgesia has been achieved, because if the patient feels pain while doing exercises he is not likely to cooperate with the therapist.

Care of Drainage Tubes and Catheters after Surgery

The patient may have a variety of tubes, drains, and equipment attached to the body immediately after surgery.

- *Drainage tubes:* In thoracotomy, a pair of chest drainage tubes are placed within the pleural cavity on completion of surgery. When the surgeon opens the chest wall, the normal negative intrapleural pressure, which keeps the lung expanded, is lost. To reinflate the lung, a chest tube is put in the upper part of pleural space (apical drain), between the lung and chest wall linings, to draw out the trapped air. The other tube is placed at the base of the pleural cavity (basal drain) to collect blood and secretions that ooze out after the surgery. Both tubes are hooked to drainage bottles that collect trapped air, fluid and blood (Fig. 4.2).

  Traditionally, under water sealed drainage system, under suction, is used for draining trapped air and fluid from the pleural space. The drainage tubes, with glass end piece, end under water within draiage bottles, connected to suction by another glass tube above water. Suction

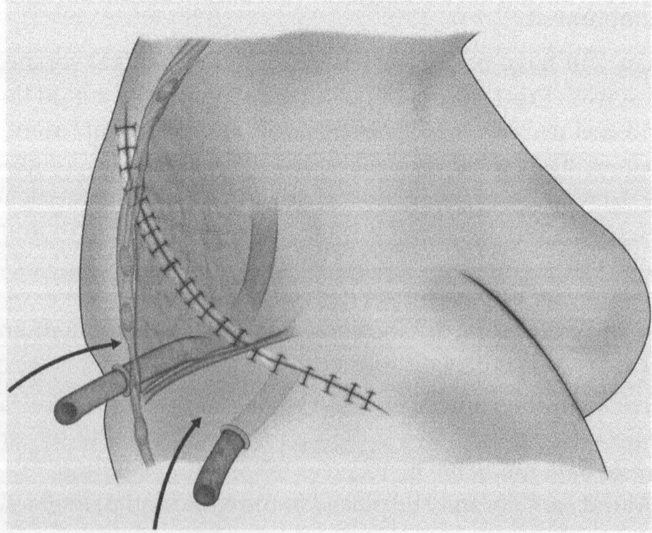

Fig. 4.2: Position of drainage tubes after thoracotomy

helps to draw out the air trapped in the pleural space. The water in the bottle prevents air from re-entering the chest cavity. This type of drainage bottles are placed on the floor below the hospital bed to allow the gravity to draw out the surgical exudates.

Points to Ponder

- Usually a patient of thoracotomy is nursed on sound side lying. This keeps the operated side uppermost. This allows for free access to the operation site for monitoring and dressing the wound, as well as prevents the drainage tubes from being squeezed.
- However the patient may need to be turned to the opposite side lying while giving percussion and vibration to the chest. This needs the drainage bottles to be shifted to the opposite side.
- The therapist has to be especially careful about handling drainage systems while turning the patient from one side to other. The drainage tubes must be first clamped with artery forceps and then lifted over the patient to place it on the floor on the opposite side, preferably behind the patient. The clamping is essential to prevent water from the bottle from siphoning back into the thoracic cavity.

Nowadays drainage systems with built in vacuum suction is used. These drainage systems are very compact, easy to use and change. They are taped to the side of the chest in such a manner that the patient can change sides without any risk of the exudates siphoning back into the thoracic cavity.

The chest tubes remain in place for 2–6 days. Most people go home within 24 hours after the chest tube is removed. The surgeon decides to remove the chest drain when the lung is reinflated, which is detected through daily chest X-ray.

- An intravenous (IV) catheter delivers nutrients, electrolytes and medicine through fluid medium directly to the blood stream of the patient. Once the patient starts eating and drinking and able to take oral medication, the IV may be removed.
- Oxygen is given through a mask or a small plastic nasal cannula.
- A Foley catheter drains urine from the bladder into a collecting bag. It is removed as soon as the patient is able to use the bed pan.
- An ECG monitor may be used for a few days to watch the heart rate and rhythm.

How to do Self-care of the Lungs?

The patient must be encouraged to deep breathe, cough, and use the 'lung exerciser' called an incentive spirometer as frequently as he can. This helps toning muscles of inspiration, open up the alveoli in the lungs and keeps airways clear of secretions.

How to Restore Normal Activity?

It is important that the patient becomes active as soon as possible, since this is the best antidote for most of the secondary complications. The physiotherapist is the key person in planning the return of the patient to fullest possible activity. However the extent of activity allowed will depend on the clinical background of the patient and presence of any complication. Usually on the day of surgery, the patient will be allowed to sit up in bed. The 1st postoperative day the patient may be allowed out of bed to walk a few steps around the bed. On the 2nd postoperative day he may be allowed to walk within the ward. From 3rd day onwards he walks longer and longer distances, till by the time stiches are removed and he goes home on 7th–10th day, he should be able to walk in the hall 3–4 times a day, as well as climb up and down one flight of stairs.

How to Care at Home?

When the patient goes home he may need help from a home health nurse or a relative for the first week, mainly for the care of the incision, management of pain, maintain activity level and self care.

Care of the incision: The incision may look slightly red for several days. It should be watched for signs of infection.

Points to Ponder

- If the stitches look swollen, tender or red, or if the patient has a temperature greater than 100°F, the surgeon must be informed.
- The incision must be kept clean and dry.
- Patient may be allowed to take shower, but do not take baths or swim until the wound has healed completely.
- The incisions must not be rubbed because this prevents healing. Pat them dry.
- Other than those prescribed by the surgeon no lotions or powders should be applied on the incision area.
- Once healed, sunscreen should to be applied when in the sun because the incision is at risk for sunburn.

When the patient goes home, the incision may have all or a few of the staples or stitches in place. Sometimes, small pieces of sterile tape are placed after the staples are removed. It is okay if these tape strips fall off, but do not pull them off. In 1–2 weeks, the doctor will remove remaining staples or stitches that are left.

Management of pain: The patient will have some pain for two to three weeks after the surgery. Pain is more likely to increase as he becomes more active. When in pain, the patient must take pain medication as prescribed. All pain killers have side effects. Self-medication of these pills or alteration of dosage must be avoided. If the pain is sharp and constant or suddenly increases in intensity the doctor must be informed.

Maintaining activity level: During first few days or weeks at home the patient may feel tired and sore, and may need someone to help with ADL. One must stay active and do necessary ADL, but pace oneself carefully to avoid fatigue.

Points to Ponder

- Patient should avoid using the affected side arm for streneous exercises or activities like pulling, pushing and lifting weight greater than 10 pounds within 4 weeks after surgery. It is okay to use the arm on the operated side for nonstrenuous activity.
- Patient should not drive for 4 weeks, especially if taking narcotic pain pills.
- *Sexual activity:* As the patient feels better, he may resume having sex. At first, he may not have the energy or may worry about the incision or about becoming short of breath. These are normal feelings and should not be allowed to inhibit oneself.

Smoking: If a smoker, the patient needs to quit smoking to prevent further damage to his lungs.

Common Surgeries of the Heart

Most common surgeries of the heart in an adult concern with the:

- Removal of a blockage in the coronary arteries and restoring normal circulation
- Repair and replacement of defective heart valves
- Transplanting a severely damaged heart with a healthy heart from a recently dead individual.

In children heart surgeries are done mostly to:

- Repair congenital defects in the heart septa (muscular partitions between chambers of the heart)
- Dilate narrowed heart valves
- Correct malposition of the great vessels (the aorta and the vena cava) of the heart.

Since physiotherapy techniques, applicable in any patient who has under gone heart surgery, remains largely uniform irrespective of the type of surgery, in following section, I have focused on the most common heart sugery of them all—the coronary artery bypass graft surgery; as an example to illustrate the techniques of physiotherapy applied in rehabilitation following cardiac surgery in an adult.

CORONARY ARTERY BYPASS GRAFT SURGERY (CABG) (Other Term: Open Heart Bypass Surgery)

Introduction to Arteries of the Heart

To better understand how coronary artery disease affects the heart, a review of basic heart anatomy and function is necessary.

The heart is basically a pump. The heart is made up of specialized muscle tissue, called the myocardium. The heart's primary function is to pump blood throughout the body, so that the body's tissues can receive oxygen and nutrients and have waste substances taken away in the blood stream.

Like any other pump, the heart needs fuel in order to work. The myocardium requires oxygen and nutrients, just like any other tissue in the body, to work efficiently. The myocardium receives oxygen and nutrients from the blood flowing in through the coronary arteries. The coronary arteries lie on the outer surface of the heart and supply oxygenated blood to the heart muscles through numerous branches that penetrate deep within the heart. Trouble, in the form of coronary artery disease (CAD), strikes when blood flowing through the coronary artery network is blocked or slowes down due to Atherosclerosis. Atherosclerosis causes progressive narrowing of the coronary arteries due to deposition of plaques of fat that stick to the inner walls of the artery. As a result the heart muscles do not receive adequate amount of blood. When the heart muscle (myocardium) does not receive an adequate blood supply, it recieves less than normal ammount of oxygen and nutrient and therefore it cannot function as well as it should. If the myocardium's blood supply is decreased for a length of time, an irreversible ischemia develops, causing degradation of heart muscle tissue. Cardiac ischemia decreases the heart's pumping ability, because the heart muscle is weakened due to a lack of food and oxygen.

For many years, coronary artery disease (CAD) was known as "hardening of the arteries" and in spite of many advances have been made in the diagnosis and treatment of cardiac diseases, it is still not easily treated other than by physically restoring blood supply to heart muscle through surgery, bypassing the blocked arteies.

What is Coronary Artery Bypass Graft Surgery?

Coronary artery bypass graft (CABG) surgery is a procedure used to treat coronary artery disease. The blocked or narrowed coronary arteries are simply bypassed, replacing the blocked portion of the coronary artery with a piece of patent blood vessel taken from any other less sensitive area of the body. Such vascular grafts, used for the CABG procedure, may be pieces of a vein taken from the legs or mammary artery in the chest. One end of the graft is attached above the blockage and the other end is attached below the blockage. Thus, the blood is rerouted around, or bypasses the blockage through the new graft to reach the heart muscle.

Description of the Procedure

Traditionally, in order to bypass the blocked coronary artery in this manner, the chest is opened through a vertical midsternal incision to expose the heart. In order to open the chest, the sternum is cut in half vertically along the midline (median sternotomy) and spread apart with retractors. The heart is stopped (fibrilated) for a time with a mild electric shock, so that the surgeon can perform the bypass of the blocked coronary artery using a piece of vascular graft (Artery/Vein). Once the heart is stopped, tubes are inserted into the heart at the point of inflow and outflow so that the blood can be diverted and continue to be pumped through the body during the surgery using a cardiopulmonary bypass machine (heart-lung machine). The heart lung machine has an inbuilt oxygenator and a pump. The oxygenator oxygenates and extracts carbodioxide from the blood, doing the job of the lungs and the pump circulates the blood through the body. This way the vital organs of the body like the brain, liver, kidney continue to recieve a steady supply of oxygen and nutrients, keeping them healthy.

Recent Advance in CABG

While the traditional "open heart" procedure is still performed and often preferred in many situations, newer, less invasive techniques have been developed to bypass blocked coronary arteries. "Off-pump" or "Beating Heart" procedures, in which the heart does not have to be stopped, were developed in the 1990s.

Other minimally-invasive procedures, such as keyhole surgery performed through very small incisions and robotic procedures performed with the aid of a programmable mechanical device, are in final stages of development.

Two other surgical advancements for persons undergoing CABG are endoscopic vein harvesting and endoscopic radial artery harvesting. In both of these procedures surgeons use an endoscope (thin flexible fiber-optic surgical tube with a light and camera at the tip) to locate blood vessels that will be used for bypassing the blocked coronary arteries. Veins are generally harvested from the inner thigh and calf areas of the legs, while the mammary artery from the chest or radial artery from the wrist is harvested.

Traditional (open) harvesting approaches involve making long surgical incisions down the inner thigh and/or calf. As compared to the traditional vein harvesting approaches, endoscopic harvesting methods have fewer complications, less leg pain, and shorter hospital stay.

Preoperative Investigations

Investigative procedures that may be used to assess and /or treat the heart include resting or exercise electrocardiogram (ECG), Holter monitor, signal-averaged ECG, cardiac catheterization, chest X-ray, computed tomography (CT scan) of the chest, echocardiography, electrophysiological studies, magnetic resonance imaging (MRI) of the heart, myocardial perfusion scans, percutaneous transluminal coronary angioplasty (PTCA), radionuclide angiography and ultrafast CT scan.

Indications for CABG

Coronary artery bypass surgery is performed to treat a blockage or narrowing of one or more of the coronary arteries, thus restoring the blood supply to the heart muscle.

Symptoms of coronary artery disease may include the following:

- Chest pain
- Fatigue
- Palpitations
- Shortness of breath.

Unfortunately, there may be no symptoms of early coronary artery disease, yet the disease will continue to progress until sufficient artery blockage exists to cause symptoms and problems. If the blood supply to the heart muscle continues to decrease as a result of increasing obstruction of a coronary artery, a myocardial infarction, or heart attack, may occur. If the blood flow cannot be restored to the particular area of the heart muscle affected by ischemia, the muscle tissue in that area will die.

Risks of the Procedure

Possible risks associated with coronary artery bypass graft surgery include the following:

- Bleeding during or after the surgery
- Blood clots entering blood stream that can cause embolism leading to heart attack, stroke, or lung problems
- Infection at the incision site
- Pneumonia
- Breathing problems
- Cardiac dysrhythmias /arrhythmias (abnormal heart rhythms).

Patients who are allergic to or sensitive to medications, contrasts dyes, iodine, shellfish, or latex should notify their physician.

There may be other risks associated with certain specific pre-exisiting medical condition, such as hypertension, renal insufficiency, hypothyroidism and diabetes.

Preoperative Preparations

- The surgeon will explain the procedure and answer any questions that the patient might have before obtaining a written consent to do necessary tests, give anesthesia and perform the operation.
- In addition to a complete medical history, the surgeon may perform a complete physical examination including complete battery of tests as detailed above to ensure that the patient is suitable for the procedure.
- The patient will have to fast the night before the procedure.
- The patient should notify the physician if there is a history of bleeding disorders or if he is taking any anticoagulants such as aterovastatin or aspirin, medications that affect blood clotting. A blood test is done to determine how long a patient bleeds from a pinprick (bleeding time or BT) and how long it takes for the blood to clot (clotting time or CT).
- If a smoker, the patient will have to stop smoking as soon as possible prior to the procedure. This will improve the chances for a successful recovery from surgery and benefit overall health status of the patient. Full profile lung function tests are some times needed, though usually the surgeon is satisfied with a preoperative exercise tolerance and respiratory efficiency test done by the physiotherapist.
- Based upon the clinical background of the patient, the physician may require other specific preparation, such as a regimen of insulin in a diabetic patient to control the blood sugar or a course of bronchodilators and vigorous chest physiotherapy in a patient of long-standing COPD.

During the Procedure

Generally, a coronary artery bypass surgery or any other open heart surgery follows the following steps:

1. The patient is asked to remove any jewelry and clothing and will be given a gown to wear and asked to empty the bladder prior to anesthesia. Patient has to be fasting with nil oral food or water for 12 hours atleast before surgery.
2. An intravenous (IV) line is started in the vein of forearm, elbow or dorsum of the hand to infuse glucose and electrolyte solutions and if required for transfusion of blood and plasma. Central venous pressure catheters (CVP) is inserted in the jugular vein in the neck region to monitor the status of the heart and blood pressure, as well as for obtaining blood samples. Cardiac catheters may be introduced in the subclavian artery under the collarbone area or the femoral artery at the groin.
3. The patient is positioned in supine position on the operating table.
4. The anesthesiologist, standing at the head end of the operating table will continuously monitor the heart rate, blood pressure, breathing,

and blood oxygen and carbon dioxide saturation along with electrolyte levels during the surgery.

5. Once the patient has been deeply sedated, an endotracheal tube is inserted into the airway through the mouth and the patient connected to a positive pressure ventilator, which will breathe for the patient as long as the patient remains under the influence of general anesthesia during and for sometime after the surgery, till he is completely regains the ability to breathe spontaneously.
6. A catheter is inserted into the bladder before to drain urine into an urine bag.
7. The skin over the surgical site is shaved and cleansed with an antiseptic solution.
8. Once all the IV tubes, catheters and monitors are in place, incisions may be made in one or both legs to obtain a section of any superficial vein to be used as grafts. Recent techniques tend to harvest the internal mammary artery for use as a bypass graft. The grafts thus harvested are preseved in cool normal sanline till they are put to use.
9. The surgeon will make an incision down the center of the chest from the manubrium sterni to just above the navel, cutting through the skin, fascia and the bridging aponeurosis of the pectoralis major muscle on both side and upper part of the rectus sheath. No muscle is divided in such midsternal or median sternotomy incision.
10. The sternum is divided in two halves vertically and they are spread apart with a retractor to visualize the heart.
11. The pericardial membrane is cut and the surface of the heart is exposed.

CABG-on-Pump Procedure

1. In order to sew the grafts onto the very small coronary arteries, the heart must be stopped to allow the surgeon to perform the very delicate procedure under an operating microscope.
2. Once the blood input and output vesseles to and from the heart has been diverted into the heart-lung machine for oxygenation and pumping, the heart beat is stopped by injecting it with a cold solution.
3. Once the heart has been stopped, the surgeon performs the bypass graft procedure by sewing one end of a section of vascular graft over a tiny opening made in the coronary artery just above the blockage, and the other end over a tiny opening made in the coronary artery just below the blockage.
4. A patient may have more than one bypass graft performed, depending on how many blockages he has and where they are located. After all the grafts have been completed, the surgeon examines them to make sure they are working as desired.
5. Once the bypass grafts have been completed, the blood circulating through the bypass machine is allowed back into the heart and the tubes

to the machine is removed. Then the heart is restarted (Defibrillated) with an electric shock.

6. Temporary electrode wires for pacing the rhythm and rate may be inserted into the heart. These wires can be attached to a pacemaker outside the body and the heart can be paced, if needed, during the initial recovery period.

CABG-off-Pump Procedure

1. Once the heart has been exposed, the area around the artery to be bypassed is stabilized with a special type of instrument.
2. The rest of the heart continues to function and pump blood through the body.
3. The cardiopulmonary bypass machine and the perfusionist who runs it, may be kept on stand-by should the procedure need to be completed on bypass.
4. The surgeon performs the bypass graft procedure by sewing one end of a section of vein over a tiny opening made in the coronary artery just above the blockage, and the other end over a tiny opening made in the coronary artery just below the blockage.
5. Before the chest is closed, the surgeon examines the grafts to make sure they are working optimally.

Procedure Completion, Both Methods

1. The sternum is pushed back together and sewn together with small wires.
2. The skin, fascia and pectoral aponeurosis over the sternum is sewn back in layers. A sterile bandage/dressing is applied over the sutures.
3. Tubes are inserted into the mediastinal space to drain blood and other fluids from around the heart. These tubes will remain connected to a suction device to suck fluids away from arround the heart.
4. A Ryle's tube is inserted through the mouth or nose into the stomach to drain stomach fluids as they form.

Recovery after the CABG

In the hospital:

Coronary artery bypass surgery requires an in-hospital stay of seven days or longer in case of complications.

Immediately after the surgery the patient is kept in the recovery room for two to three hours, before being shifted to the intensive care unit (ICU) to be closely monitored. Alternatively, the patient may be taken directly to the Surgical ICU from the operating room.

In the ICU the patient is connected to a bank of monitors that constantly display the electrocardiogram (ECG or EKG) tracing, blood pressure, CV pressure readings, breathing rate and oxygen saturation level.

The patient will most likely have an endotracheal tube in airway so that breathing can be assisted with a ventilator until stable enough to breathe on his own. As the patient wakes up from the anesthesia and start to breathe on his own, the ventilator will be weaned off to allow the patient to take over more of the breathing voluntarily. When the patient is awake enough to breathe completely on his own and is able to cough, the endotracheal tube will be removed. The Ryle's tube will also be removed at this time.

Initially the patient will be on multichannel IV drips to help feed, hydrate and give medication for controlling blood pressure, heart rhythm and rate, and to control any problems with infection or bleeding. As the condition stabilizes, these drips will be gradually decreased and turned off as patient's condition allows.

Once the breathing and stomach tubes have been removed and patient's condition has stabilized, he may start liquids to drink.

Role of the Physiotherapist

After the endotracheal tube is out, the physiotherapist will assist the patient to cough and take deep breaths every two hours. This will be uncomfortable due to soreness of the incision, but it is extremely important that the patient do this in order to keep mucus from collecting in the lungs and possibly causing pneumonia. The physiotherapist must show the patient how to hug a pillow tightly against the chest while coughing to stabilize the sternal ends to ease the discomfort. An elastic chest binder is very effective in this matter and should be requisitioned by the therapist as per patient's size before the surgery. While applying the chest binder the therapist must take care not to squeeze the drainage tubes and kink the temporary pacemaker leads coming out of the surgical wound.

The surgical incision may be tender or sore for several days after a CABG procedure. The physiotherapist can reduce this pain by utilizing TENS. Disposable TENS electrodes are fixed over the prepared skin at either ends or on both sides of the suture line and connected to the TENS unit. Chest binder may be applied over the TENS electrodes to hold them firmly in place. TENS using burst mode may be applied for as long as eight hours or if needed continuously. It is important to note that TENS is most effective in patients not receiving narcotic analgesics. (For details refer to "Handbook of Practical Electrotherapy" by the author).

The patient may also get narcotic pain reliever as per preference of the surgeon. In such case the therapist may time his two hourly visits to the patient half an hour after the pain medication has been administered. This way patient will be able to better comply with breathing and mobility exercises to be done by the therapist.

Usually by the third postoperative day the surgeon may decide that the patient is ready to be shifted to a surgical ward. The physiotherapist will continuously regulate the activity level allowed, which will be gradually increased from the fourth postoperative day as the patient gets out of bed till he walks around for longer periods of time by the seventh postoperative day. The patient is usually discharged by the seventh to tenth day after the stitches have been removed.

Care at home: Once the patient is home, it will be important to keep the surgical area clean and dry. The surgeon or the nurse will give the patient specific bathing instructions if the sutures or staples are in place. The sutures or surgical staples will be removed during a follow-up visit, in the event they were not removed before leaving the hospital.

The patient should not undertake vigorous activity or drive until the physician tells him to. Other activity restrictions may apply depending upon the cardiac competence of the patient. The physician must be notified immediately if any of the following occur after going home:

- Fever and/or chills
- Redness, swelling, or bleeding or other drainage from the incision site
- Increase in pain around the incision site.

Cardiac Rehabilitation after Heart Surgeries—an Overview

Ideally the therapist should continue to visit the patient on alternate days at home for at least three weeks after discharge from the hospital. The therapist at this stage should draw out a patient specific rehabilitation plan with the knowledge and concurrence of the cardiologist, to restore the patient to a lifestyle that is desirable medically and acceptable to the patient. The basic principle behind any cardiac rehabilitation is that the heart has to be subjected to a level of exercise stress which increases its rate by ten to twenty beats per minute from the resting rate, without triggering any arrhythmia or chest pain. Slight shortness of breath and moderate amount of sweating during exercise is desired. However, while exercising the heart the therapist must be alert for any signs of undue fatigue or chest pain/tightness. The golden rule to remember in cardiac rehabilitation is that "the recovery to resting heart rate is more indicative of cardiac fitness than the peak heart rate achieved". Therefore, while training a patient to achieve cardiac fitness after CABG or for that matter any cardiac surgery, the therapist should gradually acclimatize the patient to progressively higher levels of exercise stress, always ensuring that the patient is able to recover the resting heart rate within two minutes of stopping the exercise. The essential tools for this purpose is a wristband monitor showing heart rate, rhythm and blood pressure recordings on a real time basis. The exercises can be designed with progressive levels of stress, starting from mat activity like rolling, bridging and pelvic shifting on bed. Stretching of the upper extremities, with particular attention to shoulder horizontal abduction, abduction-elevation and scapular bracing exercises must be done next. This may be followed up with walking on level surface with gradually increasing distance and speed. The Bruce's protocol may be used to grade the cardiac competence by plotting the speed of walking against ambient heart rate. In patients with painful knee, a static cycle or a stepper may be used to give endurance exercises instead of walking. Once the patient has achieved adequate exercise tolerance to perform all ADL within the home without assistance, it is time to shift his rehabilitation process to a dedicated cardiac fitness training center. Here many patients with similar level of cardiac fitness are put through their paces under close supervision of a trained cardiophysiotherapist. The aim of such group therapy session is to provide an element of competition among patients to motivate themselves and for the psychological support generated through interaction among a peer group affected in the same manner by a disease common among all of them.

PHYSICAL THERAPY AFTER CARDIOTHORACIC SURGERIES

Introduction

Physical therapy is essential to the treatment of patients admitted for major surgery of the heart and lungs, including patients with critical illness in intensive care units.

Physical therapy contributes towards assessing and treating various aspects of respiratory disorders such as airflow obstruction, mucus retention, alterations in ventilatory pump function, dyspnea, impaired exercise performance and quality of life.

This section discusses airway clearance techniques, breathing retraining, exercise training and peripheral and respiratory muscle training, in relation to a variety of conditions affecting the respiratory system after a major cardiothoracic surgery.

Principles of Physical Reconditioning

Impaired exercise tolerance is a common finding in patients with chronic respiratory disease, especially after a major cardiothoracic surgery. Factors, such as peripheral and respiratory muscle weakness and deconditioning, are now recognized as important contributors towards reduced exercise tolerance.[1,2]

Randomized controlled studies have reported that carefully planned and executed pulmonary rehabilitation has produced significant improvements in walking distance and exercise tolerance after cardiothoracic surgeries, including improved quality of life and reduced symptoms.[3,4]

Endurance training involves a larger muscle mass working at moderate intensity for a period of time. For patients with more advanced disease or after surgery of the heart or the lungs, reducing the impact of exercise on the cardiopulmonary system, can be done by shortening the exercise duration and/or reducing active muscle mass.

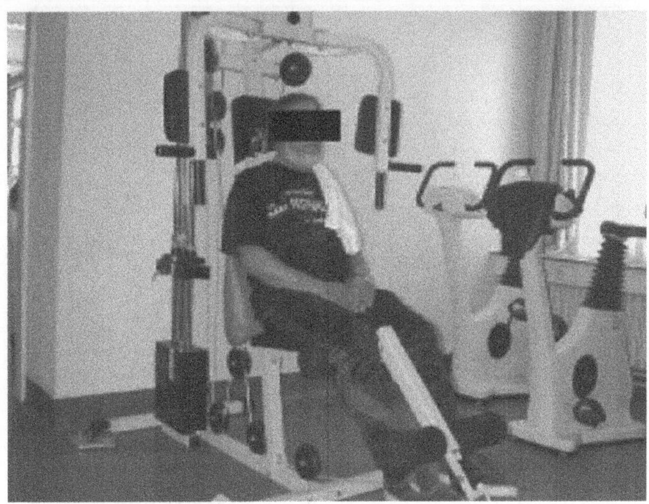

Fig. 4.3: Resisted exercises are effective in optimizing respiratory competence in COPD or postoperative cases

Resisted exercises, done against moderate resistance for the lower limbs are appropriate and effective for exercise training in patients with compromised cardiorespiratory function (Fig. 4.3).[5,6]

Recently, neuromuscular stimulation of lower limb muscles in patients with severe COPD has been shown to improve muscle strength, exercise performance and quality of life (Fig. 4.5).[7,9]

Principles of PT in Physical Reconditioning

- Early mobilization enhances oxygen transport, muscle function, joint mobility and coordination of movement.
- Prevention of muscle atrophy is best achieved with active muscle contractions, but critically-ill patients are often unable to perform voluntary contractions. Under these conditions, active or passive cycling or pedocycling done on bed (Fig. 4.4) has been shown to prevent muscle fiber atrophy and protein loss, in comparison with twice-a-day passive stretching of less than five minutes per session.[8,10]
- Electrical stimulation of the quadriceps (Fig. 4.5) not only gives active limb mobilization but also enhances muscle strength and decreases the number of days needed to transfer from bed to chair.[11]

Dysfunction of the Respiratory Pump

Surgeries of the heart and the lungs create serious compromise of the respiratory pump. Disruption of the integrity of the chest wall, postoperative inhibition of the diaphragm due to pain and resultant disuse weakness of the major respiratory muscles are the main cause of this dysfunction. Pre-existing COPD only worsens the postoperative clinical picture. Outcome of such dysfunction are as follows:

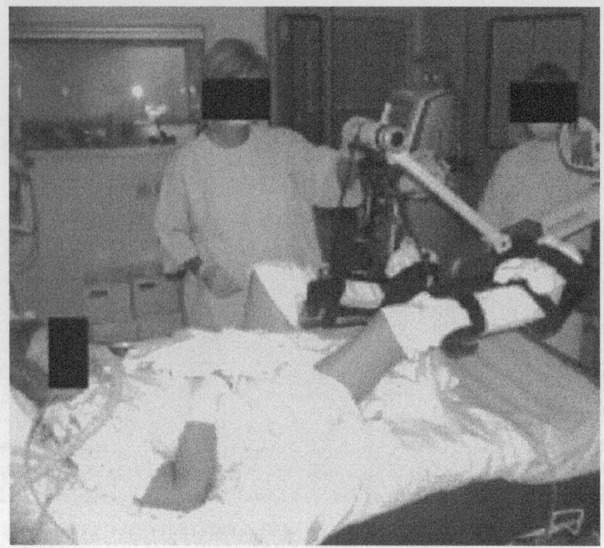

Fig. 4.4: Bed cycling exercises

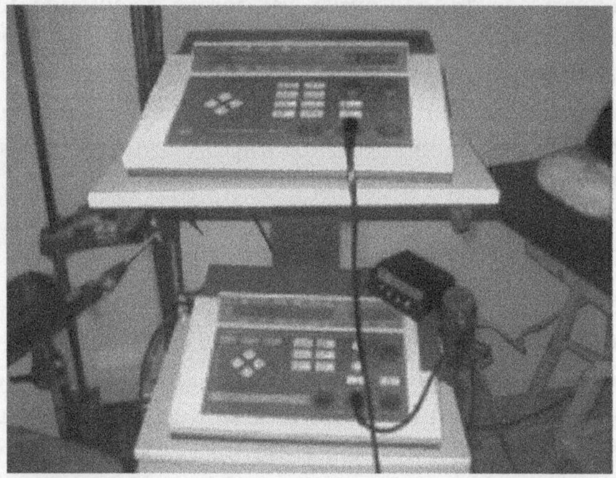

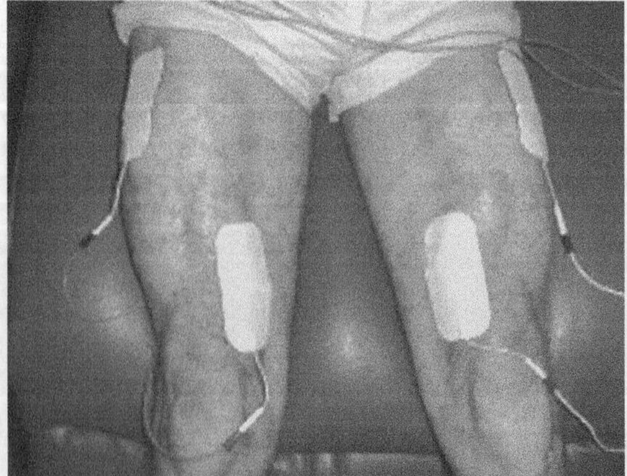

Fig. 4.5: Electrical stimulation of quadriceps muscles

Dyspnea or shortness of breath (SOB): Dyspnea is an important and debilitating symptom seen in patients after major heart and lung surgeries, with or without pre-exisiting COPD.[12] Several other pathophysiological factors that contribute towards dyspnea in postoperative cases are as follows:
- Fatigue, inhibition and weakness of the inspiratory muscles
- Postoperative pain and tightness of the chest wall
- After effects of general anesthesia
- Gas exchange abnormalities
- Dynamic airway compression due to bronchospasm
- Cardiovascular insufficiency
- Surgical shock
- Infection.

Controlling dyspnea is an important aim in the postoperative physiotherapy care of any major surgery and specifically after cardiothoracic surgeries. Common treatment methods are bronchodilator therapy, breathing exercise and oxygen therapy are also applied to alleviate symptoms and improve respiratory function.

"Breathing exercise" is an all-embracing term for a range of exercises including relaxation exercises, pursed lips breathing, corrective positioning, inspiratory and expiratory muscle training.

Relaxation Exercises

Relaxation exercises slow down the respiratory rate to allow more time for complete expiration to take place. One study showed that progressive relaxation resulted in an immediate decrease in heart rate, respiratory rate, anxiety and dyspnea, and long-term stabilization of the respiratory rate Renfoe[13] and Kolaczkowski et al[14] observed that the combination of relaxation exercises and manual compression of the thorax improved the excursion of the thorax and oxygen saturation significantly.

Pursed Lips Breathing

Pursed lips breathing improves expiration of trapped air from the lungs by the active and prolonged expiration through the half-closed lips. This generates back pressure of air, preventing airway collapse. Compared with spontaneous breathing, pursed lips breathing reduces the respiratory rate, dyspnea and $PaCO_2$, and improves tidal volume and oxygen saturation under resting conditions[15,16] contributing towards reduction in breathlessness.

Some COPD patients use pursed lip breathing instinctively, while other patients have to be taught the technique by the therapist. Pursed lips breathing is found to be effective in improving reducing breathlessness. Patients with loss of elastic recoil of lungs seem to benefit more from practicing this technique during exertion and to cope with episodes of breathlessness.

Breathe Reeducation to Improve Respiratory Muscle Efficiency

Endurance and strength of the inspiratory muscles are frequently reduced in chronic lung disease, after major abdominal/cardiothoracic surgeries, burn and neuromuscular disorders. This weakness in the muscles of respiration contributes towards dyspnea and exercise intolerance, and probably towards respiratory failure. Respiratory muscle function training has the aim of reducing the relative load on the muscles, i.e. the ratio between the actual pressure and the maximal pressure; PI/PImax and hence may contribute towards reducing dyspnea and increasing the maximal sustained ventilatory capacity. This might also imply improvement in exercise capacity among patients with ventilatory limitation during exercise. Breathing retraining and body positions have the aim of improving the length-tension relationship or geometry of the respiratory muscles, in particular the diaphragm, or increasing the strength and endurance of the inspiratory muscles. According to the length-tension relationship, the output from the muscle increases when operating at a greater length, for the same neural input. With breath re-training, the efficacy of intercostal muscle contraction in stabilizing the rib cage improves. Moreover, the piston-like movement of the diaphragm increases and enhances the lung volume changes during the breath cycle.

Contraction of the Abdominal Muscles during Expiration

Contraction of the abdominal muscles during expiration lengthens the diaphragm, thus allowing it to operate close to its optimal length. In addition, active expiration will increase the elastic recoil pressure of the diaphragm and rib cage. The release of this pressure after relaxation of the expiratory muscles will assist the next inspiration. In healthy subjects, this mechanism is brought into play only with increased ventilation. However, in patients with severe COPD, contraction of abdominal muscles invariably becomes linked to resting breathing.[17] Active expiration increases the transdiaphragmatic pressure (P di) and PImax. The additional effects of active expiration on exercise training among patients with severe COPD were studied by Casciari et al.[18] They observed a significant increase in maximum oxygen uptake during a bicycle ergometer test, if the test was done after a period of breathing retraining, as a part of a training program on a treadmill, in comparison with the treadmill program without breathing retraining.

Body Position

Relief of dyspnea is often experienced by patients in different body positions. Forward leaning has been shown to be very effective in reducing SOB in COPD[19] and is probably the body position most adopted by patients with lung disease (Fig. 4.6). The effect of this position seems to be unrelated to the

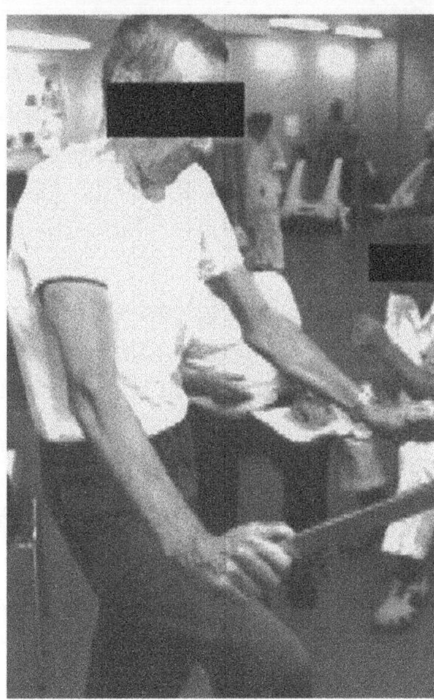

Fig. 4.6: Forward lean position offloads the accessory muscle of respiration and helps control shortness of breath

severity of airway obstruction, changes in minute ventilation or improved oxygenation.[19] Reduction of hyperinflation and paradoxical abdominal movement have also been controlled effectively in the forward leaning position resulting in reduced SOB.[19] Further, forward leaning has been associated with significantly reduced electromyographic (EMG) activity in the scalene and sternomastoid muscles, increased trans-diaphragmatic pressure and significantly improved thoracoabdominal movements.[19] From these studies, it can be concluded that the subjective improvement in dyspnea achieved in patients with COPD was the result of the more favorable position of the diaphragm on its length-tension curve. In addition, forward leaning with the upper girdle resting on arm support allows accessory muscles of respiration to contribute significantly towards inspiration, due to passive stabilization of the rib cage and off loading the accessory muscles by passive elevation of the upper girdle.

Abdominal Belt

The "abdominal belt" was developed as an aid to support diaphragmatic function. Early studies reported on its use on patients with emphysema, but it has only been successfully used on patients with spinal cord injury, for whom it improves vital capacity.[20] However, increased expiratory flow and expiratory pressures during abdominal strapping have not been consistently observed in such patients.[21]

Respiratory Muscle Training

Recent studies on patients with COPD have shown natural adaptations of the diaphragm at cellular level with increased proportion of type I fibers and subcellular level with shortened sarcomeres and increased mitochondria concentration, which contributes towards greater fatigue resistance and better functional muscle behavior.[22] Despite these cellular adaptations, both functional inspiratory muscle strength and inspiratory muscle endurance are compromised in COPD cases. Inspiratory muscle training may further enhance these spontaneous adaptations.

Three types of training are practiced at the present time:

1. Inspiratory resistive training (IRT)
2. Threshold loading (ITL)
3. Normocapnic hyperpnea (NCH) during which the patient is asked to ventilate maximally for 15–20 minutes (Fig. 4.7).

In a randomized controlled trial, NCH was shown to enhance respiratory muscle endurance and exercise capacity, as well as quality of life, in COPD patients.[23] During inspiratory resistive breathing, the patient inspires through a mouthpiece and adapter with an adjustable diameter or "threshold loading". Most studies have observed that breathing against an inspiratory load (at least 30% PImax) increased maximal inspiratory pressure and endurance of the inspiratory muscles. A recent study on COPD patients has shown significant gain in the proportion of type I fibers and the size of type II fibers in the external intercostals following IMT.[25] Dyspnea[26] and nocturnal desaturation time[27] also decreased, while exercise performance tended to improve.[24] Inspiratory muscle training in

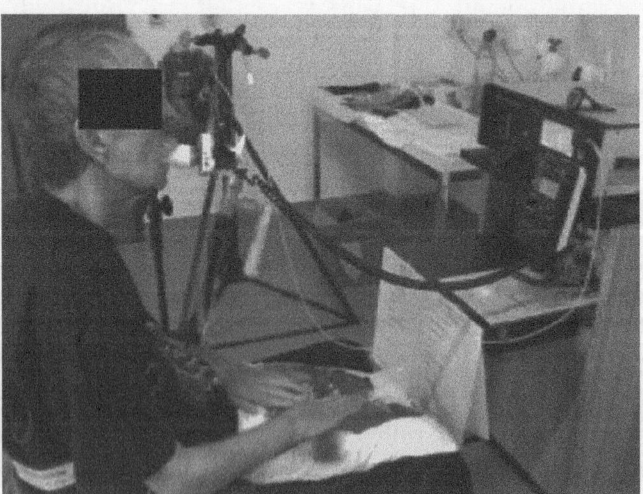

Fig. 4.7: Training for normocapnic hyperpnea—during resisted inspiration the patient inspires through a mouthpiece and adapter with an adjustable diameter or "threshold loading"

addition to exercise training has been shown to improve exercise capacity more than that is achieved by exercise training alone.[28,29] The additional beneficial effect of IMT on exercise performance seems to be related to the presence of inspiratory muscle weakness.[24] At present there are no data to support resistive or threshold loading as the training method of choice. Threshold loading enhances the velocity of inspiratory muscle shortening.[30] This might be considered an important additional beneficial effect, as this shortens inspiratory time and increases the exhalation and relaxation time.

It may therefore be concluded that, in postoperative cases with active COPD and inspiratory muscle weakness, well-controlled and carefully guided inspiratory muscle training exercises improves inspiratory muscle function, thereby reducing dyspnea and nocturnal desaturation time, resulting in potential improvement in exercise tolerance. Training intensity should be at least 30 percent of the maximal inspiratory pressure for 30 minutes per day.

In quadriplegic patients, respiratory muscle training has also been shown to enhance inspiratory muscle function, improve pulmonary function and control dyspnea.[31,32] In patients with neuromuscular disease (NMD), respiratory muscle dysfunction is more complex and dependent on the precise disease and its stage. It seems that NMD patients, for whom more than 25 percent of the predicted pulmonary function still remains, are still trainable.[33] Although inspiratory muscle function is commonly affected in these diseases, expiratory muscle function is often more impaired in quadriplegia and multiple sclerosis. Expiratory muscle training has also been shown to be beneficial in the latter condition.[34] In the long-term, the progressive nature of most neuromuscular disorders affecting muscle function impedes the beneficial effects of training.

Finally, respiratory muscle weakness is a frequent cause of failure to wean a patient from ventilator support.

Respiration training during the weaning period could facilitate the weaning process.[35,36] Biofeedback of breathing patterns can be given to such patients to accelerate the weaning process.[37]

BREATHING RETRAINING TO OPTIMIZE THORACOABDOMINAL MOVEMENTS

Alterations in chest wall motion are common in patients after cardiothoracic surgeries, as well as, in asthma and COPD. Several studies have described increased rib cage contribution towards chest wall motion and/or asynchrony between rib cage and abdominal motion in these patients.[38,39] The mechanisms underlying these alterations have not been fully understood, but it appears to be related to the degree of airflow obstruction, rigidity of the rib cage, changes in diaphragmatic function and increased contribution of accessory inspiratory muscles towards chest wall motion. Indeed, increased firing frequency of single motor units of the scalene and parasternal muscles,[40] and also that of the diaphragm,[41,42] have been observed in COPD patients as compared with age-matched normal persons used as control. The activity of accessory muscles has been positively associated with the sensation of shortness of breath (SOB), whereas diaphragm activity has been negatively related to this sensation.[43] Consequently, diaphragmatic breathing, or slow and deep breathing, is commonly applied in physical therapy practice, in an attempt to correct abnormal chest wall motion and decrease the work of breathing, accessory muscle overload and SOB.

Diaphragmatic Breathing

During diaphragmatic breathing, the patient is told to move the abdominal wall predominantly during inspiration and to reduce upper rib cage motion. All studies have shown that, with appropriate commands from the therapist during diaphragmatic breathing exercises, COPD patients are able to voluntarily change their breathing pattern to more abdominal movement and less thoracic excursion.[44,45] However, diaphragmatic breathing may be accompanied by increased asynchronous and paradoxical breathing movements, while no permanent changes in breathing pattern are observed. Although abdominal and thoracic movement clearly changes, no changes in ventilation distribution has been observed.[45] In addition, in some cases dyspnea has been found to worsen during diaphragmatic breathing, while increased work of breathing, increased oxygen cost in breathing and reduced mechanical efficiency of breathing have been found in patients with severe COPD.[46]

In conclusion, there is no evidence from controlled studies to support the use of diaphragmatic breathing in COPD patients.

Slow and Deep Breathing

Since, for a given minute ventilation, alveolar ventilation improves when breathing at a slower rate and higher tidal volume, this type of breathing should be encouraged for patients with impaired alveolar ventilation. Several authors have reported a significant drop in respiratory frequency, and significant rise in tidal volume and PaO_2 during imposed low frequency breathing at rest in patients with COPD. Slow and deep breathing practiced during pulmonary rehab training helps the patient achieve more efficient breathing during exercise and hence reduce the ventilatory demand and dyspnea.[47]

In summary, slow and deep breathing improves breathing efficiency and oxygen saturation at rest. A similar tendency has also been observed during exercise.

IMPAIRED AIRWAY CLEARANCE AND LUNG INFLATION

Hypersecretion and impaired mucociliary transport are important pathophysiological features of obstructive lung diseases like cystic fibrosis and chronic bronchitis, as well as in patients with acute lung disease, i.e. atelectasis and pneumonia. Hypersecretion is associated with rapid decline of pulmonary function and higher mortality in patients with COPD.[48] In patients with advanced neuromuscular disease, mucus retention and associated respiratory complications contribute significantly towards morbidity and mortality.[49] Although a cause and effect relationship between mucus retention and lung dysfunction has not been conclusively proven, under present circumstances, improvement of airway clearance is considered to be an important aim in treating such patients.

Medication and physical therapy are commonly effective in enhancing mucus transport by improving the fluidity of the mucus layer, thus stimulating or compensating weak ciliary action or by using compensatory physical mechanisms such as pull of gravity as in postural drainage, two-phase gas-liquid interaction through the interaction and energy transfer between the high airflow velocity and the mucus layer, vibration, oscillation or airway compression.[50,51]

Forced expiratory maneuvers such as huffing and coughing are considered to be the cornerstone of forced expiratory airway clearance techniques and thus an essential part in every combination of treatment methods.

Forced Expiration Techniques

The idea behind therapeutic forced expiratory maneuvers is to enhance mucus transport through the interaction and energy transfer between the high airflow velocity and the mucus layer or two-phase gas-liquid interaction. The effectiveness of this transmission and hence of mucus transport depends on the thickness of the mucus layer and airflow velocity. A thicker mucus layer is easier to move, as more kinetic energy is transmitted to the mucus layer.[49] Huffing, coughing, and also ventilation at rest or during exercise, induce higher airflow velocities that effectively stimulates mucus transport from the central and intermediate lung zones.[51-53] However, in patients with airway instability as in emphysema, forced expiratory maneuvers may result in airway collapse and impair mucus transport. Indeed, manual chest wall compression during forced expiration has been found to decrease the peak cough flow rate in patients with severe COPD.[54] However, in neuromuscular disease, the reduced expiratory muscle strength limits effective huffing and coughing. Manual assistance with chest wall compression enhances the peak cough flow rate in patients with neuromuscular disease, without scoliosis or similar chest and spinel deformities, but has not been beneficial in patients with chest wall deformities.[54] In addition, deep lung inflation increases maximum peak cough flow in patients with progressive neuromuscular disease.[53] Mechanical hyperinflation using an ambu bag and manually assisted coughing are effective and safe for facilitating airway clearance.[54] Glossopharyngeal breathing has been shown to increase vital capacity and expiratory flow rates and is a treatment option for patients with high spinal cord injury.[55]

Exercise

During exercise, increased ventilation and release of mediators in the airways may be effective in enhancing mucus transport.[56] Increased mucus transport has been observed to occur during exercise in healthy subjects and patients with chronic bronchitis,[57] but it has been found to be less effective than conventional chest physical therapy in patients with cystic fibrosis.[58] When exercise is combined with chest physical therapy, significantly more sputum volume has been found to be expectorated than during chest physical therapy alone.[59]

Postural Drainage and Body Position

During postural drainage, the major bronchi are positioned appropriately to allow gravitational forces to promote mucus transport to the central airways. Studies investigating the efficacy of postural drainage using radioaerosol tracer have not shown any additional improvement in mucus transport following postural drainage[60] but, in patients of bronchiectasis with excessive mucus production, postural drainage alone enhanced mucus transport and expectoration significantly.[61]

Body position has also been shown to affect oxygenation, though This effect has not always been acknowledged in clinical practice. In patients with unilateral lung disease, the side lying position with the unaffected side down generally improves oxygenation.[62] In patients with acute respiratory distress syndrome, the prone position increases arterial PO_2. Alterations in ventilation-perfusion inequality have been suggested as the main reason for improved oxygenation in these body positions.[63]

Percussion and Vibration

Manual or mechanical percussion and vibration are based on the assumption that the oscillatory forces are transmitted to the bronchi. Although such oscillations are observed during bronchoscopy in the central airways, it is believed that absorption of the forces by air and by the lung parenchyma prevents transmission to smaller and intermediate airways. This probably explains the lack of additional effect on mucus transport from adding chest percussion and vibration to breathing retraining, postural drainage and coughing.[64] Another explanation might be the frequency dependence of the effects of vibration and oscillation. The optimal frequency-enhancing mucus transport appears to be around 12–17 Hz.[65]

POSITIVE EXPIRATORY PRESSURE MASKS BREATHING (BI-PAP) AND FLUTTER BREATHING

Positive expiratory pressure mask breathing (Fig. 4.8) can be introduced to prevent airway collapse and improve collateral ventilation, and thus to enhance mucus transport Falk et al[66] showed that the addition of this technique to forced expiration or postural drainage increased the mucus expectoration in cases with retention of secretion. It has been demonstrated that positive expiratory pressure therapy is superior to standard treatment in preserving pulmonary function over the long-term.[67]

Flutter breathing is the addition of a variable, oscillating expiratory pressure and airflow at the mouth, to facilitate mucus clearance. Konstan et al[68] observed a fivefold increase in expectorated mucus using this method in patients with cystic fibrosis, in comparison with coughing or postural drainage.

Chest Expansion and Lung Inflation

Mechanically ventilated patients are often unable to perform forced expiratory maneuvers effectively, due to unconsciousness. "bag squeezing"—manual hyperinflation using an Ambu-Bag followed by "chest squeezing"— forced expiration with chest wall compression (Fig. 4.9) is frequently applied in unconscious patients, and this improves oxygenation, lung compliance, and facilitates secretion removal.[69-71] Potential adverse lung issues—such as emphysema must be taken in consideration when applying manual hyperinflation.[72]

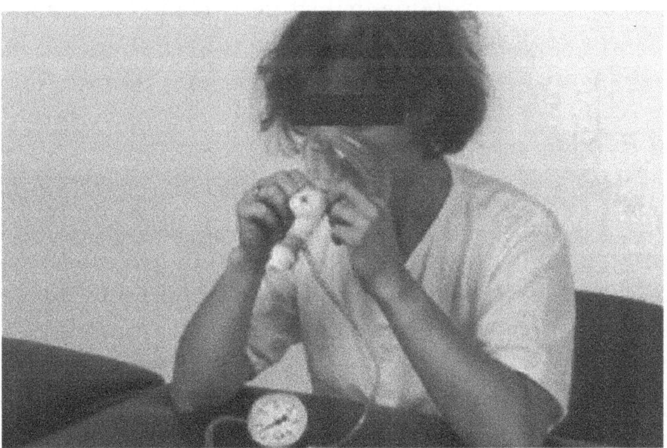

Fig. 4.8: Breathing exercises using positive expiratory pressure mask

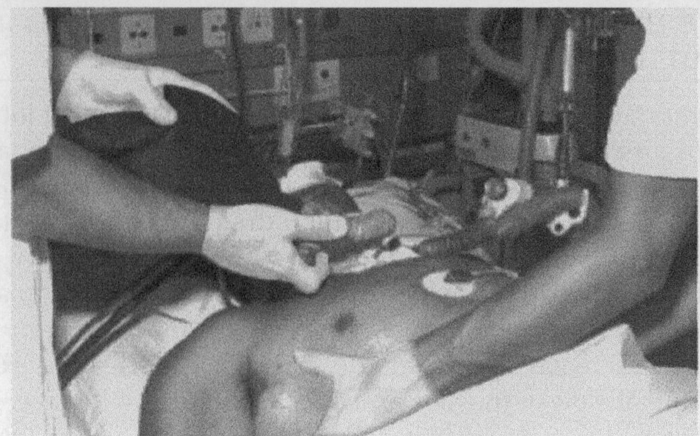

Fig. 4.9: Manual hyperinflation using Ambu-Bag followed by chest wall compression in ventilated patient

CONCLUSION

It is now well-established that postoperative pulmonary complications following thoracic and abdominal surgery remain a major cause of morbidity and mortality. Early mobilization is very effective in preventing pulmonary complications. Evidence for the effectiveness of chest physical therapy in preventing postoperative pulmonary complications following abdominal surgery is provided by randomized controlled trials.[73,74] In addition, absence of preoperative physical therapy has been found to be an additional factor associated with higher risk of postoperative pulmonary complications in patients with lung surgeries.[74]

In addition to deep breathing exercises, coughing and early mobilization; incentive spirometry can also promotes reductions in pulmonary complications. Following abdominal surgery, Hall et al[75] concluded that incentive spirometry was as effective as chest physical therapy in both low and high-risk patients.

Points to Ponder

- Chest physical therapy is important in the supportive treatment of patients with acute and chronic respiratory disease, being managed with or without surgery.
- In addition to its traditional role in treating airflow obstruction and mucus retention, other aspects of respiratory disorders such as ventilatory pump dysfunction, dyspnea, impaired exercise performance and quality of life are also benefitted by chest physical therapy interventions.
- Exercise training, peripheral and respiratory muscle training, airway clearance techniques, lung expansion maneuvers such as huffing and assisted coughing, breathing retraining through pursed lips breathing

and active prolonged expiration techniques in spontaneously breathing patients and bag squeezing in mechanically ventilated patients, all have been shown to be effective in patients with postoperative complications affecting the respiratory system.

- Assessment of patients is critical, to identify clinical characteristics that allow appropriate selection of treatment modalities for providing optimal effectiveness and efficacy.

REFERENCES

1. Gosselink R, Troosters T, Decramer M. Peripheral muscle weakness contributes to exercise limitation in COPD. Am J Respir Crit Care Med 1996;(153):976-80.
2. Saey D, Debigare R, Leblanc P, et al. Contractile leg fatigue after cycle exercise: A factor limiting exercise in patients with chronic obstructive pulmonary disease. Am J Respir Crit Care Med 2003;(168):425-30.
3. Lacasse Y, Brosseau L, Milne S, et al. Pulmonary rehabilitation for chronic obstructive pulmonary disease. Cochrane Database Syst Rev [CD-ROM] 2002.
4. Troosters T, Casaburi R, Gosselink R, et al. Pulmonary rehabilitation in chronic obstructive pulmonary disease. Am J Respir Crit Care Med 2005;(172):19-38.
5. Vogiatzis I, Nanas S, Roussos C. Interval training as an alternative modality to continuous exercise in patients with COPD. Eur Respir J 2002;19.
6. Spruit M, Gosselink R, Troosters T, et al. Resistance vs endurance training in patients with COPD and peripheral muscle weakness. Eur Respir J 2002;(19):1072-8.
7. Neder JA, Sword D, Ward SA, et al. Home based neuromuscular electrical stimulation as a new rehabilitative strategy for severely disabled patients with chronic obstructive pulmonary disease (COPD). Thorax 2002;(57):333-7.
8. Griffiths RD, Palmer A, Helliwell T, et al. Effect of passive stretching on the wasting of muscle in the critically ill. Nutrition 1995; (11): 428-32.
9. Zanotti E, Felicetti G, Maini M, et al. Peripheral muscle strength training in bed-bound patients with COPD receiving mechanical ventilation: Effect of electrical stimulation. Chest 2003;(124):292-6.
10. Renfroe KL. Effect of progressive relaxation on dyspnea and state of anxiety in patients with chronic obstructive pulmonary disease. Heart Lung 1988; (17):408-13.
11. Kolaczkowski W, Taylor R, Hoffstein V. Improvement in oxygen saturation after chest physiotherapy in patients with emphysema. Physiotherapy 1989; (41):18-23.
12. Breslin EH. The pattern of respiratory muscle recruitment during pursed-lips breathing in COPD. Chest 1992;(101):75-8.
13. Ingram RH, Schilder DP. Effect of pursed lips breathing on the pulmonary pressure-flow relationship in obstructive lung disease. Am Rev Respir Dis 1967;(96):381-8.
14. Ninane V, Rypens F, Yernault JC, et al. Abdominal muscle use during breathing in patients with chronic airflow obstruction. Am Rev Respir Dis 1992;(146):16-21.
15. Casciari RJ, Fairshter RD, Harrison A, et al. Effects of breathing retraining in patients with chronic obstructive pulmonary disease. Chest 1981;(79):393-8.

16. Sharp JT, Druz WS, Moisan T, et al. Postural relief of dyspnea in severe chronic obstructive pulmonary disease. Am Rev Respir Dis 1980;(122):201-11.
17. Goldman JM, Rose LS, Williams SJ, et al. Effect of abdominal binders on breathing in tetraplegic patients. Thorax 1986; (41): 940-5.
18. Estenne M, Van Muylem A , Gorini M, et al. Effects of abdominal strapping on forced expiration in tetraplegic patients. Am J Respir Crit Care Med 1998;(157):95-8.
19. Levine S, Kaiser L, Leferovich J, et al. Cellular adaptations in the diaphragm in chronic obstructive pulmonary disease. N Engl J Med 1997; (337):1799-806.
20. Scherer TA, Spengler C, Owassapian D, et al. Respiratory muscle endurance training in chronic obstructive pulmonary disease: Impact on exercise capacity, dyspnea, and quality of life. Am J Respir Crit Care Med 2000; (162):1709-14.
21. Lotters F, B Van Tol B, Kwakkel G, et al. Effects of controlled inspiratory muscle training in patients with COPD: A meta-analysis. Eur Respir J 2002;(20):570-6.
22. Ramirez-Sarmiento A, Orozco-Levi M, Guell R, et al. Inspiratory muscle training in patients with chronic obstructive pulmonary disease: Structural adaptation and physiologic outcomes. Am J Respir Crit Care Med 2002:1491-7.
23. Lisboa C, Villafranca C, Leiva A, et al. Inspiratory muscle training in chronic airflow limitation: Effect on exercise performance. Eur Respir J 1997;(10):537-42.
24. Heijdra YF, Dekhuijzen PNR, Herwaarden CLA van, et al. Nocturnal saturation improves by target-flow inspiratory muscle training in patients with COPD. Am J Respir Crit Care Med 1996;(153):260-5.
25. Dekhuijzen PNR, Folgering HTM, Herwaarden CLA van. Target-flow inspiratory muscle training during pulmonary rehabilitation in patients with COPD. Chest 1991; (99): 128-33.
26. Wanke T, Formanek D, Lahrmann H, et al. The effects of combined inspiratory muscle and cycle ergometer training on exercise performance in patients with COPD. Eur Respir J 1994;(7): 2205-11.
27. Villafranca C, Borzone G, Leiva A, et al. Effect of inspiratory muscle–training with intermediate load on inspiratory power output in COPD. Eur Respir J 1998;(11):28-33.
28. Uijl SG, Houtman S, Folgering HT, et al. Training of the respiratory muscles in individuals with tetraplegia. Paraplegia 1999;(37):575-9.
29. Liauw MY, Lin MC, Cheng PT, et al. Resistive inspiratory muscle training: Its effectiveness in patients with acute complete cervical cord injury. Arch Phys Med Rehabil 2000;(81):752-6.
30. Wanke T, Toifl K, Merkle M, et al. Inspiratory muscle training in patients with Duchenne muscular dystrophy. Chest 1994; (105):475-82.
31. Gosselink R, Kovacs L, Ketelaer P, et al. Respiratory muscle weakness and respiratory muscle training in severely disabled multiple sclerosis patients. Arch Phys Med Rehabil 2000;(81):747-51.
32. Sprague SS, Hopkins PD. Use of inspiratory strength training to wean six patients who were ventilator-dependent. Phys Ther 2003;(83):171-81.
33. Martin AD, Davenport PD, Franceschi AC, et al. Use of inspiratory muscle strength training to facilitate ventilator weaning: A series of 10 consecutive patients. Chest 2002;(122):192-6.
34. Holliday JE, Hyers TM. The reduction of weaning time from mechanical ventilation using tidal volume and relaxation biofeedback. Am Rev Respir Dis 1990;(141):1214-20.

35. Sharp JT, Danon J, Druz WS, et al. Respiratory muscle function in patients with chronic obstructive pulmonary disease: Its relationship to disability and to respiratory therapy. Am Rev Respir Dis 1974;(110):154-68.
36. Sharp JT, Goldberg NM, Druz WS, et al. Thoracoabdominal motion in COPD. Am Rev Respir Dis 1977;(115):47-56.
37. Gandevia SC, Leeper JB, McKenzie DK, et al. Discharge frequencies of parasternal intercostal and scalene motor units during breathing in normal and COPD subjects. Am J Respir Crit Care Med 1996; (153): 622-8.
38. De Troyer A, Leeper JB, McKenzie DK, et al. Neural drive to the diaphragm in patients with severe COPD. Am J Respir Crit Care Med 1997; (155):1335-40.
39. Sinderby C, Beck J, Spahija JA, et al. Voluntary activation of the diaphragm in health and disease. J Appl Physiol 1998;(850):2146-58.
40. Breslin GH, Garoutte BC, Celli BR. Correlations between dyspnea, diaphragm, and sternomastoid recruitment during inspiratory resistance breathing. Chest 1990;(98):298-302.
41. Sackner MA, Gonzalez HF, Jenouri G, et al. Effects of abdominal and thoracic breathing on breathing pattern components in normal subjects and in patients with COPD. Am Rev Respir Dis 1984;(130):584-7.
42. Grimby G, Oxhoj H, Bake B. Effects of abdominal breathing on distribution of ventilation in obstructive lung disease. Clin Sci Mol Med 1975;(48):193-9.
43. Gosselink RAAM, Wagenaar RC, Sargeant AJ, et al. Diaphragmatic breathing reduces efficiency of breathing in chronic obstructive pulmonary disease. Am J Respir Crit Care Med 1995;(151):1136-42.
44. Casaburi R, Porszasz J, Burns MR, et al. Physiologic benefits of exercise training in rehabilitation of patients with severe chronic obstructive pulmonary disease. Am J Respir Crit Care Med 1997;(155):1541-51.
45. Vestbo J, Prescott E, Lange P. Association of chronic mucus hypersecretion with FEV1 decline and chronic obstructive pulmonary disease morbidity. Am J Respir Crit Care Med 1996;(153):1530-5.
46. Lieberman SL, Shefner JM, Young RR. Neurological disorders affecting respiration. In: Roussos C (Ed). The Thorax. Part C: Disease. 2nd. New York: Marcel Dekker 1995;2135-75.
47. Houtmeyers E, Gosselink R, Gayan-Ramirez G, et al. Effects of drugs on mucus clearance. Eur Respir J 1999;(14):452-67.
48. Houtmeyers E, Gosselink R, Gayan-Ramirez G, et al. Regulation of mucociliary clearance in health and disease. Eur Respir J 1999;(13):1177-88.
49. Clarke SW, Jones JG, Oliver DR. Resistance to two-phase gas-liquid flow in airways. J Appl Physiol 1970;(29):464-71.
50. De Troyer A, Leeper JB, McKenzie DK, Gandevia SC. Neural drive to the diaphragm in patients with severe COPD. Am J Respir Crit Care Med. 1997; (155): 1335-40.
51. Hasani A, Pavia D, Agnew JE, et al. Regional lung clearance during cough and forced expiration technique (FET): Effects of flow and viscoelasticity. Thorax 1994;(49):557-61.
52. Hasani A, Pavia D, Agnew JE, et al. Regional mucus transport following unproductive cough and forced expiration technique in patients with airways obstruction. Chest 1994;(105):1420-5.
53. Sivasothy P, Brown L, Smith IE, et al. Effect of manually assisted cough and mechanical insufflation on cough flow of normal subjects, patients with chronic obstructive pulmonary disease (COPD), and patients with respiratory muscle weakness. Thorax 2001;(56):438-44.

54. Bach JR. Mechanical insufflation-exsufflation. Comparison with peak expiratory flows with manually assisted and unassisted coughing techniques. Chest 1993;(104):1553-62.
55. Warren VC. Glossopharyngeal and neck accessory muscle breathing in a young adult with C2 complete tetraplegia resulting in ventilator dependency. Phys Ther 2002;(82):590-600.
56. Wolff RK, Dolovich MB, Obminski G, et al. Effects of exercise and eucapnic hyperventilation on bronchial clearance in man. J Appl Physiol 1977;(43):46-50.
57. Oldenburg FA, Dolovich MB, Montgomery JM, et al. Effects of postural drainage, exercise and cough on mucus clearance in chronic bronchitis. Am Rev Respir Dis 1979;(120):739-45.
58. Salh W, Bilton D, Dodd M, et al. Effect of exercise and physiotherapy in aiding sputum expectoration in adults with cystic fibrosis. Thorax 1989;(44):1006-8.
59. Baldwin DR, Hill AL, Peckham DG, et al. Effect of addition of exercise to chest physiotherapy on sputum expectoration and lung function in adults with cystic fibrosis. Respir Med 1994;(88):49-53.
60. Rossman CM, Waldes R, Sampson D, et al. Effect of chest physiotherapy on the removal of mucus in patients with cystic fibrosis. Am Rev Respir Dis 1982;(126):131-5.
61. Sutton PP, Parker RA, Webber BA, et al. Assessment of the forced expiration technique, postural drainage and directed coughing in chest physiotherapy. Eur J Respir Dis 1983;(64): 62-8.
62. Gillespie DJ, Rehder K. Body position and ventilation-perfusion relationships in unilateral pulmonary disease. Chest 1987;(91):75-9.
63. Lamm WJE, Graham MM, Albert RK. Mechanism by which the prone position improves oxygenation in acute lung injury. Am J Respir Crit Care Med 1994;(150):184-93.
64. Van der Schans CP, Piers DA, Postma DS. Effect of manual percussion on tracheobronchial clearance in patients with chronic airflow obstruction and excessive tracheobronchial secretion. Thorax 1986;(41):448-52.
65. King M, Philips DM, Gross D, et al. Enhanced tracheal mucus clearance with high frequency chest wall compression. Am Rev Respir Dis 1983;(128):511-5.
66. Falk M, Kelstrup M, Andersen JB, et al. Improving the ketchup bottle method with positive expiratory pressure (PEP), in cystic fibrosis. Eur J Respir Dis 1984;(65):423-32.
67. McIlwaine PM, Wong LT, Peacock D, et al. Long-term comparative trial of conventional postural drainage and percussion versus positive expiratory pressure therapy in the treatment of cystic fibrosis. J Pediatr 1997;(131):570-4.
68. Konstan MW, Stern RC, Doershuk CF. Efficacy of the Flutter device for airway mucus clearance in patients with cystic fibrosis. J Pediatr 1994;(124): 689-93.
69. Jones AYM, Hutchinson RC, Oh TE. Chest physiotherapy practice in intensive care units in Australia, the UK and Hong Kong. Physioth Theory and Pract 1992;(8):39-47.
70. Hodgson C, Denehy L, Ntoumenopoulos G, et al. An investigation of the early effects of manual lung hyperinflation in critically ill patients. Anaesth Intensive Care 2000;(28):255-61.
71. Tugrul S, Akinci O, Ozcan PE, et al. Effects of sustained inflation and postinflation positive end-expiratory pressure in acute respiratory distress

syndrome: Focusing on pulmonary and extrapulmonary forms. Crit Care Med 2003;(31):738-44.

72. Singer M, Vermaat J, Hall G, et al. Hemodynamic effects of manual hyperinflation in critically ill mechanically ventilated patients. Chest 1994;(106):1182-7.
73. Fagevik O, Hahn MI, Nordgren S, et al. Randomized controlled trial of prophylactic chest physiotherapy in major abdominal surgery. Brit J Surg 1997;(84):1535-8.
74. Thomas JA, McIntosh JM. Are incentive spirometry, intermittent positive pressure breathing and deep breathing exercises effective in the prevention of postoperative pulmonary complications after abdominal surgery: A systematic overview and meta-analysis. Phys Ther 1994;(74):3-10.
75. Algar FJ, Alvarez A, Salvatierra A, et al. Predicting pulmonary complications after pneumonectomy for lung cancer. Eur J Cardiothorac Surg 2003;(23):201-8.

Chapter

Physiotherapy after Breast Surgeries

INTRODUCTION

The human breast is largely a cosmetic organ, its use as a food source for the infant limited to few months at most during an average life time of a woman. Though apparently innocuous, it's potential for creating mischief is great, which can become life-threatening at times when breast cancer develops.

RISK FACTORS

Family Connection

Breast cancer seems to run in some families and not in others. Whatever the underlying reason may be, family history definitely does play a significant role. If any woman's mother or sister—or both—have had breast cancer, the estimated risk of developing breast cancer is significantly higher in that person as compared to others without any family history of this deadly disease.

Age

Breast cancer rarely occurs in the teenage. The odds of developing it gradually increase after teenage, leveling off for a bit after menopause, and then starting to rise again.

Fertility

The longer a woman remains fertile, the greater her chances of developing breast cancer. Many researchers speculate that the factors that eventually trigger the development of breast cancer begin to work as soon as a girl enters puberty and continues until she reaches her menopause.

Late Pregnancy

Pregnancy seems to short circuit the process under certain circumstances. The earlier a woman completes her first full-term pregnancy, the less chance she has of developing breast cancer.

Breastfeeding

Widespread belief that breastfeeding naturally protects a nursing mother from breast cancer is still under scientific debate.

Removal of the Ovaries

Seems to offer some protection against breast cancer. If a woman's ovaries are surgically removed while she is still in her mid-to-late thirties, her chances of getting breast cancer can fall significantly.

Other Probable Risk Factors

Breast cancer is most common among Caucasians and occurs much less often among Asians and Negroids. Breast cancer also occurs more frequently among overweight women; city dwellers; and those who have previously had cancer of other organs such as the ovary or endometrial lining of the uterus. Women from high-income group are also at greater risk, because they eat rich, fatty foods that can raise estrogen levels in the body, thought to promote the growth of a breast cancer. Because the breast is extremely vulnerable to the effects of radiation, exposure to radiation increases the risk of breast cancer.

WARNING SIGNS TO WATCH FOR

The first indication of breast cancer is the discovery of a palpable lump in the breast. Most women discover breast lumps themselves, either by accident or while performing a monthly self-examination (Fig. 5.1) or by

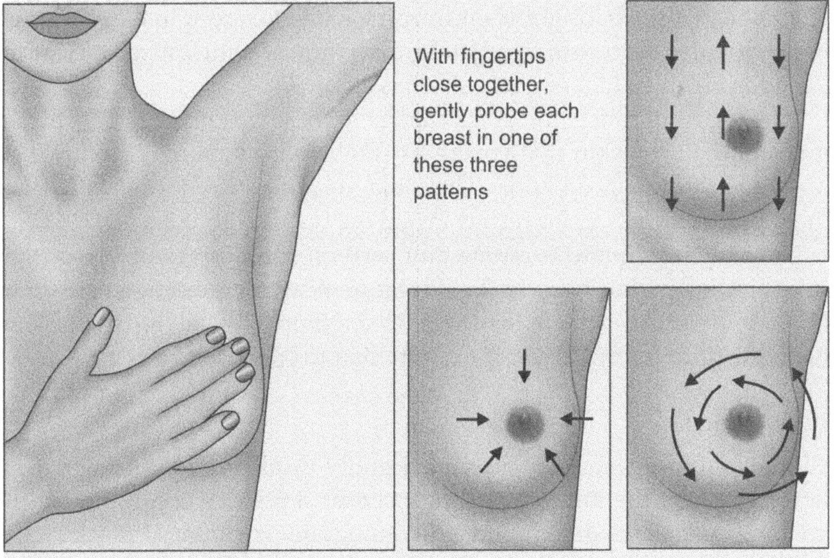

Fig. 5.1: Manual self-examination of the breast

a partner. Fortunately, most of the breast lumps discovered turn out to be noncancerous, but if someone does find a suspicious lump, it is still best to seek medical opinion right away. Because early detection is crucial for a cure, women need to learn to examine their breasts each month. Early detection of breast cancer means that smaller tumors are found which require less intensive surgery and have better treatment outcomes.

Nearly half of all lumps appear at the top of the breast on the side nearest the armpit. For some reason the lumps occur in the left breast slightly more often than in the right. It is important to remember, though, that lumps can turn up anywhere within the breast, and that in many cases breast cancer is found even if there is no lump at all.

If one does find a lump, the breast may be tender, or it may feel normal. There could be some discomfort or a "pulling sensation". Cysts, which are benign, tend to move freely within the breast, so when a lump appears to be immobile, or the skin over it is dimpled or puckered, doctors tend to suspect that the growth is malignant. However, this is not a certainty.

A discharge from *one of the nipples* is the second most common sign of a potential problem. The discharge may be clear, bloody, or colored. It is important to understand that a discharge can be perfectly normal in women who are not breastfeeding. In this case, a small amount of discharge usually comes out of several openings in *both* breasts and not from any one breast as in case of cancer.

A spontaneous discharge that occurs without squeezing the breast is a far greater cause for concern. A discharge coming from the same general location in one breast may well indicate the presence of an underlying mass. Although a bloody discharge occasionally may occur during pregnancy, it can also be a significant warning sign of cancer. In older women there is greater the possibility that the discharge is being caused by cancer. The odds are even higher if she also has a lump.

Other signs of cancer include a change in the shape or size of the breast or swelling of the skin that covers it. The breast tissue may feel thicker, even though there is no lump. There may be pain or redness of the skin. The nipple may be sore or retract inside the breast (Fig. 5.2).

The clinician should examine any sore on the nipples or breast that do not clear up after two weeks of treatment with a prescribed cream or lotion. In most cases the patient will need a biopsy by taking a sample of the tissue fluid for microscopic examination to check for cancer.

Biopsy

All lumps in the breast are presumed guilty until proven innocent, even though most of the lumps are noncancerous. Presence of a lump and/or anything suspicious detected in a mammogram, is automatically a signal for a biopsy. A biopsy must be done if a nipple is inflamed, encrusted, or

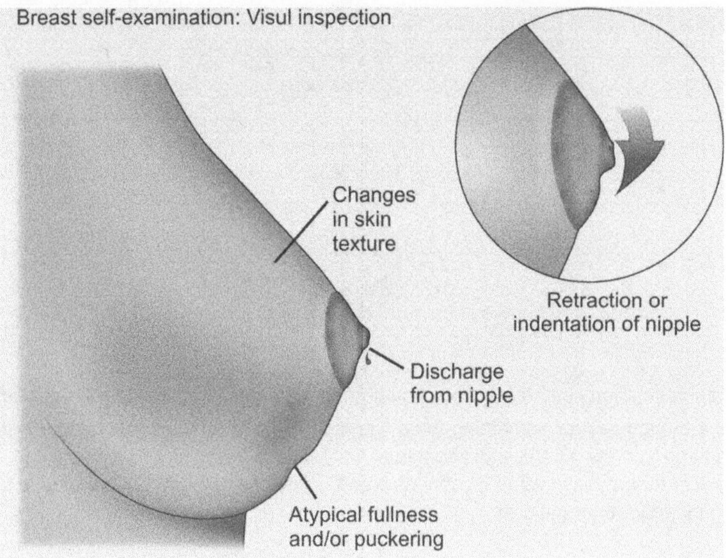

Fig. 5.2: Changes in the breast seen on visual inspection in the presence of a suspicious lump

has scaly lesions that do not go away, or if it is leaking a bloody fluid, even if there is no palpable lump detected on manual exmination.

If the patient have not yet gone through menopause and does not have any signs or symptoms that point to the possibility of cancer, the doctor may decide to wait through one complete menstrual cycle before proceeding with biopsy. During this time he or she will check to see whether the lump goes away or is in any way affected by the hormonal changes that occur before, during, and after menstruation. On the other hand, if the patient has a history of cysts, or if the physician strongly suspects the mass is a relatively harmless cyst, he or she may do a needle biopsy right in the OPD.

This procedure, also known as fine needle aspiration cytology test (FNAC), is fast, relatively painless and can help ease patient's anxiety if the lump is only a cyst and not a tumor. The doctor simply swabs the area with an antiseptic solution, then inserts a thin needle into the lump and draws off the fluid. The procedure can be done under local anesthesia (Fig. 5.3).

A cyst is little more than a fluid-filled sac (see Fig. 5.5); a mass has more substance. The needle should have no trouble penetrating a cyst, but may encounter resistance if the lump is a solid mass and potentially malignant.

Fine Needle Aspiration

If the lump is really a cyst, the sac will collapse as soon as the fluid is removed, and the lump will suddenly disappear. In this case a mammogram needs to be done just to be sure, as well as doing another physical

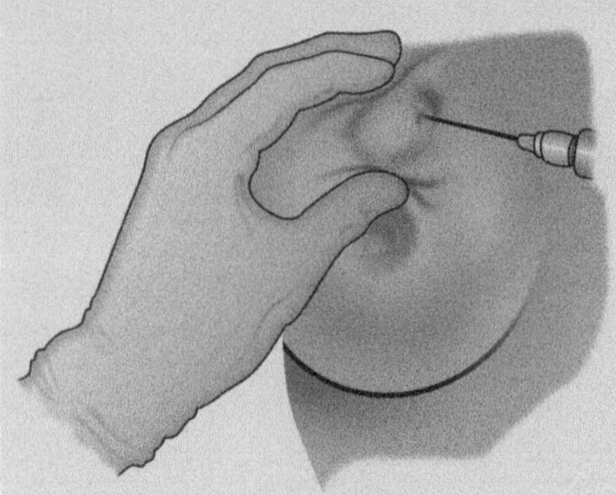

Fig. 5.3: Fine needle aspiration—this minor procedure can quickly reveal whether a breast lump is a benign cyst or something more worrisome. To find out, a thin needle is inserted into the lump to draw out the liquid contents. If the fluid is greenish or straw-colored, we are dealing with a harmless cyst. If it contains blood, smear sample on a glass slide is taken to be examined for abnormal cells

examination after a few weeks. If the lump has not returned, there generally is no further cause for concern.

However, a follow-up biopsy is always indicated if the doctor is not able to get any fluid or if the fluid is bloody or if the mass does not completely disappear after the fluid is drawn or if the "cyst" returns after two "successful" aspirations or if the mammogram is suspicious.

Another possible procedure is a core needle biopsy, which uses a larger needle to take a tissue sample from the mass. This approach, which does require local anesthesia, can be helpful for large tumors that might be difficult to remove in the OPD. However, a negative result could be misleading. In other words, even though the small sample contains no cancer cells, there is no guarantee that the entire mass is cancer free.

If there is any doubt about the results of a needle biopsy, a surgical biopsy may be considered. This is necessary because the only way to be sure of the diagnosis is to look at the abnormal tissue under a microscope. If the lump is small, the surgeon will probably do an excision biopsy, removing the entire mass. If the lump is larger, an incisional wedge biopsy can be done instead. This procedure removes a small specimen from the mass, usually providing enough tissue for a diagnosis without having to make a large incision. However, if a diagnosis cannot be made without more tissue, the surgeon may decide to do an excision biopsy and remove the rest of the lump.

Biopsies are often performed on an outpatient basis. In the old days, the woman remained in the operating room while the pathologist examined the specimen. If the diagnosis was cancer, her breast was removed immediately. Clinical studies eventually showed that there was no need to do the biopsy and surgery in a single step. In the increasingly popular two-step approach, the biopsy is done at an outpatient clinic and surgery, if necessary, is performed in a hospital a week or so later.

A short delay between biopsy and surgery does not harm a woman's chance of survival, but does allow her time to discuss the proposed treatment and possible breast reconstruction with her physician. The doctor, in turn, has time to order a chest X-ray, blood tests, and other laboratory procedures that help determine whether the cancer has spread from the breast to the bones, lungs, liver or brain. If the cancer is localized, these test results can establish a baseline against which the doctor will compare with follow-up test results done every three months after surgery.

Biopsy of a noncancerous mass may also reveal the first signs of an early cancer in the surrounding "healthy" tissue. Without a doubt, biopsy remains the best possible way to identify malignancies while the cancer is still highly curable.

As breast cancer progresses, signs and symptoms become unmistakable, including skin ulcers and extensive swelling and redness of the breast and swelling of the arm. The nipple may retract into the breast, and the breast may retract into the chest.

Mammography

Mammography is a well-known procedure, essentially a **medical imaging** procedure, used in order to detect and investigate a lump in the breast, the areas of parenchyma distortion, and microcalcifications being the key signs of cancer. This procedure requires compression of the breast between two plates and is considered to be quite uncomfortable by many women. Two views, oblique and craniocaudal, of each breast are taken. An X-ray exposure of less than 1.5 mGy used in standard mammograms is useful not only for examining a known lump, but also for detecting lumps too small to feel (Fig. 5.4).

A tumor can keep growing for many years before one can feel it; and some buried deep within the breast or in the axilla can be detected only by a mammogram. However, a mammogram can only show the size and location of a mass. To be certain about malignancy a biopsy must be done.

Ultrasonogram

Ultrasound scanning is another relatively inexpensive diagnostic tool that forms a picture by bouncing sound waves off the mass (Fig. 5.5). Ultrasound takes longer to perform than a needle biopsy, and the results are generally not as good. However, it can be helpful in locating masses in younger women whose breasts are more dense and harder to see on a mammogram. Ultrasound is most useful in evaluating masses deep within the breast and thus cannot be felt or reached with a needle.

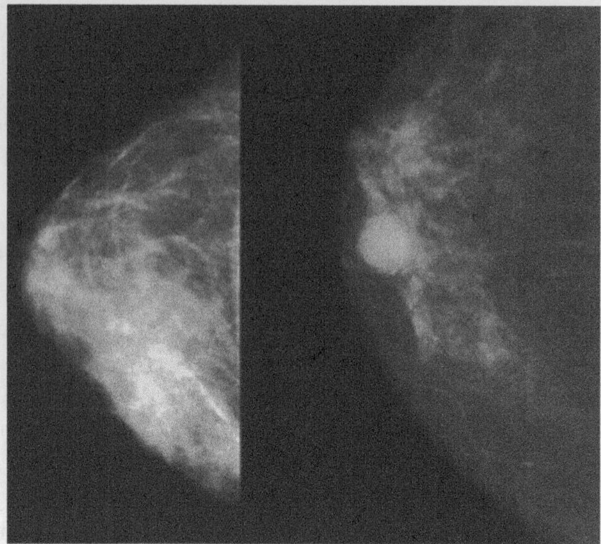

Fig. 5.4: Mammography—typical mammogram studies showing diffuse mass effect on the left, most likely to be malignant and a discrete lump on the right, most likely to be benign

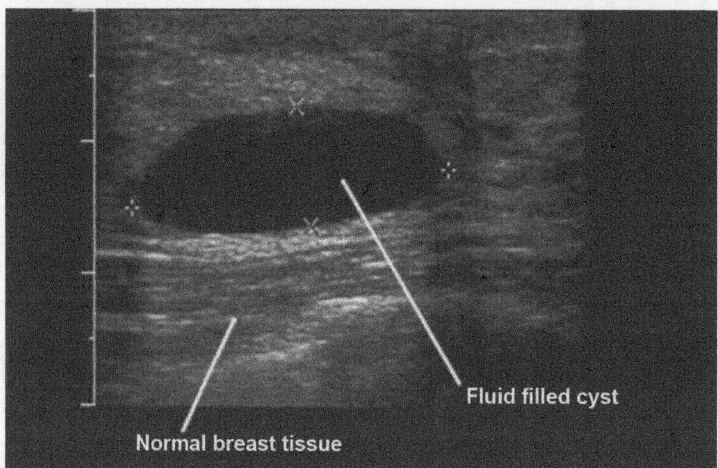

Fig. 5.5: Ultrasonogram—this ultrasound picture shows a benign cyst with normal breast tissue around it. Because this type of cyst is fluid-filled and usually does not contain any tissue or other particles, it can be drained easily

MRI Screening of the Breast

Early breast cancers, undetected by mammogram and ultrasonogram can be found when MRI is performed, hence, The American Cancer Society recommends that women with a high-risk of developing breast cancer should be screened with MRI in addition to their yearly mammogram and USG beginning at age 30. Because MRI is a very expensive test and requires

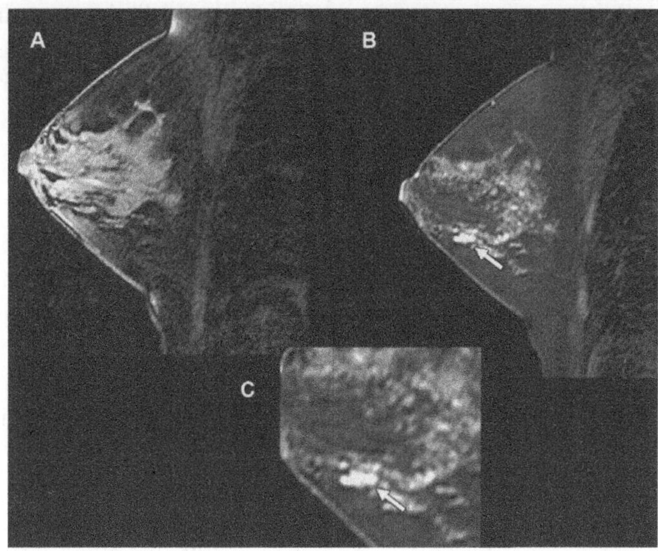

Fig. 5.6: MRI screening of the breast—this breast MRI showing focus of enhancement in left breast, see arrow, which was found to be negative on mammography and USG. FNAC has subsequently proved positive for infiltrating ductal carcinoma

Table 5.1: The four stages of breast cancer

Stage	*Extent*
I.	The tumor is no larger than 2 centimeters (about 1 inch), and the cancer has not spread beyond the breast
II.	The tumor is 2 to 5 centimeters (about 1 to 2 inches), and/or the cancer has spread to the lymph nodes of the axilla
III.	The tumor is larger than 5 centimeters (two inches), the cancer involves more of the axillary lymph nodes, and/or the cancer has spread to other tissues near the breast
IV.	The cancer has spread to other organs in the body, most often to the bones, liver, lungs, or brain

intravenous contrast, it is recommended for screening the approximately two percent of women at very high-risk for breast cancer (Fig. 5.6).*

STAGING THE SPREAD OF BREAST CANCER

With the diagnosis of breast cancer firmly established, the focus shifts on determining whether the cancer has spread, and, if so, how far. This evaluation, or "staging", involves ranking the cancer from Stage I (early cases) to Stage IV (advanced cases). For the precise description of each stage, see the (Table 5.1). There is no single "best" operation or treatment for breast cancer. Much depends on whether the disease is localized to only in the breast or spread to other parts of the body as well, the phenomenon called

*Source: Wendie A Berg, et al. American Radiology Services, Johns Hopkins, Green Spring Station in Lutherville, MD, USA

Metastasis. Unfortunately, it is often difficult to tell whether the cancer has spread to other parts of the body or not. There is no definitive laboratory test for metastasis or spread of cancer, and many women do not show any symptoms at all.

TREATMENT: ASSESSING THE OPTIONS

Prompt treatment is essential. Without surgery, radiation, or chemotherapy, a woman who has breast cancer will almost surely die. Fortunately, the chances for long-term survival and cure are excellent if the cancer is caught early enough.

Once the type of breast cancer, the size and location of the primary tumor and the extent of the disease spread has been determined, it is time to discuss the various treatment options.

The goal of treatment is to prevent the spread of cancer and to minimize the possibility of a recurrence of cancer in the future. For women whose cancer has already spread, a treatment plan called palliative therapy is needed, which eases pain or other symptoms.

SURGERY OF THE BREAST

There are many different types of surgery for breast cancer; from removing just the lump to removing the entire breast and the muscles in the chest. The surgeon in most cases also removes some or all of the axillary lymph nodes.

The lymph nodes are part of the body's lymphatic system, which filters waste from the tissues and carries fluids that help the body fight infection. The lymphatic system transports fluids very efficiently and, if invaded by cancer cells, can spread such cells throughout the body. Surgeons remove at least a sample of lymph nodes near the breast to check whether the cancer has reached the nodes. The extent of "nodal involvement", the number of lymph nodes affected by cancer, helps the physician determine how much radiation or chemotherapy a woman needs after surgery.

For many years, women went into the hospital for a biopsy not even knowing whether they even had cancer and often woke up several hours later to find that one of their breast was gone. Proponents of this one-step approach to biopsy and surgery believed that this simple procedure involved lesser risk, than waiting for days or weeks between biopsy and surgery. Treatment began immediately and the woman had less stress and anxiety because the ordeal was over much sooner. The one-step approach was also cheaper and involved only one hospitalization.

Times have changed. Many women and physicians now favor the two-step approach. The first step involves detecting cancer, confirming its type

and extent of its spread. There is a pause after the confirmation of diagnosis. This not only allows the doctor time to better evaluate the disease, but also gives the patient a chance to consider the different treatment possibilities, obtain a second opinion if she wants, make any necessary arrangements at work or at home, and get herself mentally and emotionally ready to fight the disease. The second step, the actual treatment of the cancer can then begin.

Whatever treatment option a woman chooses, it is very important for the doctor and the patient to discuss the situation thoroughly and make sure they agree on what is best. The bottom line for most women is to go for the treatment option that offers them the best chance for survival.

Mastectomy, surgical removal of the breast, offers the best chance of a cure for Stage I and II breast cancers. Surgery may also be successful for some Stage III cancers if they have not spread to other parts of the body. Women with Stage IV breast cancer may receive only palliative treatment.

The location, size, and type of tumor are of primary importance when considering breast cancer surgery options. The size of the breast is another factor the surgeon has to consider when planning for surgery. The patient's psychological outlook, as well as her lifestyle and preferences, should also be taken into account when surgical options are being decided.

Depending up on the location and nature of the tumor, extent of its malignancy and extent of cosmetic disfigurement acceptable to the patient, one may have to undergo any of the following procedures (Fig. 5.7).

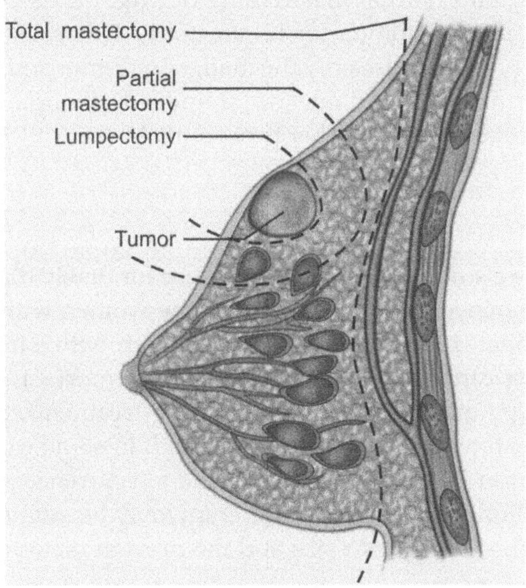

Fig. 5.7: Different types of breast surgeries

TYPES OF BREAST SURGERIES

- *Lumpectomy* just removes the tumor and a small amount of tissue surrounding it. Some lymph nodes may be removed as well.
- *Simple or total, mastectomy* has been the treatment of choice in the late 1980s and 1990s. Generally, only the breast is removed; though, sometimes, one or two lymph nodes may be removed as well.
- *Skin-sparing mastectomy* is a new surgical procedure in which the surgeon makes an incision, sometimes called a keyhole incision, around the areola. The tumor and all breast tissue are removed, but the incision is small and scarring is minimal. About 90 percent of the skin is preserved and allows a cosmetic surgeon to perform breast reconstruction concurrently with the mastectomy.
- *Modified radical mastectomy* was the most common form of mastectomy until the 1980s. The breast is removed along with the fascia over the chest muscle and all of the lymph nodes.
- *Radical mastectomy* is used only in cases where cancer cells have invaded the chest wall and the tumor is very large. The breast, muscles under the breast, and all of the lymph nodes are removed. This surgery produces a large scar and severly restricts the function of the arm on the operated side of the body.

Lumpectomy

Lumpectomy is the simplest type of surgery for breast cancer. Any amount of tissue, from, a small wedge to half of a breast, may be removed and be called a lumpectomy. Partial mastectomy or breast conservation surgery is a frequently used synonym for lumpectomy. It is considered "breast-conserving" surgery because only the malignant tumor and a surrounding margin of normal breast tissue are removed. Lymph nodes in the axilla may also be removed. This procedure is also called lymph node resection.

Indication

Lumpectomy is a surgical treatment of choice for newly diagnosed breast cancer. It is estimated that at least half of the women with breast cancer are good candidates for this procedure. Women with early stage breast cancers are best candidates for lumpectomy. In most cases, a course of radiation therapy after surgery is part of the treatment. Chemotherapy or hormone treatment may also be prescribed. In some women with late stage breast cancer or women who have had a recurrence of breast cancer after previous lumpectomies, chemotherapy may be administered before surgery to decrease the tumor size and the prevent metastasis in selected cases.

Contraindications to Lumpectomy

There are a number of factors that may prevent or prohibit a breast cancer patient from having a lumpectomy.

- The tumor itself may be too large or located in an area where it would be difficult to remove with good cosmetic results.
- Sometimes several tumors are found in one breast, so that all the tumors cannot be removed as a single lump.
- A cancer that has already attached itself to nearby structures, such as the skin or the chest wall and needs more extensive excision.
- When the surgeon is unable to remove the tumor along with a sufficient amount of surrounding normal tissue, due to "lack of clear margins".
- This surgery may not be acceptable during pregnancy because follow up radiation therapy cannot be administered to pregnant women because it may injure the fetus.

Preoperative Preparation

Preanesthetic checkup and lab investigations are done well before the surgery. Routine preoperative preparations, such as the patient kept nil orally the night before surgery, the armpits are shaved, the skin over surgical field cleaned, disinfected and draped in sterile sheet before the patient is transfered to the operation theater.

Preoperative counseling about expected outcomes and potential complications of the surgery is given to the patient before obtaining her informed consent.

If the tumor is not palpable, a preoperative localization procedure is needed. A fine wire, or other device, is placed at the tumor site as a marker, using X-ray or ultrasound for guidance.

Description of the Procedure

The surgery is usually done under general anesthetic. Local anesthetic with additional sedation may be used for some patients. An oblique incision, 3–5 cm long, is given on the skin over the lump, preferably along the skin fold and underneath the breast if possible, to expose the lump. The tumor and surrounding margin of healthy tissue is removed and sent to pathology lab for examination. The incision is then closed.

If the axillary lymph nodes are to be removed, a second vertical incision is made in the armpit along posterior axillary fold. The axillary pad of fat containing lymph nodes is removed and is sent for analysis. This portion of the procedure is called an axillary lymph node resection and is critical for determining the stage of the cancer. Typically, 10 to 15 nodes are removed. If the excision has been extensive, corrugated rubber surgical drains may be left in place in either location to prevent fluid accumulation.

Postoperative Care

The patient may stay in the hospital one or two days, or return home the same day. This generally depends on the extent of the tissue resection, the general condition of the patient, and surgeon/patient preference. The patient usually goes home with a small bandage. The inner sutures usually are done using dissolvable catgut. The skin may be sutured with silk threads; or the skin edges may be held together with sterile, thin, clear pieces of tape.

After a lumpectomy, patients are usually cautioned against lifting weights over two kilos for several days. Pain often limits shoulder motion. Over head activities may be restricted, especially if the axillary lymph nodes were removed. Women are often instructed to wear a well-fitting support bra both day and night for approximately one week after surgery.

Pain is usually well-controlled with medication. If it is not, the patient should contact the surgeon, as severe pain may be a sign of a complication. In absence of any complication, pain may be effectively controlled by TENS. A review visit to the surgeon is normally scheduled approximately ten days to two weeks after the operation.

Radiation therapy is usually started as soon as possible after lumpectomy. Other additional treatments, such as chemotherapy or hormone therapy, may also be prescribed.

RISKS OF COMPLICATIONS

The risks are similar to those associated with any surgical procedure, which include bleeding, infection, breast asymmetry, anesthesia reaction, or unexpected scarring. A lumpectomy may also cause loss of sensation in the breast. The size and shape of the breast will be affected by the operation. Fluid can accumulate in the area where tissue was removed, requiring drainage and if not drained, can form adhesion.

If axillary lymph node dissection has several potential complications. A woman may experience loss of superficial sensation, numbness, tingling, or increased skin sensitivity in the axilla. A phlebitis can occur in veins of upper extremity and injury to the brachial plexus is not unusual in axillary incisions.

There is also the risk of developing lymph edema of the arm after axillary lymph node dissection. This swelling can range from mild to very severe. It can be treated effectively in early stages with elevation of the part along with compression applied by elastic bandages, effleurage massage, intermittent compression therapy and faradism under pressure. However, once the edema becomes chronic and consolidated it is extremely difficult to treat.

Simple Mastectomy

Simple mastectomy is the surgical removal of one or both breasts. The adjacent lymph nodes and chest muscles are left intact. If a few lymph nodes are removed, the procedure is called an extended simple mastectomy. Simple mastectomy has been the standard treatment of choice for breast cancer for the past 60 years. Newer breast-sparing surgery has been gaining in acceptance since the mid-1980s.

Breast-sparing techniques are used to preserve the skin over the breast, the areola and nipple, so that cosmetic breast reconstruction can be done later using silicone prosthesis.

Indication

Removal of a patient's breast is usually recommended either when cancer is present in the breast or as a prophylactic measure when the patient has severe fibrocystic disease and a family history of breast cancer. The choice of a simple mastectomy may be determined by evaluating the size of the breast, the size of the cancerous mass, where the cancer is located, and whether any cancer cells have spread to adjacent lymph nodes or other parts of the body. If the cancer has not been contained within the breast, it calls for a modified radical mastectomy, which removes the entire breast and all of the adjacent lymph nodes. Only in extreme circumstances a radical mastectomy is indicated; which involves removal of the chest wall muscles and fascia, axillary lymph nodes along with the entire breast with the skin and areola.

A larger tumor usually is an indication of more advanced disease and will require a simple mastectomy. In addition, if a woman has small breasts, the tumor may occupy more area within the contours of the breast, necessitating a simple mastectomy in order to remove all of the cancer.

Very rapidly growing tumors usually require the removal of all breast tissue. Cancers that have spread to such adjacent tissues as the chest wall or skin make simple mastectomy a good choice. Similarly, multiple sites of cancer within a breast require that the entire breast be removed. In addition, simple mastectomy is also recommended when cancer recurs in a breast that has already undergone a lumpectomy.

Sometimes, surgeons recommend simple mastectomy for women who are unable to undergo the follow-up radiation therapy required after a lumpectomy. Radiation treatment is not allowed for pregnant women, those who have had previous therapeutic radiation in the chest area, and patients with collagen vascular diseases such as scleroderma or lupus. In these cases, simple mastectomy is the treatment of choice.

Description

During a simple mastectomy, the surgeon makes a curved incision along under side of the breast and removes the tumor and all of the breast tissue.

A few lymph nodes may also be removed. The tumor, breast tissue, and any lymph nodes will be sent to the pathology lab for analysis. If the skin is cancer-free, it is sutured in place or used immediately for breast reconstruction. One or two drains will be put in place to remove fluid from the surgical area. Surgery takes from two to five hours or longer if breast reconstruction is done.

Modified Radical Mastectomy

Modified radical mastectomy is the most widely-used surgical procedure to treat operable breast cancer with minimal loss to musculature of the chest wall. This procedure leaves the pectorals intact. Leaving this muscle in place will provide a soft tissue covering over the chest wall and a normal-appearing junction of the shoulder with the anterior chest wall. Additionally, the purpose of modified radical mastectomy is to allow for the option of breast reconstruction, a procedure that is possible, if desired, using the intact muscles around the shoulder of the affected side (Fig. 5.8).

Description

The surgeon's goal during this procedure is to:

- Minimize any chance of local/regional recurrence of cancer
- Avoid any loss of function
- Maximize options for breast reconstruction.

Incision in the shape of an ellipse is made in the underside of the breast, to avoid visibility in a low neckline dress or bathing suit. The surgeon removes the minimum amount of skin and tissue so that remaining healthy tissue can be used for possible reconstruction. Skin flaps are made carefully and as thinly as possible to maximize removal of diseased breast tissues.

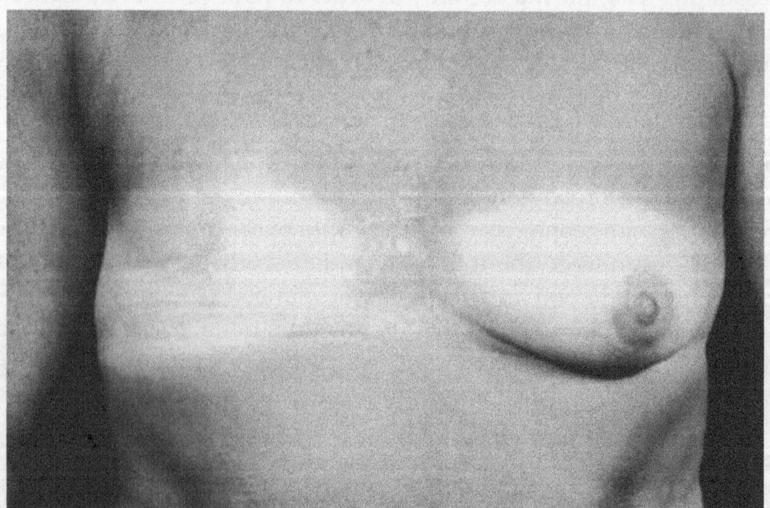

Fig. 5.8: Reconstructed right breast after modified radical mastectomy

The pectoralis major fascia is removed, after which the surgeon focuses on the axillary region, carefully identifying vital anatomical structures such as blood vessels and nerves and protecting them while removing cancerous tissue. Accidental injury to specific nerves like the medial pectoral neurovascular bundle will result in destruction of the pectoralis major muscle that this surgery attempts to preserve. After axillary surgery, breast reconstruction may be performed.

Breast Reconstruction

Breast reconstruction, especially if it is done in the same session as the simple or modified radical mastectomy, can minimize the sense of loss that women feel when having a breast removed. Although there may be other smaller surgeries later to complete the breast reconstruction, there will not be a second major operation or an additional scar.

If there is insufficient skin left over after the mastectomy, a balloon-type expander is put in place. In subsequent weeks, the expander is filled with larger amounts of saline solution to stretch the skin. When it has reached the appropriate size, the expander is removed and a permanent breast implant made of silicone is installed.

If there is enough skin, a silicone implant can be installed immediately. Alternatively, skin, fat, and muscle tissue are harvested from the patient's back or abdomen and grafted to the chest wall to form a breast (Fig. 5.8).

None of these reconstructions have nipples at first. Later, nipples are reconstructed in a separate surgery. Finally, the areola is tattooed in to make the reconstructed breast look natural. Breast reconstruction does not prevent a potential recurrence of breast cancer.

Radical Mastectomy

In a radical mastectomy, also known as the Halsted Radical Mastectomy, named after the surgeon who developed the procedure in the 1890s, the surgeon removes the entire breast, along with overlying skin and areola, as well as, all underlying chest fascia,muscles, and all of the lymph nodes and channels in the axilla. This operation was the standard procedure for breast cancer treatment until recently.

Surgeons believed that removing the entire breast was the best way to get rid of all of the cancer—assuming that the disease had not yet spread beyond the breast. Taking out all the lymph nodes made it possible to better determine the extent of any spread and to prevent it.

There are many drawbacks to such extensive surgery. Women frequently loose movement in the shoulder and experience numbness, and swelling of the arm. This surgery is also cosmetically very disfiguring. After the operation, the chest looks hollow and the scar unsightly. Breast reconstruction is possible, but very difficult.

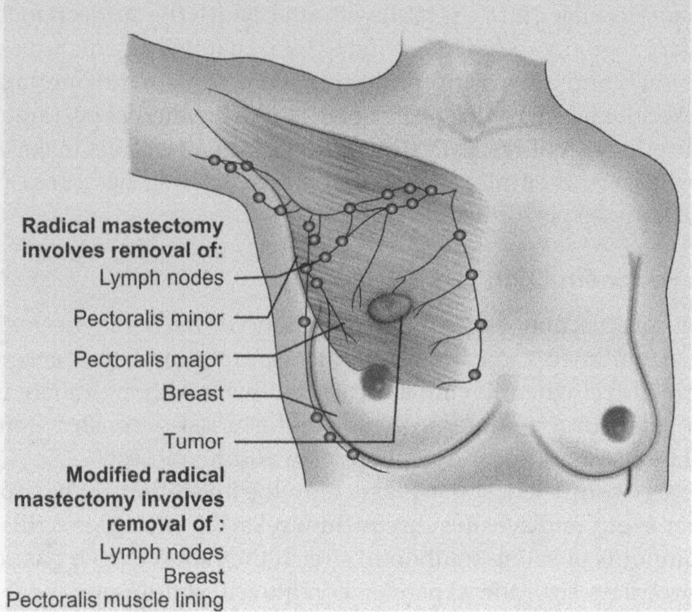

Fig. 5.9: Radical mastectomy—comparison between standard and modified procedures

Over the years, scientific studies have shown that removing the chest muscles does not improve a woman's prognosis and is not necessary if the cancer is found early. Today, surgeons seldom perform radical mastectomies. Radical mastectomy, which removes pectoral muscles along with the breast and lymph nodes, is no longer preferred except in severe cases. A modified radical mastectomy, which leaves chest muscles intact, is now considered just as effective in stopping the cancer's spread. With less muscle and nerve damage to cope with, women suffer fewer complications after the operation and find subsequent breast reconstruction to be less of a problem (Fig. 5.9).

Diagnosis/Preparation

If a mammogram has not been performed, it is usually ordered to verify the size of the lump the patient has reported. A biopsy of the suspicious lump and/or lymph nodes is usually ordered and sent to the pathology lab before surgery is discussed.

When a radical or modified radical mastectomy has been planned, preoperative tests as blood work, a chest X-ray, and an electrocardiogram is done. Blood-thinning medications such as aspirin should be stopped several days before the surgery date to avoid excessive bleeding during and after the surgery. If the patient is diabetic, medications and insulin is started well before surgery to control the raised blood sugar level. The patient is also kept nil orally the night before the operation.

Before surgery, the patient needs to sign a consent form, verifying that the surgeon has explained the purpose and risks associated with the surgery. The patient will also be checked by the anesthesiologist to review the patient's medical history and determine her suitability for anesthesia. The local area is prepared as explained above during lumpectomy.

IMMEDIATE POSTOPERATIVE CARE

The length of the hospital stay for the patient after radical or modified radical mastectomies ranges from five to seven days. If breast reconstruction has been done, the hospital stay may be longer than a week.

The surgical drains will remain in place for five to seven days. Sponge baths will be necessary until the stitches are removed, usually in a week to 10 days. It is important to avoid overhead lifting, strenuous sports, and sexual intercourse for three to six weeks. After the surgical drains are removed, stretching exercises may be started, though some physical therapists start a patient on shoulder and arm mobility exercises while in the hospital after modified radical mastectomy.

Since breast removal is often emotionally traumatic for women, seeking out a support group is often helpful. Women in these groups offer practical advice about finding well-fitting under garments, and provide emotional support because they have been through the same experience.

Finally, for women who chose not to have breast reconstruction, it will be necessary to find the proper fitting external breast prosthesis made of cloth or HDP foam. Internal prosthetic implants are made of silicone, which are created from a mould taken from the patient's other breast.

In some case, the patient may be required to undergo follow-up treatments such as radiation, chemotherapy, or hormone therapy.

RISKS ASSOCIATED WITH MASTECTOMIES

The risks involved with total/radical mastectomies are the same for any major surgery.

There is the risk of infection around the incision. When the lymph nodes are removed, lymph edema may also occur. This condition is a result of damage to the lymph system. The arm on the side nearest the affected breast may become swollen. It can either resolve itself or worsen.

As in any surgery, the risk of developing a DVT after a mastectomy is a serious matter. While in hospital, therapists use a variety of techniques to prevent blood clots from forming the deep veins of calf. These are ankle-foot pumping exercise, heel drag exercise, isometics of gluts and quads, elevation and compression of the limb using elastic bandage/hose, effleurage massage, etc. It is important for the patient to walk daily when at home.

Prognosis

The breast area will fully heal in three to four weeks time. If the patient had breast reconstruction, it may take up to six weeks to recover fully. The patient should be able to participate in all of the activities she has engaged in before surgery. If breast reconstruction is done, the patient should realize that the new breast will not have the sensitivity of a normal breast. In addition, dealing with cancer emotionally may take time, especially if follow-up radiation and chemotherapy is necessary.

Alternative Surgeries

Skin-sparing mastectomy, also called nipple-sparing mastectomy, is becoming a treatment of choice for women undergoing simple mastectomy. In this procedure, the skin of the breast, the areola, and the nipple are peeled back to remove the breast and its inherent tumor. Biopsies of the skin and nipple areas are performed immediately to assure that they do not have cancer cells in them. Then, a cosmetic surgeon performs a breast reconstruction at the same time as the mastectomy. The breast regains its normal contours once prostheses are inserted. Unfortunately, the nipple will lose its sensitivity and, of course, its function, since all underlying tissue has been removed. If cancer is found near the nipple, this procedure cannot be done.

Apart from cosmetic disfigurement, any of these procedures can affect the patient's ability to move the shoulder and arm, to take a deep breath, or to perform daily activities such as dressing, bathing, and combing hair.

Radiation's Role

Radiation therapy involves beaming X-rays at the site of the tumor to kill the growing cancer cells. X-rays will sterilize the tissue around the tumor site and keep the cancer from spreading or returning.

Although researchers are still studying the long-term success rate of radiation therapy, this treatment appears to be a promising option for early-stage cancer. Radiation is also used to shrink an especially large tumor prior to surgery or to slow down the growth of inoperable tumors.

Radiation appears to be as effective as a mastectomy in treating early-stage breast cancer and unlike surgery, it lets a woman keep her breast. However, radiation is more often used following a lumpectomy rather than as a sole primary treatment.

There are two types of radiation, a beam of concentrated booster dose at the original tumor site or implanted radioactive materials within the breast. The five-day-a week treatment usually lasts for five weeks. Some patients undergoing radiation develop a skin reaction similar to a sunburn and complain of itchy or peeling skin. However, the skin usually regains its normal appearance as soon as treatment ends.

Radiation therapy may also cause a temporary decrease in the blood's WBC count and increase the risk of developing an infection.

Follow-up Treatment

In the past few years, physicians have recognized that additional treatment may improve the survival rate in early-stage breast cancer. Earlier, it was assumed that women with no evidence of cancer in their lymph nodes had a relatively good chance of remaining cancer-free with no further treatment. Yet cancer does return in many cases and that many women undergoing treatment for "curable" tumors do not reach the 10th year survival milestone.

Since there is no way to be sure who is likely to have a recurrence, it is now strongly recommended that follow-up treatment with drugs (chemotherapy) or hormones must be done, as an insurance policy, for getting rid of any hidden cancer that may remain and preventing or at least delaying any return of the disease.

Chemotherapy

In breast cancer, the patient may need to have a combination of drugs most likely to destroy remaining cancer cells. This anticancer "cocktail" is usually administered intravenously, generally every 3 to 4 weeks for anywhere from 4 to 24 months. Some drugs may be swallowed or injected into a muscle. Chemotherapy is generally recommended if there is any spread of the cancer, even to a single lymph node, because surgery or radiation therapy usually fails to eliminate all "residual" cancer cells.

Radiation targets a specific part of the body. Chemotherapy, on the other hand, is a systemic treatment: The drugs reach every part of body. The strategy is to attack any remaining cancer cells no matter where they are found.

The problem with this strategy is that the drugs attack healthy cells and, as a result, can produce debilitating side effects such as nausea, vomiting, fatigue, and hair loss. Because chemotherapy can damage healthy cells, the body looses immunity and is unable to fight infections and other diseases.

Anticancer drug treatment can increase a woman's chance of reaching the 10-year survival mark. If the disease has already spread, chemotherapy will shrink majority of the tumors. Some of the newer drugs cause fewer and less severe side effects. Administering certain drugs before chemotherapy can help reduce nausea and vomiting. Regular laboratory tests like TC, DC and Hb are essential to monitor damaging effects of chemotherapy.

Hormonal Therapy

Studies indicate that some cancers need the female hormone estrogen or sometimes progesterone to grow. Pathologists now test the tissue removed at biopsy for the presence of estrogen receptors. If the tumor has these receptors, it means that the cancer is "receptive" to estrogen and probably will not grow as well or as quickly if deprived of the hormone.

This is how hormonal treatments work: They either block or eliminate a woman's natural supply of estrogen.

Further, if a tumor has both estrogen and progesterone receptors, there is a chance that the cancer will respond to hormone treatment.

Removing the ovaries in younger women effectively halts the body's estrogen production and produces a high rate of remission in younger women.

The Need for Follow-up Care

Follow-up care in breast cancer is crucial, especially during the first five years after the initial diagnosis.

If having breast cancer, one should schedule regular OPD visits to examine breasts, scars, chest, underarms, and neck by the doctor. From time to time, the doctor will perform a complete physical examination and may order a mammogram. Every three months or so, there will be a battery of blood and urine tests to make sure there is no sign of cancer in other parts of the body. Because breast cancer is most likely to travel to the lungs, bones, and liver, periodic chest X-rays and bone and liver scans will also be necessary.

The physical healing after breast cancer treatment takes a few weeks. The psychological scars take much longer. Many women find that it helps to meet with other cancer survivors who truly understand the fear and anger that can follow a diagnosis of breast cancer. They cope by learning to live in the present and not dwell on the unknown. And, like all women, they can take comfort in the steadily growing number of women who have fought the disease and survived.

POSTOPERATIVE CARE AFTER BREAST SURGERIES

How can Physical Therapy Help Following Breast Cancer Surgery?

Following breast surgery, limitations in range of motion may develop. Patients may have difficulty with overhead activity or fastening their bra. Pain, stiffness, weakness, swelling and loss of function in the affected side upper extremity may develop, making it useless. Most of these conditions are a result of lymphatic resection, soft tissue resection, muscle damage and atrophy, extensive scarring and fear of moving the affected arm due to pain.

These conditions may be prevented with an early short-term course of physical therapy.

Regardless of the type of mastectomy procedure undertaken, it is important to do exercises of upper limbs so that any side effects can be lessened and the patient can manage activities of independent daily living. If undergoing follow-up radiation, exercises are important to help keep the arm flexible, since this type of radiation treatment may continue to affect the arm and shoulder for six to nine months after it has been completed.

Physical therapist or occupational therapist can help design an exercise program, particularly if the patient does not regain full range of motion in the shoulder girdle and arm within three to four weeks of the breast surgery.

Some exercises should not be done until drains and sutures (stitches) are removed. However, some exercises like isometrics can be done immediately after the operation. The exercises that increase shoulder and arm motion can usually be started after a few days and the strengthening exercises are later added to the program as part of the healing process.

Wound Management and Prevention of Contractures following Mastectomies

Surgical wounds associated with mastectomies can sometimes be slow healing, leading to extensive scarring due to healing with secondary intention. This is particularly evident in patients who have had radiation therapy or in cases where the skin over the breast has been excised during radical mastectomy. Split skin or full thickness grafts are sometimes needed to cover obstinate raw area that refuses to heal by conventional measures. Therapist may take help of LPL (He-Ne low power laser therapy) or pulsed short wave or UVA exposure over the raw area to promote granulation and new skin growth.

Surgical incisions in most mastectomies are quite extensive. Such extensive wounds tend to contract as the healing progresses. Given the nature of skin and soft tissue in region of the breast and axilla, contractures are common after mastectomies. Therapists must be alert to such possibilities right from the first postoperative day. Positioning the affected side upper limb appropriately, with the shoulder held in 15–20 degrees of flexion-abduction-external rotation and the elbow, wrist and hand free to move, prevents debilitating adduction-internal rotation contracture of the shoulder following most types of mastectomies, except radical mastectomy. In first 1–2 days this position can be achieved with the help of pillows or sling suspension. Thereafter a suitable flexion-abduction splint (aeroplane splint) may be advised till the sutures are removed by 7th or 10th day. Thereafter the patient may be advised to actively position the arm in corrected position.

Initiating movements is another effective antidote for contracture. Initially, the patient may not be willing to move the part due to pain inhibition. The therapist can take recourse to relaxed passive movements (PM) within pain-free range to retain available range in the shoulder joint of the affected side. Such PMs must be done at least five repetitions twice or thrice a day in the first to third postoperative day, by which period drainage tubes are likely to be removed from the operation site. In the absence of any specific localized contraindications, active exercises are to be initiated from the third postoperative day. If pain over the operated site is still a problem, TENS in continuous or burst mode with appropriate frequency and intensity may be used.

EXERCISE PLAN FOR THE FIRST POSTOPERATIVE WEEK

Following exercises should be done for the first three to seven days after surgery, but only with the surgeon's permission. Instructions to the patient's should be as follows:

- Try to use the affected arm as one normally would when combing hair, bathing, dressing, and eating.
- Raise the affected arm above the level of the heart for 45 minutes, two or three times a day, while lying down. Put the arm on pillows so that the hand is higher than the wrist and the elbow is a little higher than the shoulder. This will help decrease the swelling that may develop after surgery.
- Exercise the affected arm while it is elevated above the level of the heart by opening and closing the fist and then flex and extend the elbow 15 to 25 times. Repeat this three to four times a day. This exercise helps reduce swelling by pumping lymph fluid out of the arm.
- Practice diaphragmatic deep breathing exercises at least six times each day. While lying supine or crook lying, take a slow, deep breath. Breathe in as much air as possible while trying to expand the chest and abdomen. Push the naval away from the spine. Relax and breathe out. Repeat this four or five times. This exercise will help maintain normal movement of the chest, making it easier for the lungs to expand. Continue to do deep breathing exercises indefinitely.
- Avoid sleeping on the affected arm or on that side.

GENERAL GUIDELINES FOR POSTOPERATIVE EXERCISES

- The patient will feel some tightness in the chest and armpit after the operation. This is normal and the tightness will decrease as one continues exercise program.

- Many women have a burning, tingling, numbness, or soreness on the back of the arm and/or chest wall. This is because the surgery has irritated some of the nerve endings. Although the sensations may increase a few weeks, patients should continue to do the exercises unless one notices unusual swelling or tenderness in the arm, shoulder girdle, upper back, chest and neck. Such incidents must be informed to the surgeon immediately. Sometimes rubbing or stroking the area with hand or a soft cloth can help "desensitize" the area.
- It may be helpful to do exercises after a warm shower when muscles are warm and relaxed.
- The patient should wear comfortable, loose clothing when doing the exercises. Do the specified movement until a slow stretch is felt. Hold each stretch at the end of the motion for a count of five. It is normal to feel some pulling as one stretches the skin and muscles that have been shortened. One should not do bouncing or jerky movements when doing any of the exercises. One should also not feel pain as she does the exercises, only gentle stretching. Do five to seven repetitions of each exercise.
- To do each exercise correctly one needs to do the same under the supervision of a physiotherapist.
- Exercises should be done twice a day until the patient regains normal flexibility and strength.
- Patient must be reminded to take deep breaths while performing each exercise.
- The following schedule of exercises are designed so that the patient can begin them lying down, move to sitting, and then finish standing.

Exercises in Lying Position

These exercises should be performed on a bed or the floor while lying on the back with knees and hips bent comfortably, feet flat on the ground.

1. *Wand exercise:* This exercise helps increase the flexion ROM of the shoulders. The patient will need a broom handle, stick, or a short lathi to perform this exercise (Fig. 5.10).
   - Hold the wand in both hands with palms facing up.
   - Lift the wand up over the head (Fig. 5.10) using the unaffected arm to help lift the wand, until the patient feels a stretch in the affected arm.

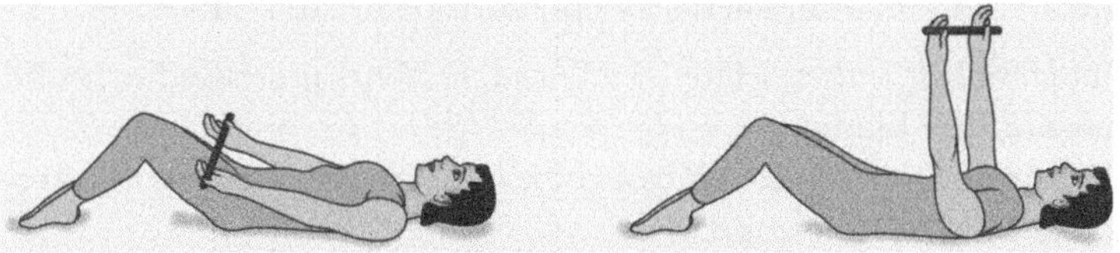

Fig. 5.10: Wand exercise

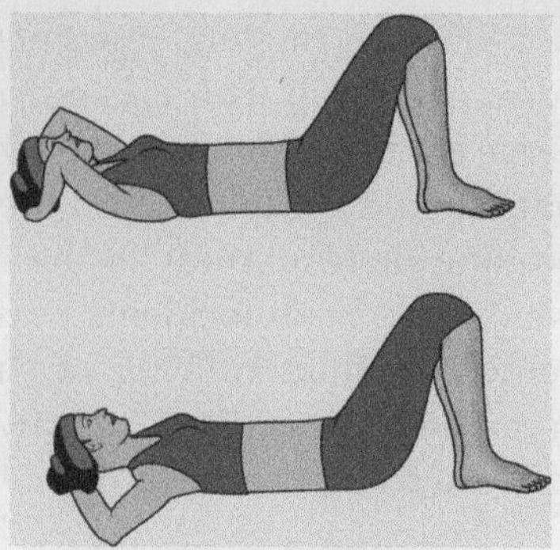

Fig. 5.11: Elbow winging

- Hold for five seconds at maximum elevation.
- Lower arms and repeat 5 to 7 times.

2. *Elbow winging:* This exercise helps increase the mobility of the structures in the front of the chest and shoulder. It may take several weeks of regular exercise before the elbows will get close to the bed (or floor) (Fig. 5.11).
   - Clasp hands behind the neck with elbows pointing toward the ceiling (Fig. 5.11)
   - Move elbows apart and down toward the bed
   - Repeat 5 to 7 times.

Exercises in Sitting Position

These exercises should be performed on a bed or the chair with support to the back with knees and hips bent comfortably, feet flat on the ground.

1. *Shoulder blade stretch:* This exercise helps increase the mobility of the shoulder blades.
   - Sit in a chair very close to a table with back against the chair back.
   - Place the unaffected arm on the table with the elbow bent and forearm pronated with palm down. Do not move this arm during the exercise.
   - Place the affected arm on the table, palm down with the elbow straight (Fig. 5.12).
   - Without moving the trunk, slide the affected arm toward the opposite side of the table. The patient should feel the scapula abduct as he do this.
   - Relax the arm after each stretch and repeat 5 to 7 times.
2. *Shoulder blade squeeze:* This exercise also helps increase the mobility of the shoulder blade.
   - Facing straight ahead, sit in a chair in front of a mirror without resting on the back of the chair.

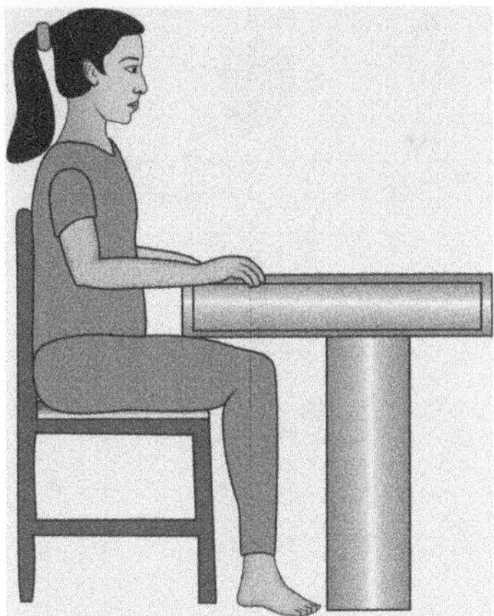

Fig. 5.12: Shoulder blade stretch

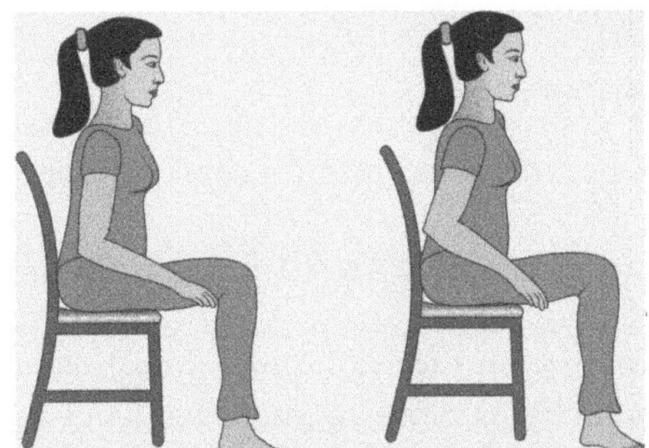

Fig. 5.13: Shoulder blade squeeze

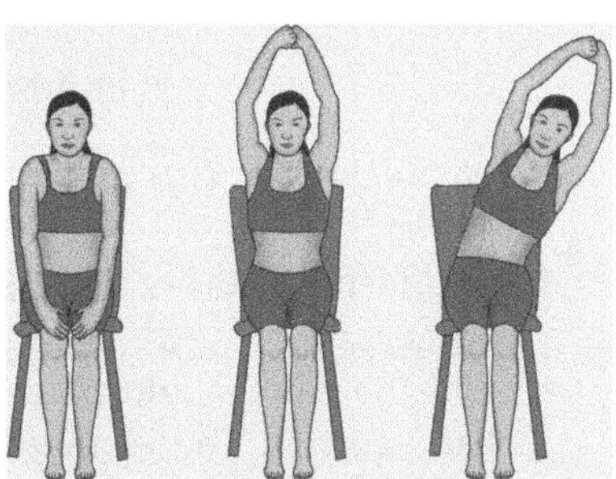

Fig. 5.14: Side bending

- Arms should be at the sides with elbows bent to 30 degrees.
- Retract the scapulae, squeezing the shoulder blades together, bringing the elbows behind to the back. Keep shoulders level as while doing this exercise. Do not lift shoulders up toward the ears (Fig. 5.13).
- Return to the starting position and repeat 5 to 7 times.

3. *Side bending:* This exercise helps increase the mobility of the trunk.
   - Clasp hands together in front and lift both arms slowly over the head, (Fig. 5.14).
   - When both the arms are overhead, bend the trunk to the right while bending at the waist and keeping both arms overhead.
   - Return to the starting position and bend to the left.
   - Repeat 5 to 7 times.

Exercises in Standing Position

These exercises should be performed standing on the floor with knees and hips straight, feet flat on the ground.

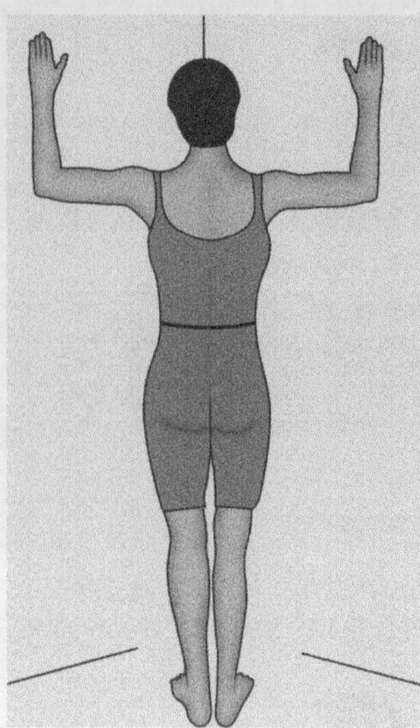

Fig. 5.15: Chest wall stretch

1. *Chest wall stretch:* This exercise helps stretch the anterior chest wall and shoulder.
   - Stand facing a corner with toes approximately 8 to 10 inches from the corner.
   - Bend the elbows and place forearms on the wall, one on each side of the corner. The elbows should be as close to shoulder level as possible.
   - Keep the arms and feet in position and lean forward, moving the chest toward the wall. The patient will feel a stretch across the anterior chest and shoulders muscles (Fig. 5.15).
   - Return to starting position and repeat 5 to 7 times.
2. *Shoulder stretch:* The following exercise helps increase the overhead mobility in the shoulder.
   - Stand facing the wall on toes approximately 12 inches away from the wall.
   - Place both hands on the wall. Use finger tips to "climb the wall," to reach as high as one can until she feels a stretch (Fig. 5.16).
   - Return to starting position and repeat 5 to 7 times.

Points to Ponder

It is important to exercise to keep muscles working as well as possible, but it is also important to be safe. The patient should talk with the therapist about exercise plan for her condition, and then set realistic goals for increasing overall activity level.

The patient should begin exercising slowly and progress gradually as she is able. However, if any complication develops after surgery one should

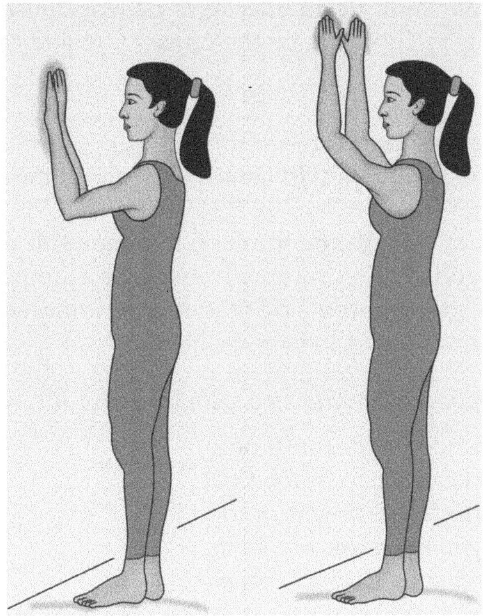

Fig. 5.16: Shoulder stretch

stop exercising and notify the surgeon, particularly if following symptoms are felt:

- Have unusual swelling in the arm, or swelling gets worse
- Have pain that gets worse
- Have heaviness in the arm
- Getting weaker, start losing balance, or start falling
- Have headaches, dizziness, blurred vision, numbness, or tingling in arms or chest.

MANAGEMENT OF LYMPHEDEMA FOLLOWING RADICAL MASTECTOMY

Lymphedema is a common complication of radical mastectomy and/or radiation therapy for breast cancer. It occurs after surgical excision and scarring of the axillary lymphatic system on the affected side. Lymphedema has important pathological and clinical consequences in many cases of mastectomy.[1]

Recognizing Symptoms of the Onset of Lymphedema (Stage I)

The following are a list of symptoms and signs which a person with a "limb-at-risk" should note:

- An increase in the size of the limb
- A feeling of heat in the limb
- A bursting sensation of the limb

- Red patches may indicate an infection—patients must see their physician immediately. This may be the cause of, or indicate the onset, of lymphedema
- Puffiness
- Pitting of the skin if pressed
- Aching limb (or shoulder, particularly the back of the shoulder area in the afternoon)
- Any swelling, or heat, in the trunk on the same side as the operation; and enlarged and at times warmer breast after a lumpectomy
- A swelling of the opposite side (e.g. if after a mastectomy the other breast or chest walls start to increase in size).

Signs of Lymphedema Progressing (Stage II and III)

- Any of the previous signs for its onset
- A compression garment gets too tight
- Pins and needles in the fingers or toes
- Lack of feeling in any areas of a limb
- Leaking areas (fistulae) start to occur.[2]

Do's and Don'ts

Patients with limb "at-risk", or with frank lymphedema should always be advised the following precaution:

- Keep the affected limb clean. When drying use a soft towel and be gentle but thorough, a hair-dryer may help for difficult areas. Make sure underclothes and compression garments are regularly washed. Keep the skin supple with a good moisturizer, particularly over skin grafts, if any.
- Avoid any trauma, sunburn, insect bites. Be careful while cutting nails, do not cut the cuticle or push back too hard as this can injure it and allow bacteria to enter, thus leading to infection. When sewing, wear a thimble; if gardening, wear a glove and long sleeves.
- Keep the limb as cool as possible in hot weather. Be careful of the water temperature in showers and spas. If traveling for a long time in a car, drape a white shirt over limb in the sun. Move it if possible when you have to sit for a long time, flex and stretch fingers.
- Do not pick up heavy loads with an arm "at-risk", e.g. a case or heavy shopping. Do not carry a heavy bag or handbag on this arm.
- Do not allow anyone to measure blood pressure, to take blood sample, or to give an injection in the affected limb.
- If traveling by air it is a good precaution to wear a compression garment or pressure bandages. Bandages may be used on fingers and hand if necessary.
- There should be no redness or indentation when clothing are removed; otherwise it is stopping some of the surviving lymphatic drainage.

- Do not to lie on an arm at risk when sleeping or resting.
- A normal balanced diet is best. Lymphedema is a high-protein edema but eating too little protein will not help. Rather it weakens the connective tissue, thus making an edema worse. Dieting will not reduce lymphedema, but nor will if a patient is overweight.
- If stressed, concentrate on relaxing the shoulders, back and neck. Extend the spine and "stand straight". Constant tension in these areas will worsen lymphedema. In Stage I lymphedema, the swelling consists of protein-rich fluid and may become temporarily reduced by simple elevation of the limb. If it remains untreated for long, the lymphedema causes a progressive hardening of the affected tissues, due to proliferation of connective tissue, adipose tissue and scarring, i.e. Stage II lymphedema.[3]

Stage III lymphedema is characterized by a tremendous increase in volume, hardening of the dermal tissues, hyperkeratosis and papillomas of the skin. Infections such as cellulitis, erysipelas or lymphangitis frequently develop in patients suffering from chronic lymphedema. Infections are most common in Stage II and III of lymphedema, each infection resulting in a worsening of the condition and necessitating frequent hospitalizations. The most effective treatment for lymphedema is Manual Lymph Drainage (MLD) and Combined Decongestive Therapy (CDT).[4]

Manual Lymph Drainage (MLD)

Manual lymph drainage (MLD) is a gentle manual technique involving centripetally directed effleurage massage, an effective way to activate the lymphatic system, especially when the transport capacity of the lymph system is reduced because of prior surgery and/or radiation therapy. The affected extremity is positioned in elevation, the level of its proximal end being higher than the level of the heart. Effleurage massage with moderate pressure is administered to the swollen upper extremity with the palm and fingers of the hand being in full contact to the skin. For best results, the proximal part of the extremity from elbow to shoulder is drained at first, using five to ten slow strokes. This empties drainage channels in the proximal part of the extremity. Thereafter the distal part from hand to elbow is massaged in similar fashion to push trapped fluid into the proximal half of the limb. The procedure is again repeated on the proximal segment to completely drain the extremity of fluid. The strokes should be slow and firm and as far as possible encompass the entire girth of the limb. If MLD is carried out as an isolated treatment for lymphedema, the results may be very temporary and lasting evacuation of lymph fluid from a swollen limb will not be possible. As such application of compressive modalities such as tailor made pressure garments must be applied on the extremity immediately after the massage. This will to some extent prevent reaccumulation of edema for some period of time at the least. Additional advantage may be gained by applying Faradism under pressure after the pressure garment has been put on the extremity.

Combined Decongestive Therapy[5]

Combined decongestive therapy (CDT) is a combination of manual lymph drainage, remedial exercises, compression bandaging or compression garments in the maintenance phase and therapeutic skin care. It may also include breathing and aquatic exercises, adjunct therapies such as low-level laser for skin lesions, as well as dietary measures.

Combined decongestive therapy (CDT) is the most successful treatment for chronic extremity lymphedema.

Postmastectomy lymphedema and other related conditions respond extremely well to this gentle, noninvasive and highly effective therapy. CDT is sometimes referred to as Combined Decongestive Therapy or Complete Decongestive Physiotherapy (CDP) or Complex Decongestive Physiotherapy.

Combined decongestive therapy (CDT) is usually divided into a two-phase program that first involves an intensive treatment phase, followed by a maintenance program that the patient continues at home. When carried out with great care, consistency and the expertise of a well-trained therapist, CDT is the treatment of choice for chronic extremity lymphedema. Even in advanced lymphedema, CDT can be used without side effects with great success. Because CDT is labor intensive, time consuming and requires patient compliance, many patients have difficulty committing to the program at first. Nevertheless, because the results of CDT are superior to other available treatments, most patients undergo CDT treatment and are then able to maintain the reduction of their limbs by diligently participating in a home-based self-care program.

Initial Phase

Patients undergo a medical assessment by a physician and are referred to a certified therapist. After a thorough evaluation to determine the best treatment plan, patients are advised of the treatment choices, which are customized to the individual needs.

During this initial phase, CDT is usually required 5–6 times per week and treatment may last anywhere from 2–4 weeks typically.

Depending on the condition, each session typically lasts one hour and involves daily assessment of the patient's condition. Skin and wound care may be undertaken (Fig. 5.17).

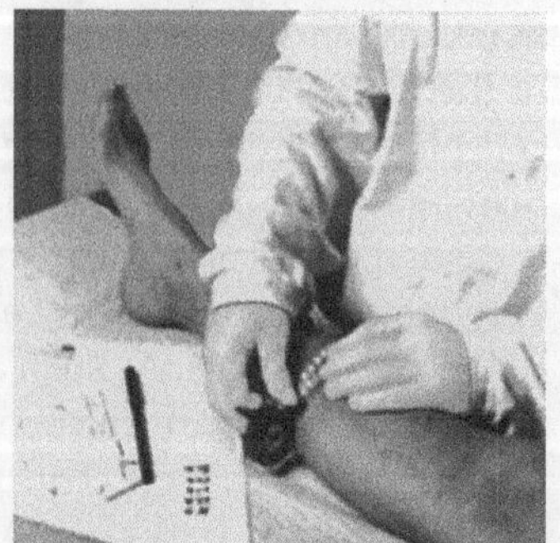

Fig. 5.17: Skin care regime

This is followed by manual lymph drainage. This hands-on part of the treatment usually lasts about 45 minutes and is followed by compression bandaging.

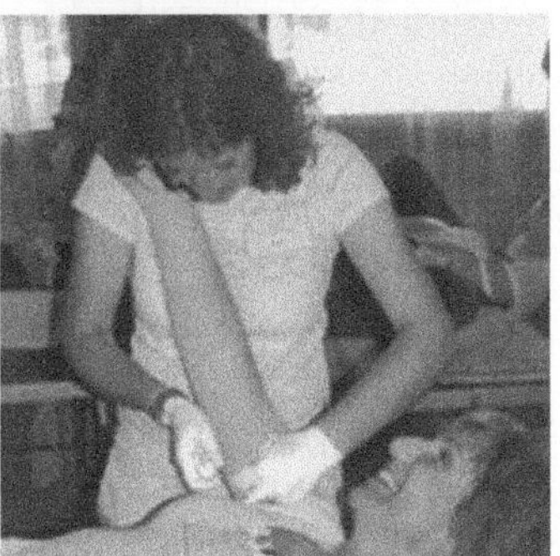

Fig. 5.18: Massage regime

The bandages are applied exactly to conform to the patient's tissues and are reapplied on a daily basis. They are short-stretch crepe bandages that resist muscle contraction, apply inward pressure and are applied with comfortable padding underneath. The bandages help to maintain the reductions achieved with MLD and may even cause further reduction (Fig. 5.18).

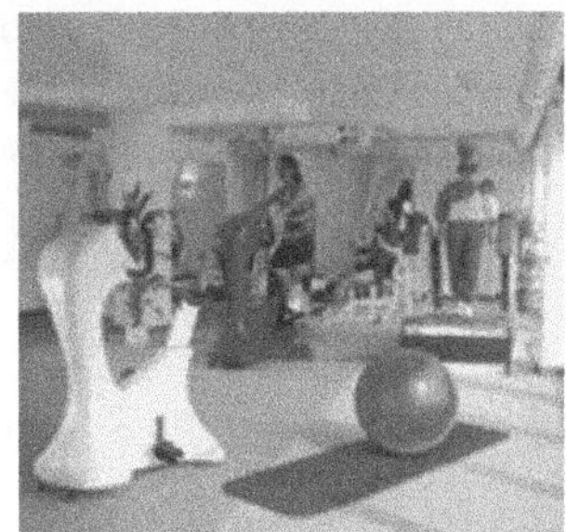

Fig. 5.19: Exercise regime

After bandaging, therapeutic exercises may be demonstrated that the patient can easily perform. These also help in further reducing the limb. Patients may join a group exercise class or be shown individual exercises (Fig. 5.19).

Reductions in limb volumes vary, dependent on many factors such as age, weight, extent of the edema, skin condition and comorbidities. Typically patients might expect a 40–50 percent reduction in limb volume although it may be more or less than this. Sometimes improvement in other measurable factors such as tissue hardness, pain and mobility may be more significant to patient than volume reduction.[6]

Maintenance Phase

Towards the end of the initial phase, volume reduction starts to stabilize and the therapist will usually recommend that the patient is fitted for a compression garment. For edematous limbs, the optimal material to use for these garments is a flat knit, low-stretch material that is similar to the short-stretch crepe bandages. Aquatic exercise performed with the edematous part submerged in water is also effective in assisting and maintaining reduction of edema, particularly in lower limbs, due to hydrostatic pressure[7] (Fig. 5.20).

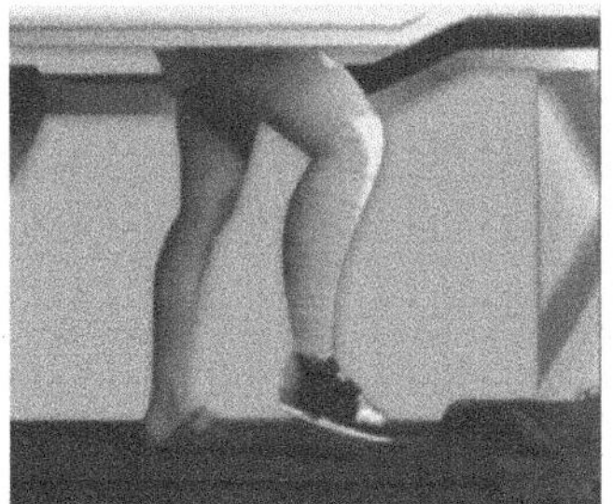

Fig. 5.20: Underwater walking exercises

A treatment plan is devised for the maintenance phase and this may require weekly, monthly or six-monthly visits to the therapist. Patients continue to wear their compression garments, continue to do exercise and home care as well as monitor their condition carefully. MLD may also be used during these visits.

Successful maintenance of the reduced limb is essential to prevent further problems developing. With correct therapeutic intervention using CDT, patients can successfully manage their lymphedema.

REFERENCES

1. RH Harris. Dr Vodder's Manual Lymph Drainage. Hand in Hand, Journal of the Canadian Massage Therapist Association. Winter 1991.
2. RH Harris. The Vodder Method, an introduction to manual lymph drainage. Massage Therapy Journal 1992;31,1.
3. RH Harris. Edema and its treatment in Massage Therapy. Journal of Soft Tissue Manipulation 1994; 1 # 4.
4. RH Harris, Neil Pille. Advances in Lymphology in Australia. British Columbia Massage Practitioner 1994; 14 # 1.
5. P Hutzschenreuter et. al. Postmastectomy Arm Lymphedema: Treated by Manual lymph Drainage and Compression Bandage Therapy. European Journal of Physical Medicine and Rehabilitation 1991;1,6.
6. SK Johannsen et. al. Effects of Compression Bandaging with or without Manual Lymph Drainage Treatment in Patients with Postoperative Arm Lymphedema. Lymph Link, Publ. by National Lymphedema Network, San Francisco, CA. 2000;12,1.
7. SK Johansson. Lymphedema and Breast Cancer, A Physiotherapeutic Approach. Studentlitteratur, Lund University, 2002.

Chapter

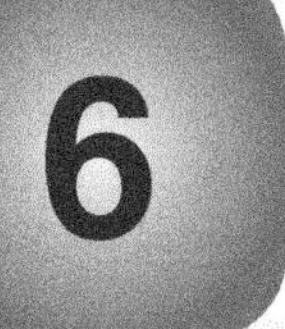

Physiotherapy in Burn and Plastic Surgeries

INTRODUCTION TO BURN INJURY

A burn injury can be defined as "damage to the skin and underlying tissues caused by unprotected exposure to extreme energy source, such as heat, cold, chemicals, electricity or radiant energy".

Until recently, survival was the only measure of success in managing serious burn injuries. More recently, the objective of burn care has become successful reintegration of the patient as a productive memeber in the workplace, at home and in the community. This revised objective has extended the traditional role of the physiotherapist beyond hospital based caregiver and into the settings of workplace, home, and community.

Three broad aspects are involved in this effort: Reconstruction, rehabilitation and reintegration. The importance of early and active focus on long-term rehabilitation goals must be emphasized in any care plan for the burn patients.

Modern burn care may be divided into the following four general phases:

- The *first phase*, initial evaluation and resuscitation, occurs on days 1–3 after the burn and requires an accurate assessment for adequate fluid resuscitation and thorough evaluation for associated injuries to nerves, muscles and bones and systemic comorbidities such as cardiorespiratory, hepatic and renal failure.
- The *second phase*, initial wound excision followed by wound closure using biological skin/artificial skin as temporary cover. This is done by a series of operations within the first few days after injury.
- The *third phase*, final wound closure, involves replacement of temporary wound covers with a definitive cover; there is also reconstruction of small surface wound area with higher complexity, such as the face and hands.
- The *final phase* of care is rehabilitation, reconstruction, and reintegration. This begins with simple positioning and movements during the resuscitation period and progressively becomes more complex and time-consuming, incorporating multidisciplinary involvement toward the end of the hospital stay.

Events associated with a burn incident, such as smoke inhalation, jumping from a burning building, being struck by debris, or being victim of a motor vehicle or air crash, may cause other associated secondary injuries such as TBI, fractures, spinal injuries and respiratory distress, all of which contribute to the overall morbidity, outcome of treatment and final mortality of the burn injury.

PHASE 1

Acute Care of Burn

First Aid: COOL, COVER and CALL

Burn is one of those emergencies that can occur any time of the year in or out of the house. First aid of a burn injury helps minimize pain and provide relief before the specialized professionals takeover. It should always include:

For Thermal Burns

- Cool all burns with tepid to cool water, regardless of degree. Continue flushing the area for up to 15 minutes. Do not apply ice, ointments, butter or other "home remedies". Remove all clothing and jewelry to reduce the contact time with hot items.
- Burn injuries are sterile to begin with. Cover affected areas with a clean dry cloth, towel or blanket to protect the burn from contamination and to minimize pain. Keep blisters intact. Do not apply unsterilized dressings.
- One should seek medical attention if burn is larger than the victim's hand size, particularly if the victim is a child or elderly person. (refer to Criteria for hospitalization).

For Chemical Burns

- "The solution to pollution is dilution". Wash the chemical burn wound profusely with running water for 20 minutes.
- Monitor for hypothermia while irrigating.
- Preserve victim's clothing for chemical analysis to identify the chemical agent responsible for causing the burn.

Emergency Treatment of Burns: Points to Ponder

- Prehospital burned patients must be removed from the source of injury and the burning process stopped
- Inhalation injury must always be suspected and 100 percent oxygen given by facemask.
- Burning clothing, all rings, watches, jewelry, and belts are removed because they retain heat and can produce a tourniquet-like effect.

- Water at room-temperature can be poured on the wound within 15 minutes of injury to decrease the depth of the wound, but any subsequent measures to cool the wound should be avoided to prevent hypothermia during resuscitation.

Stabilization, Wound Care and Transport: Points to Ponder

- The patient should be wrapped in a sheet or blanket to minimize heat loss and for temperature control during transport.
- The first step in diminishing pain is to cover the wounds to prevent contact with exposed nerve endings.
- Small doses of intravenous (IV) morphine may be given after complete assessment of the patient and once it is determined to be safe by an experienced practitioner.
- Mode of transport needs to be of appropriate size with emergency equipment available, along with nurses, physicians, paramedics, or respiratory therapists who are familiar with trauma patients.

Primary Care in the Hospital ER

The arrival of the victim of a burn accident at the emergency department is one of the most dramatic events in a hospital. The suddenness of the accident, visibility of the damage, the pain, fear and the reaction of the patient's relatives all combines to create an atmosphere charged with tension.

The immediate need of resuscitation and pain relief may interfere with assessment of the patient, particularly with history taking and physical examination. The history of mechanism of burning is of major importance in assessing its severity. In the event the patient is unable to provide history of the injury, any relative/eyewitness/passerby may provide necessary inputs. The severity of the burn is primarily estimated from the surface area of the burnt skin and the depth of the burn wound.

Initial Assessment

Initial assessment involves primary and secondary survey.

- In the primary survey, immediately life-threatening conditions are quickly identified and treated.
- In the secondary survey, a more thorough head-to-toe evaluation of the patient is undertaken.

On arrival, a burn patient should be treated as any other trauma. ABC of trauma care, i.e. checking the airway, breathing and circulation applies as usual.

Assessing Airway Damage

The upper respiratory tract may be damaged due to exposure to heated gases and smoke. Direct injury to the upper airway results in edema, which together with the generalized whole-body edema associated with a severe burn, may obstruct the airway. Airway injury must be suspected with facial burns, singed nasal hairs, carbonaceous sputum, and rapid shallow breathing. Progressive hoarseness is a sign of impending airway obstruction, and endotracheal intubation needs to be done immidiately before edema distorts the upper airway.

Assessing Breathing

The chest is exposed in order to assess breathing pattern; airway patency alone does not ensure adequate ventilation. Chest expansion and equal breath sounds in both lungs ensure adequate air exchange.

Assessing Circulation

Blood pressure may be difficult to measure in burned patients with edematous or charred extremities. Pulse rate as an indirect measure of circulation, which in most burned patients remain rapid even with adequate resuscitation. Pulse oxymeter signals taken from the finger/toe tip is sufficient until better monitors for circulation, such as arterial pressure and urine output can be recorded.

Assessing Associated Injuries

In patients who have been in an explosion or road accident, the possibility of spinal cord injury exists. Appropriate spinal stabilization must be accomplished by whatever means necessary, including the use of body boards/cervical collars to keep the spine immobilized until it has been evaluated by an expert.

If there is burn around the nose and mouth, possibility of smoke and flame inhalation must be considered. Laryngeal edema can develop and lung function may deteriorate rapidly. Endotracheal intubation should be considered early, before laryngeal edema sets in. If laryngeal edema has already develops endotracheal intubation is difficult and at times impossible. Then a surgical airway, i.e. tracheostomy will be needed immediately.

Checklist for ER

Respiratory

- Assess the airway, respiratory rate and rhythm.
- Note chest wall expansion, especially if full thickness burns that are circumferential to the trunk.
- Administer 100 percent (humidified) oxygen by non-rebreather mask.
- For a compromised airway—consider chin lift or jaw thrust or oropharyngeal airway for the unconscious patient.

Circulatory

- Assess peripheral pulsation, blood pressure, pulse rate and skin color.
- Elevate extremities. Fluid shifting in burn patient's causes edema and volume loss.

LOC (Level of Consciousness)

- Determine level of consciousness by AVPU method; alert, verbal/ painful stimuli, unresponsive. Burn patients should be initially alert and oriented. If not, consider brain trauma or other associated injuries.
- Obtain a complete history of the events; time, open or enclosed space, last meal, medications, allergies, past medical history and any other pertinent data.

Physical examination

- Conduct a thorough head-to-toe examination of the patient, noting any deformities, irregularities, as well as calculating out the total burn surface area.
- A widely-used clinical rule, the rule of nine acts as a rough guide to the body surface involvement. As a general rule an adult with more than 20 percent of the burn surface area involvement, or a child with more than 10 percent of the body surface area involvement will require intravenous fluid replacement. However an intravenous line may be necessary to achieve adequate analgesia for much smaller burn and in children fluid replacement may be required because of vomiting.
- The prognosis depends upon the percentage of body surface area burned. A rough guide is that, if the sum total of the age and percentage of burned is 100 or above, then the burn is likely to be fatal.

Assessment of the Burn Injury

In order to treat a burn injury the primary requirement is a detailed assessment of the damage to the skin. Clinicians need to classify burns according to strict, widely-accepted parameters to facilitate planning treatment. The parameters used to classify the extent of burn injury to the skin and underlying tissue damage are:

1. Agent of burn.
2. Depth of skin thickness affected by the burn.
3. Percentage of total body surface area (TBSA) involved in the burn.

Classification Based on Agents of Burn

- *Thermal burn:* Caused by flame, causing damage from superheated, oxidized air or scald due to contact with hot objects, liquids and steam are the most common causes of burns.

- *Cold burn:* Caused by exposure to very cold air, contact to very cold objects or even unregulated therapeutic application of ice/coolant spray.
- *Chemical burn:* Caused by corrosive chemicals like acids, coming in contact with the skin, are in effect similar to thermal burns.
- *Electrical burn:* Caused by the passage of high voltage electric current through the body.
- *Radiation burn:* Caused by exposure to radioactive source or very bright sunlight.

Thermal, cold and chemical burns usually affect the skin, which sustains most of the damage. However, severe surface burns may penetrate to deeper body structures, such as fat, fascia, muscle or bone.

An electrical burn on the other hand affects deeper structures such as blood vessels and nerves, because these structures provide pathway of minimum impedance for the electric current to flow. The damage to the skin is restricted only to the points of entry and exit of the electrical current.

Radiation burns are far more insidious, affecting the vitality of the skin and the underlying tissues gradually, leading to progressive skin breakdown, peeling and ulceration.

Structure of Human Skin

To understand the extent of the primary assault caused by a burn injury on the human body, one must begin by understanding the structure of the human skin, since it is the skin, being the outermost protective covering of the body, bears the brunt of the injury caused by burn.

Skin is the largest organ in the human body. It has the highest rate of metabolic turnover and is endowed with a rare ability to regenerate and repair itself at an astonishing rate. It is also the body's first line of defense against a hostile environment. It prevents entry of pathogens such as bacteria and virus, protects the underlying tissues from injury due to friction, heat and corrosive chemicals, and helps regulate the body temperature and excretion of body waste through sweating.

The skin contains three distinct layers, the outer epidermis, the middle dermis and the lowest subcutaneous layer (Fig. 6.1).

The epidermis has top four layers made of only dead skin cells and a lowermost layer made up of living and continuously multiplying cells, called the stratum germinativum. The dead cells from the outermost layers of the epidermis are being shed continuously as a result of friction from clothing, scratching, washing, etc. These cells are replenished continuously from below by new cells being produced by the stratum germinativum. As a result the skin can maintain its optimum thickness in spite of continuous loss of top layer of dead cells.

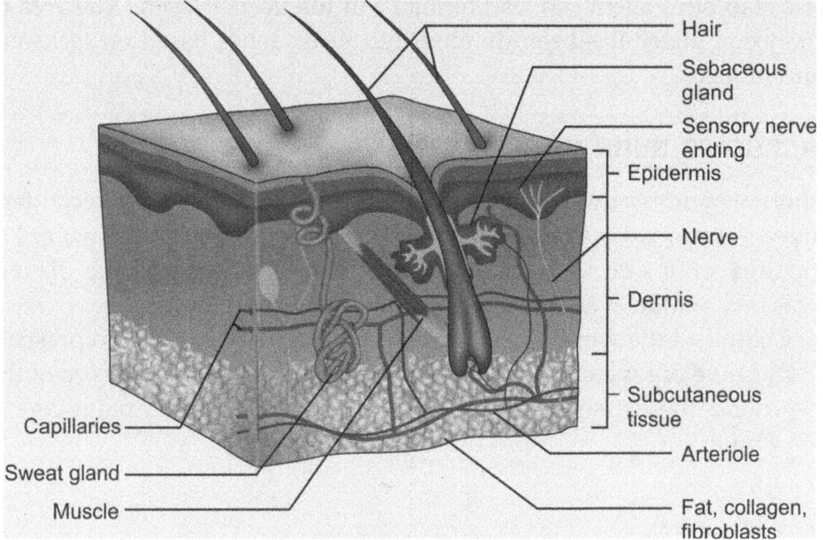

Fig. 6.1: Cross section of skin

- The middle layer of the skin, the dermis begins just below the stratum germinativum, the lowest layer of epidermis. The dermis contains vital skin structures such as sweat glands, sebaceous glands, muscles controlling the hair, blood capillaries and sensory nerves whose ending penetrate outward up to lower level of epidermis.
- Below the dermis lies the lowest subcutaneous layer, consisting of collagen, fat and fibroblasts forming a dense but resilient matrix through which the skin as a whole is anchored to the underlying tissues of the body.

Nature of Burn Injury

- *The primary injury:* It is the immediate damage caused by the burn. Little can be done to limit the primary injury in most cases of burn. However a prompt removal of the heat source and rapid cooling of the burn limits the extent of primary injury.
- *The secondary injury:* It is the deleterious effect resulting from the primary injury. A major burn can result in loss of fluid, secondary infection, endogenous and exogenous release of toxins, powerful inflammatory response, fluid shift, tissue coagulation, edema and constriction of blood vesseles caused by burn eschar.

PART—I

The skin provides a robust barrier to transfer of energy to deeper tissues; much of the burn injury is confined to this layer. The response of local tissues to burn agent can lead to injury in the deeper layers. The area of cutaneous injury has been divided into three zones based on Jackson's burn model:

JACKSON'S BURN MODEL

A burn wound is a dynamic entity and is subject to the effects of secondary injury. A burn wound may deepen if the blood supply of the wound is impaired or if infection occurs. Jackson's model describes the distinct areas seen within every burn wound (Figs 6.2A to C).

a. Central to the wound lies the zone of coagulation, which represents the zone of severe damage caused by primary injury—the core of the wound; these tissues will not recover and will slough off in due course of time.

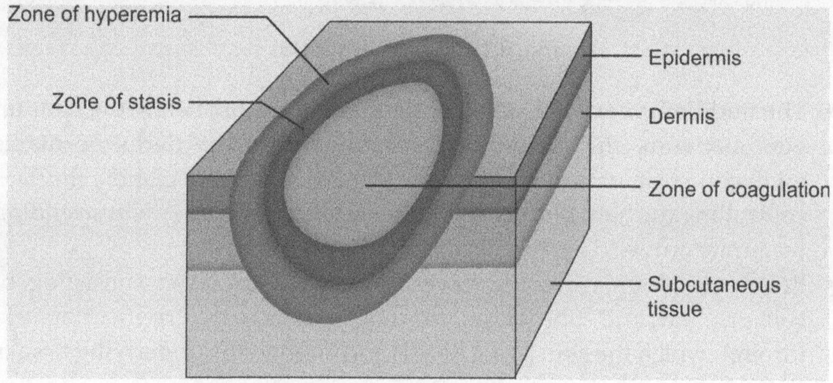

A. Schematic representation of zones of tissue damage in burn injury

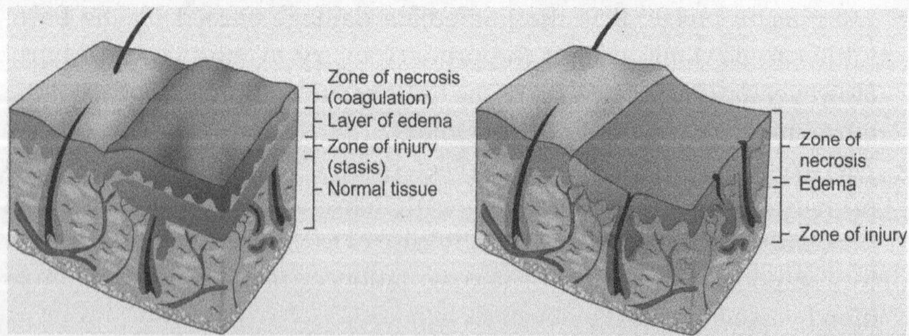

B. Schematic representation of a superficial partial thickness and
C. Deep partial thickness burns

Figs 6.2A to C: Jackson's burn model

b. Surrounding the zone of coagulation is the zone of stasis, which comprises of less damaged tissue surrounding the core of the wound, in which inflammation occurs and vascularity is impaired. Tissue in this zone have the potential to recover under correct conditions.
c. The outer layer is the zone of hyperemia comprising of tissue with intense vasodilatation and increased blood flow. These usually recover spontaneously unless severely infected. The margins between the zones are not static as they are influenced by local and systemic factors like reduced blood flow, excessive edema which tends to extend the zone of coagulation and hence increase the area of tissue necrosis. In favorable conditions the margin of the central zone remains static and the zone of stasis shrinks as it is replaced by the zone of hyperemia.

Classification Based on Depth of Burn

The depth of injury from a burn is described as first, second, third or fourth degree, depending on the layers of skin affected from outermost epidermis progressing deeper into the body surface:

First Degree Burn

This is possibly the most common type of burn; usually indicated by redness to the skin without blistering, pain, slight swelling of the affected area. First-degree burns are the most superficial, affecting only the outer most layer of the skin, i.e. the epidermis.

The skin becomes painful, red and blanches to the touch. The usual cause of first degree burn is sunburn or steamburn. Figure 6.3 shows first degree sunburn on the lower back, with the skin appearing blotchy red and swollen over the sacrum and steamburn over the forearm, with the skin looking red. This finding is characteristic of first-degree burns, occurring without blisters but with significant amount of pain, swelling and local tenderness.

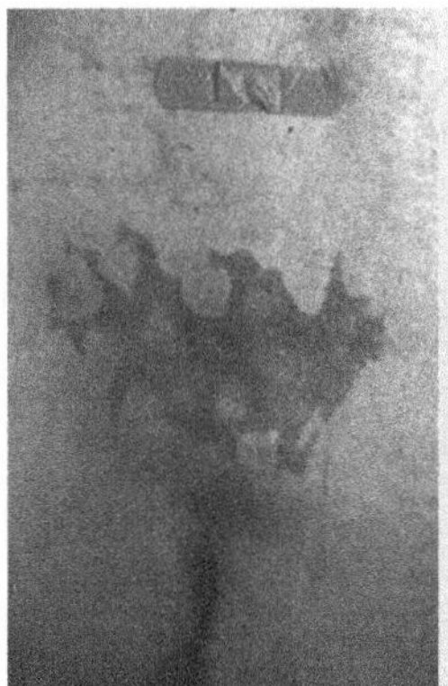
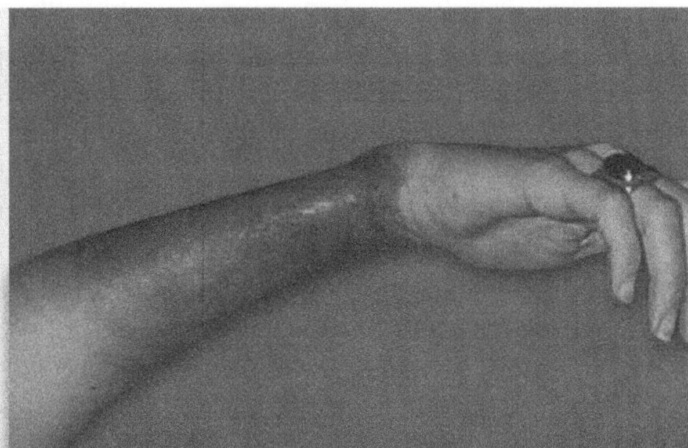

Fig. 6.3: First degree burn over the sacrum (left) and forearm (right)

First degree burn injury is usually self-limiting and self-curing in nature. It heals within a span of three to seven days. Cold water bath and local application of Calamine lotion with Aloe Vera or Lidocaine gel helps reduce skin irritation and pain. Simple NSAIDs such as ibuprofen may also be given.

Prevention of sunburn is simple. One may use a sun block with a minimum of SPF 30. Cover the body as best as possible with light-colored long sleeve clothing and full pants when the sun is exceptionally hot.

Second Degree Burn

A second degree burn is indicated by redness or whiteness to the skin, intense pain, and swelling of the affected area as well as blisters. Second degree burns can range from severe sunburn to burns from flame, steam or corrosive chemicals like acids. Prevention can be difficult due to the wide range of causes. Caution is always advised when dealing with fire or dangerous chemicals. Should someone else become burned quickly flush the burned areas with lots of water. Once you think you have flushed the area enough flush it some more. An adage that fire fighters learn is, "the solution to pollution is dilution". This also applies to chemical burns. Though certain chemicals may react with water to cause a more intense burning, but even so enough water will wash off any chemicals that may be causing the burn. Remove any jewelry from the body as the metal can become hot and cause further burns as well. After flushing the burned area, the wound must be quickly air dried and covered with dry gauze. Do not use any type of burn cream or ointment on the burn as they can actually cause harm with severe burns.

Second degree burns (also called partial-thickness burns) extend into the middle layer of skin, i.e. the dermis. Second degree burns appear pink or red, swollen, and painful, and they develop blisters that may ooze a clear fluid. The burned area may blanch when touched.

Second degree burns are further classified as:

- Superficial partial thickness burns, which are red, painful, and blanch to touch and often may form blister (Fig. 6.4). It involves the entire epidermis and superficial part of the dermis, sparing patches of the stratum germinativum (layer of growing skin cells between epidermis and dermis), hair follicles, sebaceous and sweat glands. Healing takes place spontaneously in 7 to 14 days in absence of any secondary infections, usually by primary intention, without any scar formation but with slight discoloration over the long term. The skin grows back from surviving stratum germinativum retained in epidermal structures like the skin ridges, hair follicles, and sweat glands.
- Deep partial thickness second degree burn involving both the superficial and the deep parts of the dermis, appear more pale and mottled, do not blanch to touch and remain painful to pinprick. These burns heal

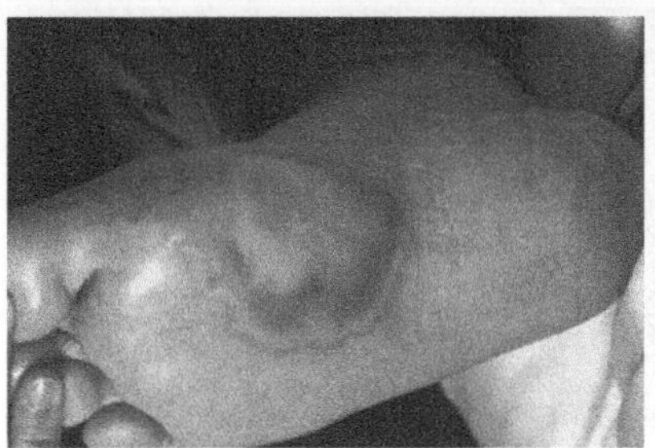
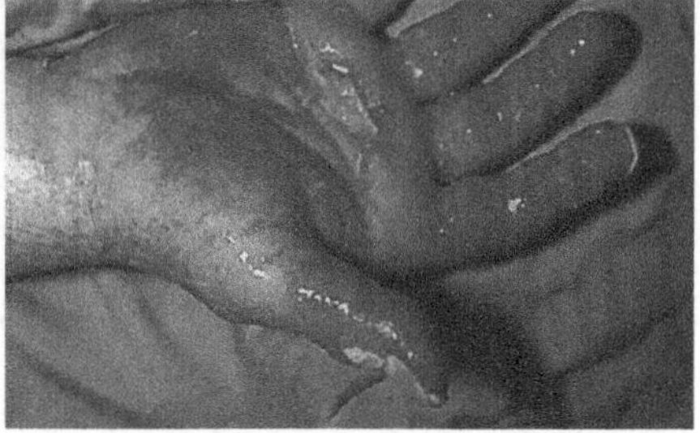

Fig. 6.4: Second degree burn of the foot with blister and the palm without blisters

in 14 to 35 days by re-epithelialization from hair follicles and sweat gland keratinocytes, often with severe scarring as a result of the loss of dermis. Infection is almost inevitable in most cases of deep partial thickness burns and that causes the wound to downgrade rapidly to third degree burn. All surviving patches of growing skin cells may be destroyed due to the infection and therefore the healing can take place only by secondary intention, with extensive scar formation.

Second degree burns are characterized by severe pain due to damage caused to the superficial sensory nerve endings. Treatment of superficial partial thickness burn consists of aggressive pain management, burn dressing, antibiotic cover and fluid-nutrition replenishment. In deep partial thickness burn the same treatment is complimented by artificial or split skin graft to cover the raw area. The purpose of wound cover is to minimize fluid loss, protect the delicate surviving pockets of growing skin cells from infection and external trauma and allow them to grow back to the maximum possible extent and promote revascularization of the new skin. In the later stage of wound healing any small residual raw area may need a full thickness skin graft.

Third Degree (Full Thickness) Burns

This is an extremely severe burn injury and requires immediate medical care. These types of burns usually occur with explosions or fires, which are fueled by highly inflammable chemicals such as gasoline or alcohol. These burns are indicated by charred black and even waxy white flesh. Blisters and redness occurs typically around the edge of the burns and sometimes can be completely pain-free within the burn area and painful only around the edges. The initial treatment for this type of burn is the same as a second degree burn, i.e. remove all jewelry, flush with lots and lots and lots of water, dry and cover with dry gauze. The victim will however need to go immediately to a hospital emergency room and from there to a burn center. In fact it is often recommended that they go directly to the emergency room of a hospital with an active Burn Center.

Third degree burns, also called full-thickness burn, involve all three layers of skin (epidermis, dermis, and subcutaneous fat layer),

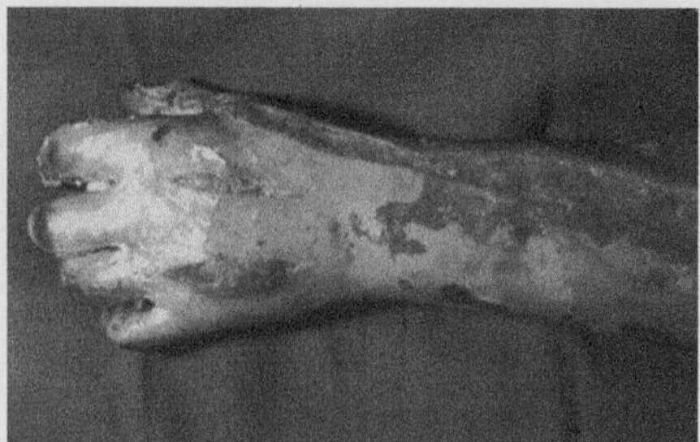
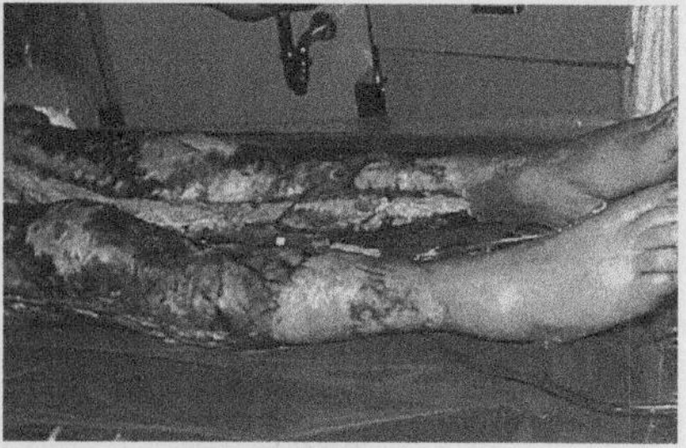

Fig 6.5: Third degree burn of the dorsal surface of hand and both legs

characterized by a hard, leathery eschar that is painless and black, white, or cherry red (Fig. 6.5).

Since these burns penetrate the dermis, nerve endings have been destroyed, and the patient has no feeling in the burned area. No epidermal or dermal appendages remain; thus, these wounds must heal by re-epithelialization from the wound edges. Deep dermal and full-thickness burns require eschar excision with skin grafting to heal the wounds in timely fashion.

Fourth Degree Burns

Fourth degree burns or charring involves carbonization of other tissues beneath the skin, such as muscle, bone, and brain and helps control shortness of breath.

Calculating Percentage of Total Body Surface Area (TBSA) Affected by Burn

The skin is the largest structure in the body. It isolates a patient's inside from his outside, chemically, thermally, mechanically and biologically.

A burn destroys these functions, so that treatment is mainly an attempt to restore them. A severe burn is a three dimensional rather than a two dimensional lesion. It opens up a huge surface through which the body loses water, electrolytes, proteins, and heat, and across which bacteria and drugs can enter. To determine the severity of a burn, one has to estimate what percentage of the body's surface has been damaged, specifically in second or third or fourth degree burns using Berkow formula (beŕko).

Berkow formula is a method for determining the percentage of total body surface affected by a burn derived from the rule of nines.

Rule of nines is a method of estimating the extent of burns in an adult, expressed as a percentage of total body surfaces. In this method, the body is divided into sections of 9 percent, or multiples of 9 percent, each: head and neck, 9 percent; anterior trunk, 18 percent; posterior trunk, 18 percent; upper limbs, 18 percent; lower limbs, 36 percent; genitalia and perineum,

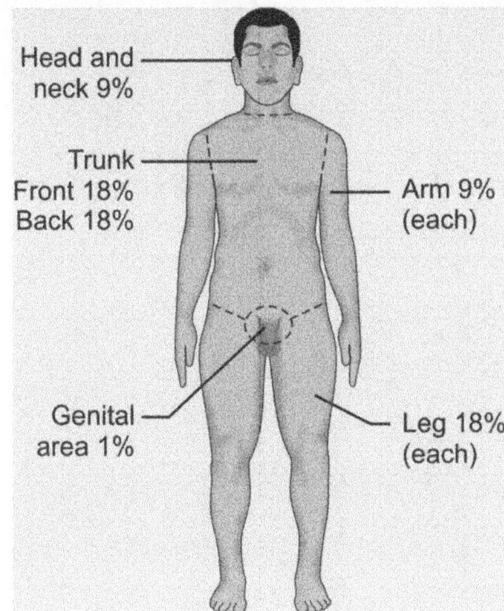

Fig. 6.6: Calculating TBSA of burn based on the rule-of-nine

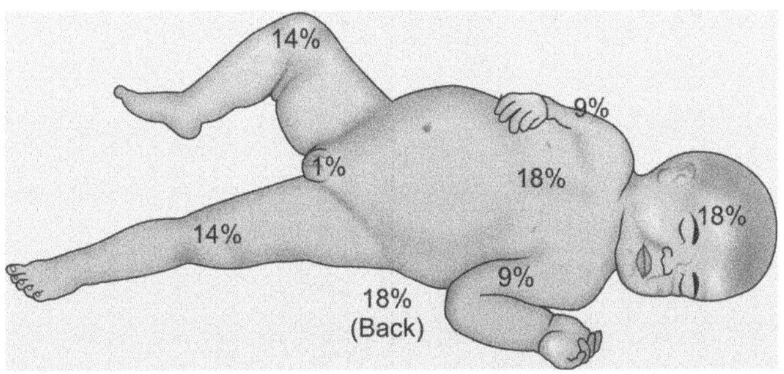

Fig. 6.7: Lund-Browder chart for TBSA estimation in children

1 percent (Fig. 6.6). The rule of nines is fairly accurate for adults but does not allow for differences in proportion in children, for whom Lund-Browder chart is used.

Lund-Browder charts that adjust TBSA percentages according to the child's age (Fig. 6.7). Adjustment is needed because different areas of the body in a child grow at different rate and therefore the TBSA of the head-neck is larger than those of the lower limbs.

Alternatively, one may also use the rule of sevens in case of children. Unlike an adult nine, in a child the unit is 7 percent, body segments are assigned percentage of surface area in multiples of seven and his proportionally larger head makes up 28 percent (Fig. 6.8).

Findings of the clinician can be arranged in an composite burn diagram based on Berkow formula (Fig. 6.9). Such diagram incorporates the depth, the body surface area and the position of the burn in a single chart, providing a much more holistic picture of extent of burn damage.

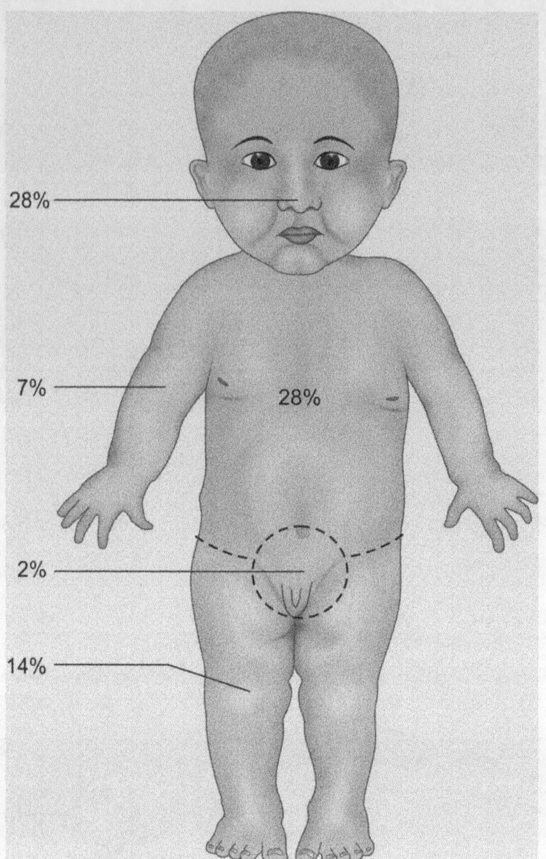

Fig. 6.8: Rule-of-seven—the head 28%, each arm 7%, trunk front and back 28%, each lower limb 14% and the perineum 2%

The area of a burn determines the volume of fluid lost and the volume of fluid that must be given to a patient in the first few hours to replace it and prevent shock. The depth of the burn determines how it should be treated, and especially, if it needs a skin graft. Its position determines how the patient should be nursed and especially to prevent contractures. Between them the area, depth, and position of a patient's burn determine what will be the final outcome.

As a general rule an adult with more than 20 percent of the burn surface area involvement, or a child with more than 10 percent of the body surface area involvement will require intravenous fluid replacement. However, an intravenous line may be necessary to achieve adequate analgesia for much smaller burn and in children fluid replacement may be required because of vomiting.

The prognosis depends upon the percentage of body surface area burned. A thumb rule is that, if the age and percentage of burned is added together and the score of 100 or above than the burn is likely to be fatal.

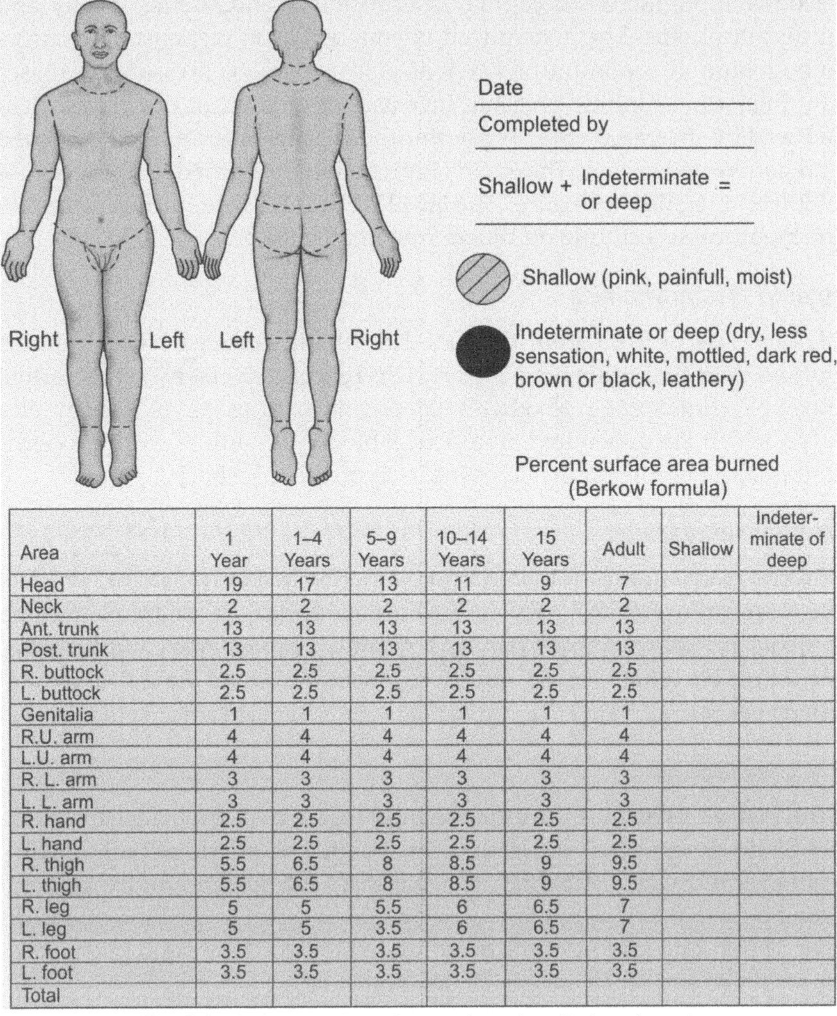

Area	1 Year	1–4 Years	5–9 Years	10–14 Years	15 Years	Adult	Shallow	Indeter-minate of deep
Head	19	17	13	11	9	7		
Neck	2	2	2	2	2	2		
Ant. trunk	13	13	13	13	13	13		
Post. trunk	13	13	13	13	13	13		
R. buttock	2.5	2.5	2.5	2.5	2.5	2.5		
L. buttock	2.5	2.5	2.5	2.5	2.5	2.5		
Genitalia	1	1	1	1	1	1		
R.U. arm	4	4	4	4	4	4		
L.U. arm	4	4	4	4	4	4		
R. L. arm	3	3	3	3	3	3		
L. L. arm	3	3	3	3	3	3		
R. hand	2.5	2.5	2.5	2.5	2.5	2.5		
L. hand	2.5	2.5	2.5	2.5	2.5	2.5		
R. thigh	5.5	6.5	8	8.5	9	9.5		
L. thigh	5.5	6.5	8	8.5	9	9.5		
R. leg	5	5	5.5	6	6.5	7		
L. leg	5	5	3.5	6	6.5	7		
R. foot	3.5	3.5	3.5	3.5	3.5	3.5		
L. foot	3.5	3.5	3.5	3.5	3.5	3.5		
Total								

Fig. 6.9: Composite burn diagram based on Berkow formula

Pathophysiology of Burn

Following systemic changes takes place in the human body following a burn injury:

- Inflammation and edema
- Altered hemodynamics
- Immunosuppression
- Hypermetabolism
- Decreased renal flow
- Increased gut mucosal permeability.

Inflammation and Edema

Burn injury causes massive release of inflammatory mediators which produce first vasoconstriction of the skin capillaries followed by rebound vasodilatation, increased capillary permeability and edema, locally and in distant organs. The generalized edema occurs in response to changes in both burned and unburned skin as plasma osmotic pressure decreases and interstitial osmotic pressure increases as a result of the protein loss induced by increased capillary permeability, edema forms in the burned and nonburned tissues. The edema is greater in the burned tissues because of lower interstitial pressure. The swelling in the tissue further compress the blood vessels cutting off blood flow in the tissues.

Altered Hemodynamics

Massive loss of fluid from the blood results in reduced blood volume, putting excessive strain on the heart. This reflects adversely on the normal metabolic functioning of other vital organs such as lungs, kidney and lever, which are dependent on a critical blood pressure to work properly. In this situation the patient goes into a hypovolemic shock.

Immunosuppression

There is global depression of immune function in a burn patient, which is the reason allograft skin survives on burn wounds for a long time. Burned patients are thus at a great risk for a number of infectious complications, including bacterial wound infection, pneumonia and fungal and viral infections.

Hypermetabolism

Burn injury sets off massive inflammatory reactions due to which the metabolic rate shoots up as the body tries to fight the effects of pain, inflammation and tissue destruction. This increases the demand for oxygen and blood flow to the tissues, with associated increase in respiration and heart rate. The energy reserve of the body is depleted at a very rapid rate to keep up with this suddenly increased metabolic rate.

Renal System

Renal system dysfunction is caused by diminished blood volume and cardiac output, resulting in decreased renal blood flow and glomerular filtration rate. Other stress-induced hormones and mediators such as angiotensin, aldosterone, and vasopressin further reduce renal blood flow immediately after the injury. This result in oliguria, which if left untreated will cause acute tubular necrosis and renal failure. Early fluid replenishment therapy decreases chances of renal failure and improves the associated mortality rate.

Gastrointestinal System

Gastrointestinal system dysfunction is highlighted by mucosal atrophy, changes in digestive absorption and increased intestinal permeability.

Infection and Septicemia

Loss of skin cover, even if partial, can lead to infections because of damage to the skin's protective barrier. Ideally small, shallow burns may need only to be kept clean and to have an antibiotic cream applied for it to heal. However, onset of secondary infection, even in a superficial shallow burn may lead to down gradation of the wound. Infected burn wounds end up with deep and extensive skin loss which may aggravate.

In addition, damaged skin and other body tissues serve as excellent culture media for infective organisms. The wound is easily infected because the skin can no longer act as a barrier against invading micro-organisms. This massive invasion of pathogens into the body overwhelms the immune system and the patient may develop septicemia.

Principles Medical Management of Burns

Ideally the treatment of a burn injury should commence at the site of the incident. Earlier the intervention the better will be the outcome. Paramedics who respond to such emergencies must have adequate training to undertake basic treatment procedures. This in the long-term will minimize complications and hasten recovery.

Hospital Treatment of Burn Injury

Hospitalization is often necessary for optimal care of moderate to severe burns. This is particularly essential in situations where the patient has sustained a massive assault to his physiology due to the burn injury and needs intensive medical care to cope with it. For example, transfusing blood, plasma and fluids through intravenous route, monitoring the vital signs like BP, ECG and prevention of secondary infections, etc. can be achieved under specialized care in a hospital setting only. Elevating and compression splinting a severely burned arm or leg above the level of the heart to prevent swelling is more easily accommodated in a hospital. In addition, burns can prevent people from carrying out essential daily functions (ADL), such as selfcare, toilet, dressing or eating, which make hospitalization a necessary and sensible step. Severe burns such as deep second-and third-degree burns involving more than 30 percent TBSA in an adult or more than 10 percent TBSA in the very young or the very old individuals, and burns involving the hands, feet, face, or genitals are usually best treated at burn centers. Burn centers are hospitals that are specially equipped and staffed to care for burn victims. Figure 6.10 shows a schematic representation of the level of support a patient with severe burn needs in a hospital setting.

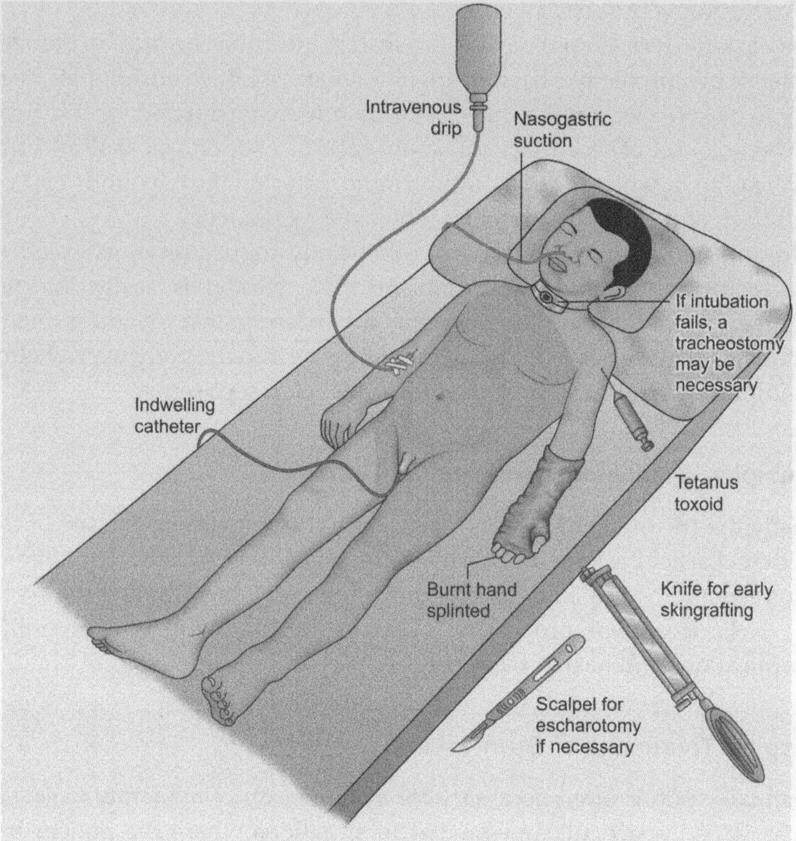

Fig. 6.10: While treating a severely burnt patient following are essential: (1) An Intravenous drip for early and rapid transfusion of fluids, colloids and blood; (2) A catheter for monitoring his urine output; (3) Knives for early escharotomy or skin grafting; (4) Nasogastric tube for gastric lavage; (5) Endotrachial intubation or tracheostomy for bronchial toilet and providing patent airway

Criteria for Hospitalization: Points to Ponder

The criteria for hospital transfer recommended by American Burn Association are as follows:

- Second- or third-degree burns greater than 10 percent total body surface area (TBSA) in patients younger than 10 years or older than 50 years
- Second- or third-degree burns greater than 20 percent TBSA in persons of other age groups
- Second- or third-degree burns that involve the face, hands, feet, genitalia, perineum, or major joints
- Third degree burns greater than five percent TBSA in persons of any age group

- Electrical burns, including lightening injury
- Chemical burns
- Inhalational injury
- Burn injury in patients with pre-existing medical disorders IHD, renal failure, diabetes mellitus, etc. that could complicate management, prolong recovery, or affect mortality
- Any burn patient with associated injury, e.g. fracture or head injury, in which the burn injury poses the greatest risk of mortality. In such cases, if the trauma poses the greater immediate risk, the patient may be treated initially in a trauma center until stable before being transferred to a burn center.
- As a general rule an adult with more than 20 percent of the burn surface area involvement, or a child with more than 10 percent of the body surface area involvement will require intravenous fluid replacement. However, an intravenous line may be necessary to achieve adequate analgesia for much smaller burn and in children fluid replacement may be required because of vomiting.
- The prognosis depends upon the percentage of body surface area burned. A rough guide is that, if the age and percentage of burned is added together and the score of 100 or above than the burn is likely to be fatal.

Resuscitation: Points to Ponder

- Resuscitation depends on establishment and maintenance of reliable IV access.
- Delays must be minimized.
- Venous access is best attained through short peripheral catheters in unburned skin.
- Veins in burned skin can be used and are preferable to no IV access.
- Superficial veins are often thrombosed in full-thickness injuries and are therefore not suitable for inserting IV cannula.
- Saphenous vein cut-down is useful in patients with difficult access and is used in preference to central vein IV cannula because of lower complication rates.

Fluid Replacement Therapy

Intravenous infusion of Colloidal isotonic solution @ 4 ml/kg per percent TBSA burn total fluid = 4 × body wt × TBSA ½ of which is given in first 8 hours from the point of injury

Next half is given in the next 16 hours (According to Brooks formula).

Escharotomy[1]

When deep second and third-degree burn wounds encompass the circumference of an extremity, peripheral circulation to the limb can be

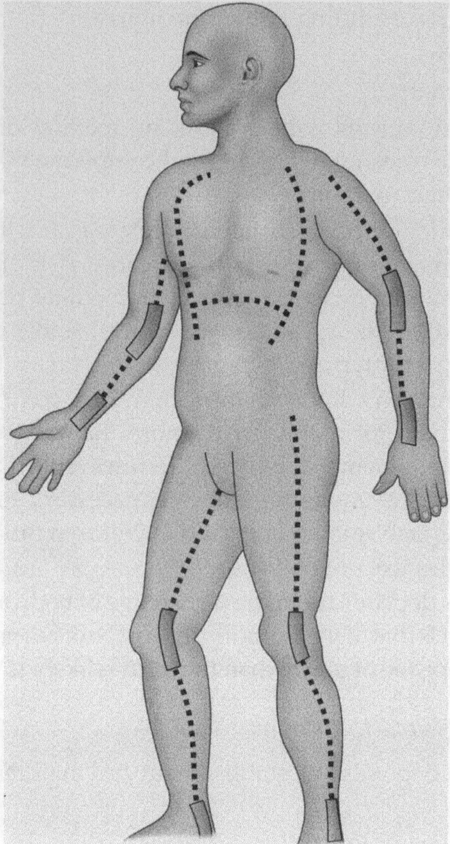

Fig. 6.11: Common sites for escharotomy

compromised by hard, unyielding layer of dead dermis and subcutaneous tissue, called the eschar. Eschar impedes venous outflow and eventually affects arterial inflow to the distal beds. Eschar complication is recognized by numbness and tingling in the limb and increased pain in the digits. Such patients require escharotomy, which consist of release of the eschar at the bedside by incising the lateral and medial aspects of the extremity with a scalpel (Fig. 6.11).

Smoke Inhalation Injury

It is one of the major factor contributing to death in burn injury patients. Smoke damage adds another inflammatory focus to the burn and impedes the normal gas exchange vital for critically-injured patients. Airway injury is principally chemical in nature, except in high-pressure steam inhalation, which has 4000 times the heat-carrying capacity of dry air. Direct thermal damage to the lung is seldom seen because of dispersal of the heat in the pharynx. The response to smoke inhalation is an immediate dramatic increase in blood flow in the bronchial arteries to the bronchi along with edema formation and increases in lung lymph flow.

Hallmark features of inhalation injury are:

- Separation of ciliated epithelial cells from the basement membrane, followed by the formation of exudates within the airways.
- Exudates coalesces to form fibrin plugs.
- Fibrin plugs are hard and sticky and can be difficult to clear with standard airway suction techniques. Bronchoscope removal could therefore be required.
- Fibrin plugs add to air pressure injury to localized areas of lung by producing a ball-valve effect thereby preventing the inhaled air from escaping.
- Increasing residual volume leads to localized increases in intrapulmonary pressure causing complications such as pneumothorax and decreased lung compliance.

The clinical course of patients with inhalation injury is divided into three stages.

1. The first is acute pulmonary insufficiency. Patients with severe lung injury may begin to show signs of pulmonary failure from the time of injury, such as asphyxia, carbon monoxide poisoning, bronchospasm, and upper airway obstruction. Clinical signs of parenchymal damage with hypoxia are not common during this phase.
2. The second stage occurs 72 to 96 hours after injury associated with hypoxia and the development of diffuse lobar infiltrates. Clinically similar to the adult respiratory distress syndrome (ARDS) that occurs in nonburned injured and critically-ill patients.
3. In the third stage, clinical bronchopneumonia dominates. These infections generally occur 3 to 10 days after inhalation injury and are associated with the expectoration of large mucous casts formed in the tracheobronchial tree. Early pneumonia usually caused by penicillin-resistant Staphylococcus species, whereas after five to seven days, the changing flora of the burn wound is reflected in the appearance of gram-negative species in the lung, especially Pseudomonas. Ball-valve effects and ventilator-associated barotrauma are also hallmarks of this period.

Management of Inhalation Injury: Points to Ponder

- Management of inhalation injury is directed at maintaining open airways and maximizing gas exchange while the lung heals.
- A coughing patient with a patent airway can clear secretions effectively, and effort is made to manage patients without mechanical ventilation if possible.
- If respiratory failure is imminent, endotrachial intubation is done, followed by frequent vibration, percussion and suctioning to remove secretions.
- Frequent bronchoscopy may be needed to clear mucus-fibrin plugs.

- Mechanical ventilation is used to provide gas exchange with as little air pressure damage (barotrauma) as possible.
- Permissive hypercapnia and the current ARDS Network ventilation protocols can be used lower ventilatory rates and volumes to maintain arterial pH at greater than 7.25.
- This minimizes positive airway pressure delivered by the ventilator.
- Ventilator volumes and rate are decreased in a graduated manner until the patient can be extubated.
- This process may take several weeks.

Inhalation Treatments

Inhalation treatments are effective in improving the clearance of tracheobronchial secretions and decreasing bronchospasm.

Intravenous infusion of heparin has been shown to reduce tracheobronchial mucofibrin cast formation, improve minute ventilation, and optimize peak inspiratory pressure after smoke inhalation.

Heparin may also be administered directly to the lungs in a nebulized form to dissolve mucofibrin plugs without causing reduced systemic coagulation. N-acetyl cysteine treatments are added to nebulized heparin in burned children with inhalation injury, reintubation rates and mortality rates are decreased. Adequate humidification plus treatment of bronchospasm with β-agonists is also indicated.

Steroids have not been shown to be of benefit in inhalation injury and are not given unless the patient was steroid dependent before the injury or had bronchospasm resistant to standard therapy.

Novel Ventilator Therapies

Novel ventilator therapies devised to minimize barotraumas include high-frequency percussive ventilation. This method combines standard tidal volumes and respirations (ventilator rates of 6–20/min) with smaller high-frequency oscillations (200–500/min). This permits adequate ventilation and oxygenation in patients who have failed conventional ventilation and recruits more alveoli at lower airway pressure. This ventilator method may also have a percussive effect that loosens secretions and improves pulmonary toilet. In the absence of advanced equipments suitable for novel ventilation, therapists may use a heavy duty large cup vibrator to apply vibrations at desired frequencies over the chest wall during slandered mechanical positive pressure ventilation.

PHASE 2

Acute Care of Burn Wound[1]

Management: Initial copious irrigation with clean water, the burned area is treated immediately with copious 2.5 percent calcium gluconate gel.

These wounds are generally extremely painful. Intradermal injection of 10 percent calcium gluconate/intra-arterial injection of calcium gluconate into the affected extremity, or both may be required to alleviate symptoms. If after the airway is assessed and resuscitation is under way, attention must be turned to the burn wound. Treatment depends on the characteristics and size of the wound. All treatments are aimed at rapid and painless healing. Current therapy directed specifically toward burn wounds can be divided into three stages: Assessment, management rehabilitation.

Points to Ponder

Each wound is dressed with an appropriate covering that serves several functions.

- First, it protects the damaged epithelium, minimizes bacterial and fungal colonization, and provides splinting action to maintain the desired position of function.
- Second, the dressing is occlusive to reduce evaporative heat loss and minimize cold stress.
- Third, the dressing needs to provide comfort over the painful wound.

Choice of Dressing

Initial dressing is aimed at holding bacterial proliferation in check and providing occlusion until surgery is performed

- First degree burns require no dressing and are treated with topical salves to decrease pain and keep the skin moist.
- Second degree wounds can be treated with daily dressing changes and topical antibiotics, cotton gauze, and elastic wraps.
- Alternatively, the wounds can be treated with a temporary biologic or synthetic covering to close the wound.
- Deep second degree and third degree wounds require excision of dead tissue-eschar and skin grafting for sizable burns.

Antibiotic Creams or Gels

- Antibiotic topical agents with cream or gel base are used for burn dressing because these are water-soluble and therefore easily absorbed by the wound surface.
- Silversulfadiazine (Silverex)—a broad-spectrum antibiotic, painless and easy to use; does not penetrate eschar; may leave black tattoos from silver ion; mildly inhibits growth of new skin cover on the raw area (Re-epithelialization).
- Mafenide acetate (Sulfamylon)—a broad-spectrum antibiotic, penetrates eschar; may cause pain in sensitive skin of the nomans land area on the periphery of the burn; wide application may cause metabolic acidosis; mildly inhibits growth of new skin cover on the raw area (Re-epithelialization).

- Neomycin—ease of application; painless; antibiotic spectrum not as wide.
- Nystatin (Mycostatin)—effective in inhibiting most fungal growth; cannot be used in combination with mafenide acetate.
- Mupirocin (Bactroban)—more effective staphylococcal coverage; does not inhibit growth of new skin; expensive.
- In noninfected raw wound with fresh granulation, sterile vaseline gauze impregnated with gentamycine (Gentamycine Tulle) is used as a primary cover. The oily layer prevents the dressing from sticking to the delicate granulation tissue. This minimizes bleeding and destruction of the granulation during dressing changes.
- Combined gel of metrogyle (antibiotic) and sucral (granulation stimulator) may also be used for healing wounds to promote rapid granulation under antibiotic cover.

Alternative Treatment

Review of previous medical research has shown that honey can be an effective treatment for superficial and partial-thickness burns. Honey used in the treatment of superficial and partial thickness burns produces significantly more healing at 15 and 21 days than alternative dressing treatments. In most studies unprocessed honey covered by sterile gauze was compared with silver sulphadiazine-impregnated gauze. Honey has been shown to have antibacterial properties due to the presence of hydrogen peroxide which is released by the action of peroxidase, an enzyme that is added by bees to the nectar they collect. But some honey, such as some of New Zealand's manuka-based harvest, also contains additional bactericidal agents such as bioflavinoids from the flowers. Some biologically active manuka honey has been shown to have significant antibacterial activity against a few antibiotic-resistant "super bugs". Honey can also form a physical barrier on a wound, preventing bacterial penetration, and providing a moist healing environment, while preventing newly formed tissue from tearing when the dressing is removed.

Synthetic Coverings: Points to Ponder[1]

- *Op-Site:* Provides a moisture barrier, inexpensive, decreases wound pain, use complicated by accumulation of transudate and exudate requiring removal. Has no antibiotic properties.
- *Biobrane:* Provides a wound barrier associated with decreased pain. Its use is complicated by accumulation of exudates, risking invasive wound infection, has no antibiotic properties.
- *Transcyte:* Provides a wound barrier associated with decreased pain and accelerated wound healing. Its use complicated by accumulation of exudates, has no antibiotic properties.

- *Integra:* Provides complete wound closure. The integra dressing is a porous matrix of cross-linked bovine tendon collagen, glycosaminoglycan and a layer of silicone. Integra is made for onetime use, is indicated for a variety of wounds, including partial-and full-thickness wounds; pressure, venous, surgical, diabetic and chronic vascular ulcers; and surgical and trauma wounds. Integra a study cites 158 ulcers in which 92 percent of 107 patients achieved complete healing either with integra alone or with small subsidiary flaps.

Biologic Coverings[1]

Excision and grafting: Early excision of eschar followed by grafting is currently done by most burn surgeons. Attempts are made to excise tangentially to optimize cosmetic outcome. Rarely, excision to the level of fascia is required to remove all nonviable tissue, or it may become necessary at subsequent operations due to infectious complications.

- Autograft uses skin and tissue harvested from the patients own body to cover open wounds or reconstruct body surface. Such grafts may consist of:
  - *Split skin grafts*: Consisting of the upper layers of the epidermis, this graft is useful only as a temporary cover for the raw area following second degree burn. It protects the delicate cells of the surviving stratum germinativum, which is expected to grow new skin. This graft needs no blood supply since it consists of only dead cells. It is held in position with pressure bandage and usually sloughs off after 3 weeks. Routine mobilizing exercises and splinting can be done but no heat/cold/friction modality to be applied over the grafted area.
  - *Partial thickness grafts*: Consisting of the whole of epidermis and the upper layers of the dermis is harvested from anterior abdominal wall or thigh to cover the raw area not larger than 30 cm sq, following deep second degree of third burn. This graft may be a permanent cover for the raw area where the skin is not expected to grow back. Blood supply to the graft grows from the underlying subcutaneous layer; hence it must not be disturbed for at least 4 weeks. The graft is held in position with pressure bandage. Routine mobilizing exercises and splinting can be done after 4 weeks but no heat / cold / friction modality to be applied over the grafted area.
  - *Full thickness graft*: Consisting of the whole of the epidermis, dermis and part of the subcutaneous layer of collagen and fat including capillary network and nerve endings is harvested from anterior abdominal wall or thigh to cover the raw area not larger than 10 cm sq, following deep second degree of third burn. This graft is used as a permanent cover for the raw area after escharectomy. Blood supply to the graft grows into the underlying subcutaneous layer; hence it must not be disturbed for at least 6 weeks. The graft is held in position

with sutures applied to the edges of the wound. Routine mobilizing exercises and splinting can be done after 6 weeks but no heat/cold/ friction modality to be applied over the grafted area.

- *Pedicle grafts*: Consisting of the whole of the epidermis, dermis, subcutaneous layer and underlying soft tissue including subcutaneous layer of collagen and fat including capillary network and nerve endings is harvested in the form of a tube from anterior abdominal wall to reconstruct lost segment such as nose, ear, hands, feet, etc. following third or fourth degree burn. Blood supply to the graft grows into the underlying subcutaneous layer from either ends of the tube; hence it must not be disturbed for at least 6–8 weeks. The graft is held in position with sutures applied to the edges of the wound at either end of the tube. The tube or pedicle is transferred after maturity, in stages from the donor site to the recipient site. Routine mobilizing exercises and splinting can be done after 6 weeks but no heat/cold/friction modality to be applied over the grafted area. Some body segments may become stiff due to awkward positioning during stage-wise transfer, because the tube along with the attached segment has to be immobilized for at least 6 weeks in one position. The therapist must mobilize such segments as soon as the pedicle has been transferred.

- Xenograft (pig skin) consisting of the whole thickness of pig skin, used to completely close the wound, provides some immunologic benefits; must be removed or allowed to slough.
- Allograft (homograft, cadaver skin) consisting of the whole thickness of living donor/cadaver skin provides all the normal functions of skin, can be used as a dermal equivalent over short term to allow the wound to heal; epithelium must be removed or allowed to slough.

Steps for Minimizing Complications of Burn: Points to Ponder

- Early excision of dead tissue.
- Early, aggressive fluid resuscitation regimens to prevent multiorgan failure.
- An aggressive surgical approach to cover deep wounds.
- Topical and systemic antibiotic therapy to minimize infection.
- Vigilantly anticipating and aggressively treating pneumonia, which is a major cause of death in burned patients.
- Tight blood sugar control reduces stress-induced diabetes, common in burn patients.
- Early oral feeding prevents failure of the gut barrier and reduces chances of septic morbidity due to entry of bacteria from GI tract into the bloodstream.
- Renal failure may occur 2 to 14 days after resuscitation. It is indicated by progressively decreasing urine output; fluid overload, electrolyte

imbalance, elevated urea and creatinine levels. Urine output greater than 1 ml/kg/hr indicates adequate renal perfusion. If not, some form of dialysis may be necessary. Peritoneal dialysis is effective but occasionally hemodialysis is required.

- Respiratory failure is indicated by drop in oxygen saturation of the blood. This is best monitored by continuous oximetry and a decrease in saturation to less than 92 percent is indicative of respiratory failure requiring intubation. Many burned patients require mechanical ventilation to protect the airway in the initial phases of their injury. The goal is extubation as soon as possible to allow patients to clear their own airways. They can perform their own pulmonary toilet better compared to suction through an endotracheal tube or tracheostomy.
- Hepatic failure is a challenging problem in burn without many solutions. Protein concentrations of the coagulation cascade decrease to critical levels and the patient becomes coagulopathic. Toxins are not cleared from the bloodstream and concentrations of bilirubin increase. Treatment is directed at replacement of factors II, VII, IX, and X until the liver recovers. Albumin replacement may also be required.
- Hematologic failure in burned patients may develop into bleeding disorder (coagulopathic) through two mechanisms:
  - Depletion and impaired synthesis of coagulation factors associated with sepsis, common with associated head injury. With breakdown of the blood-brain barrier, brain lipids are exposed to plasma, which activates the coagulation cascade. Treatment of disseminated intravascular coagulation includes infusion of fresh frozen plasma and monitoring the concentration of fibrinogen.
  - Thrombocytopenia is frequent in severe burns as a result of depletion of platelets during excision of the burn wound. Platelet counts lower than 50,000 are common and do not require treatment. Only when the bleeding is diffuse and is noted to occur from IV sites should administration of donor platelets be considered.
- Central nervous system failure is indicated by progressive drowsiness. Worsening of LOC in a severely burned patient, not related to any sedatives, may be due to a infection. Treatment is supportive and symptomatic.

Nutrition in Burn Injury

The rate of metabolism shoots up dramatically after a severe burn. Rapid metabolism increases oxygen consumption, urinary nitrogen excretion and lipolysis (fat breakdown). The weight loss is directly proportional to the size of the burn. As the metabolic rate is so high, energy requirements are immense. Requirements are met by mobilization of carbohydrate, fat, and protein stores. Results loss of active muscle tissue and malnutrition ensue. This malnutrition is associated with functional impairment of many organs, delayed and abnormal wound healing, decreased immunocompetence altered active transport functions of the cellular membrane.[2]

Nutritional Support

Malnutrition in patients with burns can be controlled to some extent by the delivery of adequate exogenous nutritional support. The goals of nutritional support are to maintain and improve organ function and prevent protein-calorie malnutrition.

Calorie Requirement

According to "Curreri formula" calorie requirement of a burn patient is approximately 25 kcal/kg/day, plus 40 kcal per percent TBSA burned per day.[2]

Dietary Composition

Optimal dietary composition contains 1 to 2 g/kg/day of protein, which provides a calorie-to-nitrogen ratio of around 100:1 provides for the cell building needs of the patient, thus to some extent sparing the proteolysis occurring in active muscle tissue.

Nonprotein calories can be given either as carbohydrate or as fat. Carbohydrates have the advantage of stimulating endogenous insulin production, which may have beneficial effects on muscle and burn wounds as an anabolic hormone.

The diet may be delivered in two forms:

1. Either orally through Ryle's tube or
2. Parenterally through IV catheters.

Total parenteral nutrition causes increased complications and mortality. Total parenteral nutrition is reserved only for patients who cannot tolerate oral feeding. Oral feeding, however, may cause some complications that can be disastrous, such as aspiration, vomiting, and diarrhea.

Psychosocial Aspects of Burn Injury

Many of the burn treatments are directed at improving functional, psychological, and work outcomes. Though most severely burned adult patients adjust relatively well, clinically significant psychological disturbances develop in some patients, specifically somatization and phobic anxiety. Children with severe burns have similar somatization problems, as well as sleep disturbances. Major burn injuries can lead to significant disturbances in psychiatric health of the victim, such as morbid depression, denial, fear of rejection and anxiety.

Special Burn Injuries

Electrical Injuries

1. Low-voltage injury is similar to thermal burns without transmission to deeper tissues. Household voltage causes only local damage. The worst of these injuries are those involving the edge of the mouth (oral commissure), which are sustained when children chew on household electrical cords.
2. High-voltage injury consists of varying degrees of cutaneous burn at the entry and exit sites, combined with hidden destruction of deep tissue. It may have cutaneous burns associated with ignition of clothing from the electrical spark. Initial evaluation consists of cardiopulmonary resuscitation if ventricular fibrillation is induced. If the initial ECG findings are abnormal or there is a history of IHD or cardiac arrest before the injury, continued cardiac monitoring is necessary along with pharmacologic treatment of any arrhythmias.
3. Other injuries occurs being thrown by the electrical jolt falling from heights after disengaging from the electrical current. Violent tetanic muscular contractions that result from alternating current (AC) sources may cause a variety of fractures and dislocations. These patients are assessed as any other patient with blunt traumatic injuries.

Treatment of electrical burn: The most significant injury in electrical burn is within the deep tissue, and subsequent edema formation can cause vascular compromise in any area distal to the injury. Evaluation of the circulation to distal vascular beds is essential because immediate escharotomy and fasciotomy may be required and early amputation may be necessary.

Chemical Burns

Chemical burns are caused by the corrosive effect of strong alkali, acids and hydrocarbons on the skin and the body systems other than the skin.

Alkali burns: Alkali such as lime, potassium hydroxide, bleach, and sodium hydroxide cause burn. Three factors are involved in the mechanism of alkali burns:

1. Saponification (soap formation) of fat causes loss of the insulation of heat formed in the chemical reaction with tissue.
2. Massive extraction of water from cells causes damage because of the hygroscopic nature of alkali.
3. Alkalis dissolve and unite with the proteins of tissues to form alkaline proteinates, which are soluble and contain hydroxide ions (these ions induce further chemical reactions that penetrate deeper into the tissue).

Acid burns: Acid burns are treated initially like any other chemical injury: removal of all chemicals by disrobing the affected area and copious irrigation. Acids induce protein breakdown by hydrolysis, which results in a hard eschar that does not penetrate as deeply as alkalis do. Acids also induce thermal injury by generation of heat after contact with skin, thus causing additional burn is not treated in such a fashion, decalcification of the bone underlying the injury and extension of the soft tissue injury may occur.

Treatment of alkali/acid burn begins with immediate removal of the causative agent by washing in large volumes of fluid, usually tap water. Attempts to neutralize alkali agents with weak acids are not recommended because the heat released by neutralization reactions induces further injury. Particularly strong alkali are treated by lavage and consideration of the addition of wound debridement in the operating room. Tangential removal of affected areas is performed until the tissues removed are at normal pH.

Hydrocarbons

Hydrocarbons such as petroleum products promote cell membrane dissolution and skin necrosis. Erythema and blistering seen in hydrocarbon exposure on naked skin are typically superficial and heal spontaneously in most cases. If absorbed systemically, hydrocarbon toxicity can produce respiratory depression and eventual hepatic failure. Ignition of hydrocarbons on the skin produces flash or flame burn which induces a deep full-thickness injury to the skin. Any such burn above 10 percent TBSA must be treated as a medical emergency.

PHASE 3

Surgical Management of Burn[1]

Surgical reconstruction of burn injury should commence as early as possible. Acute burn surgery is the treatment of choice immediately after a burn. It is done to remove dead or devitalized skin layers through tangential or circumferential excision, as in case of escharotomy. Reconstructive burn surgery takes place after the burn wounds have healed and is generally done in two or more phases.

A surgical team that specializes in burn treatment and skin grafts performs the necessary procedures. The team may include plastic surgeon and dermatologists, as well as, nurses, nutritionist, psychiatrists, physiotherapists and occupational therapists. On call specialists such as orthopedic surgeon, neurosurgeon, cardiologists, nephrologists and internal medicine specialists are also needed to provide necessary backup to the burn team in case of complications and to manage associated injuries.

Rationale Behind Skin Graft

Skin is the largest organ in the body. In itself the skin works as an independent organ system—the integumentary system. Skin provides an outer envelope for the inner organs, primarily for protection from the environment and secondly to preserve body fluids, electrolyte and nutrients from escaping from the body. It also plays an important role in thermoregulation and excretion of wastes from the body. When skin is damaged or lost due to severe injury or burns, bacteria and other micro-organisms have easy access to warm, nutrient-rich body fluids. Loss of these vital fluids can lead to shock. Also known as hypovolemic shock, it can occur when the blood pressure in a person's arteries is too low to maintain an adequate supply of blood to organs and tissues. To treat a severe burn, surgeons first remove the burned skin and then quickly cover the underlying tissue, usually with a combination of SSG, laboratory-grown skin cells and artificial skin.

What is a Skin Graft?

A skin graft is a piece of unburned skin which is surgically removed from an unaffected area to cover a burned raw area. Skin grafting is sometimes done as part of elective plastic surgery procedures, but it is most extensively used in the treatment of burns. For first or superficial second-degree burns, skin grafting is generally not required, as these burns usually heal with little or no scarring. With deep second degree and third-degree burns, however, the skin is destroyed to its near total or full depth, in addition to damage done to underlying tissues. People who suffer such burns often require skin grafting.

Wounds such as deep second degree or third degree burns must be covered as quickly as possible to prevent infection or loss of fluid. Wounds that are left to heal on their own can contract, often resulting in serious scarring; if the wound is large enough, the scar can actually prevent movement of limbs. Nonhealing wounds, such as diabetic ulcers, venous ulcers, or pressure sores, can also be treated with skin grafts to prevent infection and further progression of the wounded area.

Types of Skin Grafts

The term "skin graft" by itself commonly refers to either an allograft or an autograft or a xenograft.

- An autograft is a type of graft that uses skin from another area of the patient's own body if there is enough undamaged skin available, and if the patient is healthy enough to undergo the additional surgery required.
- An allograft uses skin obtained from another human being, Donor skin from cadavers is frozen, stored, and made available for use as allograft.

- A xenograft is the skin taken from an animal (usually a pig) and is so called because it comes from a nonhuman species.

Allograft and xenograft provide only temporary covering because they are rejected by the patient's immune system within seven days. They must then be replaced with an autograft.

Techniques and Procedures of Skin Grafting

Preparation of the Recipient Site

The most important part of any skin graft procedure is proper preparation of the wound. Skin grafts will not survive on tissue with a limited blood supply (cartilage or tendons) or on tissue that has been damaged by radiation treatment. The patient's wound must be free of any dead tissue, foreign matter, or bacterial contamination. After the patient has been anesthetized, the surgeon prepares the wound by rinsing it with saline solution or a diluted antiseptic (betadine) and removes any dead tissue by tangential debridement. In addition, the surgeon stops the flow of blood into the wound by applying pressure, tying off blood vessels, or administering a medication (epinephrine) that causes the blood vessels to constrict. Following preparation of the wound, the surgeon then harvests the tissue for grafting from the donor site.

Procedure for Harvesting

The area where the piece of unburned skin was taken from, to be donated to a burned area, is called a donor site. After a skin graft procedure the donor sites look like a scraped or a skinned knee. The surgeon will need to decide if a split skin graft is needed to cover the donor site, depending on the depth of the skin layer harvested. The raw donor area is covered with a sterile nonadherent dressing for 5–7 days to protect it from infection. The donor area heals on its own within 2–3 weeks. Moisturizing lotion is applied to the donor site after the dressing comes off because this skin often flakes off and looks dry.

The most common donor sites to harvest skin grafts are the buttocks and inner thigh, areas which are usually hidden and therefore cosmetically less important. The graft is carefully spread on the recipient raw area to be covered. It is held in place either by gentle pressure from a well-padded dressing or by a few hidden sutures (Fig. 6.12).

Categories of Skin Graft

A split-thickness skin graft involves the epidermis and a little of the underlying dermis; the donor site usually heals within several days. The surgeon first marks the outline of the wound on the skin of the donor site, enlarging it by 3–5 percent to allow for tissue shrinkage. The surgeon

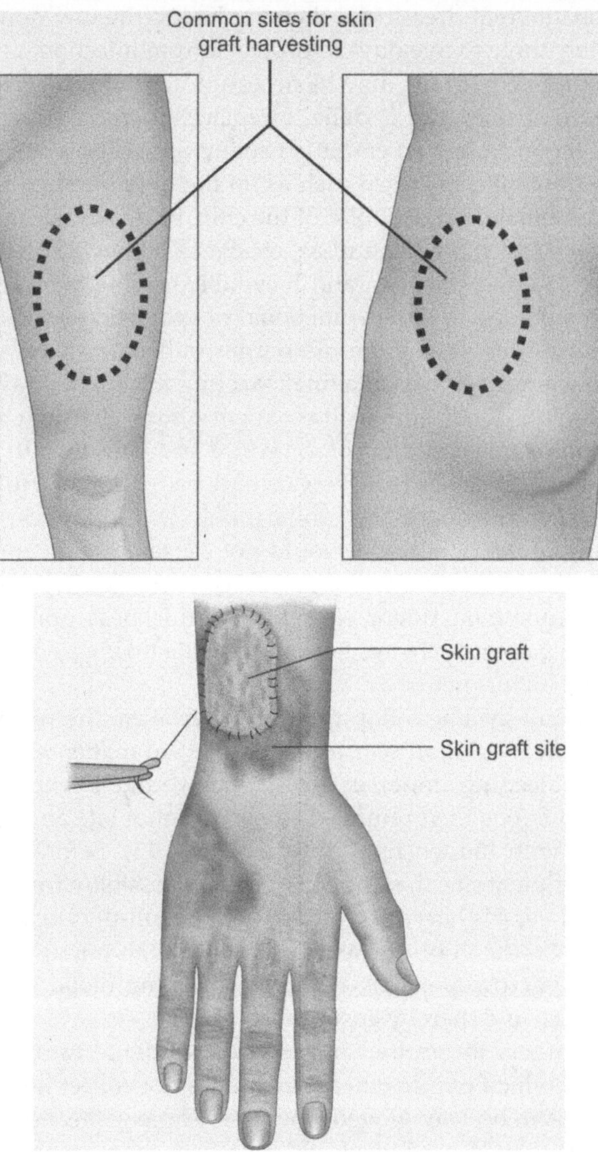

Fig. 6.12: Skin graft harvesting from donor area and being fixed on the recipient area

uses a dermatome (a special instrument for cutting thin slices of tissue) to remove a split-thickness graft from the donor site. The wound must not be too deep if a split-thickness graft is going to be successful, since the blood vessels that will nourish the grafted tissue must come from the dermis of the wound itself. The graft is usually taken from an area that is ordinarily hidden by clothes, such as the buttock or inner thigh, and spread on the bare area to be covered. Gentle pressure from a well-padded dressing is then applied, or a few small sutures used to hold the graft in place.

A sterile nonadherent dressing is then applied to the raw donor area for approximately three to five days to protect it from infection.

Full-thickness skin grafts may be necessary for more severe burn injuries. This type of skin graft is done to replace all layers of lost skin over an area not larger than 5 sq cm. It is usually opted for when a raw area persists over bony prominence such as on the dorsum of hand and feet, jaw line, submental triangle, point of the chin, bridge of the nose, orbit of the eye, cubital fossa, popliteal fossa, etc. Since no new growth of skin is expected to close the raw area and inevitable healing by scar formation is not acceptable due to either functional or cosmetic reasons or both, a full thickness of skin with epidermis, dermis, subcutaneous tissue, fat and capillary network may be used a final covering to close the raw area. The surgeon selects a donor site on the patient's body that matches closely to the skin on recipient site in color, texture and hairiness. In selecting a donor site, the surgeon has to be very careful, because after a full thickness graft being taken the donor site can heal only with thick scar formation. Such scarring of the donor site should not cause any functional impairment and is also acceptable to the patient cosmetically. The back and the abdomen are common donor sites for full-thickness grafts. However, opinion of the patient is always important while taking such critical decision. It is after all his/ her body.

Before the full-thickness flap graft is undertaken, the recipient site is meticulously cleaned of all scar tissue or infected matter with tangential excisions till bleeding undersurface of the wound is exposed. A full-thickness skin flap is then removed from the donor site and fixed on the recipient site with hidden microsutures (Fig. 6.13). Before suturing the graft on the recipient site, the surgeon makes all possible effort to reconnect delicate blood vessels harvested along with the full-thickness graft to the blood vessels on the floor of the raw area, through microsurgery under an operating microscope. This ensures continuing blood supply to the grafted skin flap and thereby ensures healing.

After the surgery the grafted area is placed under a custom made pressure garment, which ensures that edema does not collect under the graft and the graft is in no way moved from the recipient site. Special silicone pressure pads may also be used under or over the pressure garment to exert firm and accurate pressure over the graft site which in the long run help in molding the grafted skin to the desired shape of the recipient site and minimize cosmetic disfigurement.

Since these grafts involve both layers of the skin, full-thickness autografts are more complicated than partial-thickness grafts, but provide better contour, more natural color, and less contraction at the grafted site. Sometimes a flap of skin with underlying muscle and blood supply is transplanted to the area to be grafted. This procedure is used when tissue loss is extensive and deep, such as after open fractures of the lower leg,

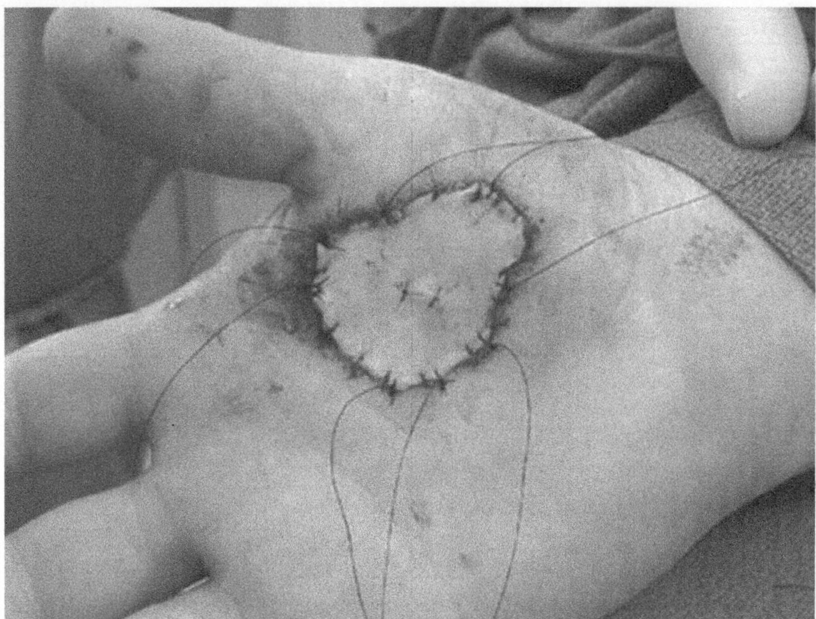

Fig. 6.13: Full thickness graft being used for reconstruction of right thumb web space

with significant skin loss and underlying infection. The main disadvantage of full-thickness skin grafts is that the wound at the donor site is larger and requires more careful management. Often, a split-thickness graft must be used to cover the donor site.

A composite skin graft is sometimes used, which consists of combinations of skin and fat, skin and cartilage, or dermis and fat.

Composite grafts are used in patients whose injuries require three-dimensional reconstruction. For example, a wedge of ear containing skin and cartilage can be used to repair the nose.

A full-thickness graft is removed from the donor site with a scalpel rather than a dermatome. After the surgeon has cut around the edges of the pattern used to determine the size of the graft, he or she lifts the skin with a special hook and trims off any fatty tissue. The graft is then placed on the wound and secured in place with absorbable sutures.

Usually, good results are expected from plastic surgery that emphasizes careful planning of incisions so that they fall in the line of natural skin folds or lines, appropriate choice of wound closure, use of best available suture materials, and early removal of exposed sutures so that the wound is held closed by buried sutures.

Care of the Grafted Skin

A pressure dressing is left on the graft site for two to five days to hold the grafted skin in place. The dressing is then changed and for next several

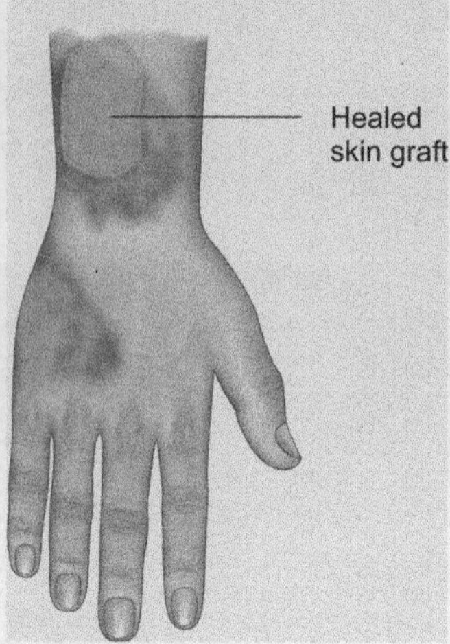

Fig. 6.14: Skin grafts, if properly cared for, heals with minimal abnormality

days the graft sites need to be kept immobilized in a plaster cast or splint and protected from rubbing or pressure. Partial thickness grafts usually heal with little scarring, and often look similar to surrounding normal skin (Fig. 6.14).

Once a skin graft has been put in place, it must be maintained carefully even after it has healed. Patients who have grafts on their legs should remain in bed for 7 to 10 days with their legs elevated. For several months, the patient should support the graft with a compression bandage or Jobst stocking. Grafts on other areas of the body should be similarly supported after healing to decrease the amount of contracture.

Grafted skin does not contain sweat or oil glands, and should be lubricated daily for two to three months with mineral oil or another bland oil to prevent drying and cracking.

Aftercare of patients with severe burns typically includes psychological or psychiatric counseling and physical rehabilitation, particularly if the patient's face and hands have been disfigured. The severe pain and lengthy period of recovery involved in burn treatment are often accompanied by anxiety and depression. If the patient's burns occurred in combat, a transportation disaster, terrorist attack, or other fire involving large numbers of people, he or she is at high-risk of developing post-traumatic stress disorder (PTSD).

Risks

The risks of skin grafting include those inherent in any surgical procedure that involves anesthesia. These include reactions to the medications, breathing problems, bleeding, and infection. In addition, the risks of an allograft procedure include transmission of an infectious disease from the donor.

The tissue for grafting and the recipient site must be as sterile as possible to prevent later infection that could result in failure of the graft. Failure of a graft can result from inadequate preparation of the wound, poor blood flow to the injured area, swelling, or infection. The most common reason for graft failure is the formation of a hematoma, or collection of blood in the injured tissues.

Usual Outcome

A skin graft should provide significant improvement in the quality of the wound site, and may prevent the serious complications associated with burns or nonhealing wounds. Normally, new blood vessels begin growing from the donor area into the transplanted skin within 36 hours. Occasionally, skin grafts are unsuccessful or do not heal well. In these cases, repeat grafting is necessary. Even though the skin graft must be protected from trauma or significant stretching for two to three weeks following split-thickness skin grafting, recovery from surgery is usually rapid. A dressing may be necessary for one to two weeks, depending on the location of the graft. Physiotherapists should be aware that exercises or activity that stretches the graft or puts it at risk for trauma should be avoided for three to four weeks. A one to two-week hospital stay is most often required in cases of full-thickness grafts, as the recovery period is longer than partial-thickness grafts.

Alternative Methods of Wound Coverage

There has been great progress in the development of artificial skin replacement products in recent years. Although nothing works as well as the patient's own skin, artificial skin products are important due to the limitation of available skin for allografting in severely burned patients. Unlike allographs and xenographs, artificial skin replacements are not rejected by the patient's body and actually encourage the generation of new tissue. Artificial skin usually consists of a synthetic epidermis and a collagen-based dermis. The artificial dermis consists of fibers arranged in a lattice that act as a template for the formation of new tissue. Fibroblasts, blood vessels, nerve fibers, and lymph vessels from surrounding healthy tissue grow into the collagen lattice, which eventually dissolves as these cells and structures build a new dermis. The synthetic epidermis, which acts as a temporary barrier during this process, is eventually replaced with a split-thickness autograft or with an epidermis cultured in the laboratory from the patient's own epithelial cells.

Several artificial skin products are available for burns or nonhealing wounds. Researchers have also obtained promising results growing or cultivating the patient's own skin cells in the laboratory. These cultured skin substitutes reduce the need for autografts and can reduce the complications of burn injuries. Laboratory cultivation of skin cells may improve the prognosis for severely burned patients with third degree burns over 50 percent of their body. The recovery of these patients has been hindered by the limited availability of uninjured skin from their own bodies for grafting. Skin substitutes may also reduce treatment costs and the length of hospital stays. In addition, other research has demonstrated the possibility of using stem cells collected from bone marrow or blood for use in growing skin grafts.

How does Artificial Skin Work?

After removing burn-damaged skin, surgeons blanket a wound with a covering like Integra, and then apply a skin graft on top of this biomaterial to encourage the growth of new skin to close the wound. Ideally, surgeons obtain skin grafts from an unburned area of skin elsewhere on the body. But when the burn is severe and covers 80 to 90 percent of a person's body surface, there is not enough skin to use for this purpose. Then only cultured skin and artificial skin cover are the only options available.

Reconstructive Surgery

Reconstructive plastic surgery is performed to correct functional or cosmetic impairments to various body caused by burns, trauma, crush fractures, congenital abnormalities, developmental anomalies, infection and cancers. Reconstructive plastic surgery is usually performed to improve function or to provide near normal appearance.

Modes of Reconstruction

Pedicle Grafts

Plastic surgeons need to harvest and transfer healthy tissue from elsewhere on the patient's body for coverage of a defect, when no local soft tissue is available to cover exposed bone, delicate tendons, nerves and blood vessels.

To obtain soft tissue to cover exposed areas and undertake reconstruction of hands, feet or face the surgeon may need to raise a pedicle graft, usually on the anterior abdominal wall of the patient. The pedicle consists of full-thickness flaps of skin along with underlying soft tissue such as fat, fascia and muscle, raised in the form of a fleshy tube.

Both ends of the tube remains initially connected to the anterior abdominal wall to ensure uninterrupted blood supply. After the sutures on the tube has healed, it is disconnected from the donor surface at one end and attached to the recipient site, say the dorsum of the hand and reconnected to a blood supply from the receptor site by suturing arteries and veins as small as 1 to 2 millimeters in diameter with the help of microsurgery under an operating microscope (Fig. 6.15).

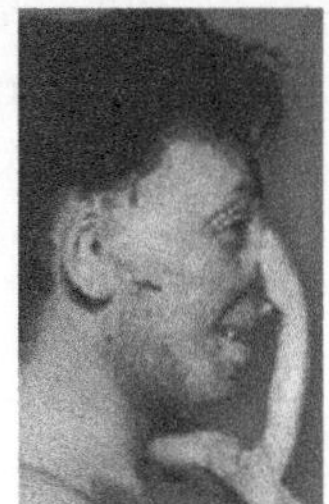
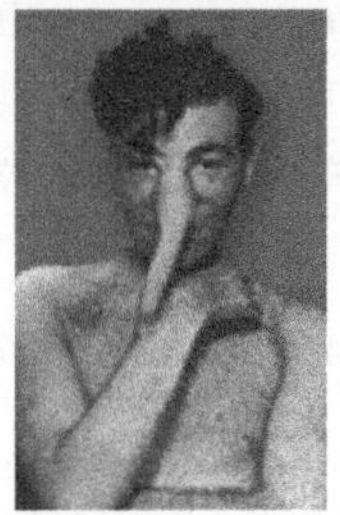

Fig. 6.15: A typical pedicle grafting for reconstruction of the nose; Royal Air Force wireless operator Jack Toper, was treated by pioneering plastic surgery at the Queen Victoria Hospital (QVH) by Sir Archibald McIndoe in 1943 after suffering facial burns when his aircraft was shot down in battle of Britain

The tube is then allowed to mature for a period of 15–21 days. Thereafter, the tube is completely detached from the donor site on the abdominal wall, split open along its length and fixed on the recipient dorsum of the hand for providing required soft tissue cover. However, before final grafting, the recipient site must be prepared carefully as explained in case of full thickness graft. Tendons, nerves and blood vessels on the hand must be freed from the scar tissue, viable ones repaired and unviable ones grafted wherever necessary. Thereafter, the pedicle is split open to provide the final outer covering over the reconstructed hand and is fixed in place with hidden microsutures. Functional outcome of pedicle grafting is usually very good since the grafted site gets back full vascular supply and sensation. However the color and the texture of the graft may not always match perfectly with that of the recipient site. After grafting the hand must be enclosed continuously in a custom made pressure gloves, with or without silicone web space retainer pads, to prevent collection of postoperative exudates under the graft, allow molding of soft tissue and prevent scar formation. This will also fix the graft firmly on the recipient site and help it "take" effectively.

Pedicle grafts raised on the anterior abdominal wall may also be transferred to remote locations such as the face. The graft is attached along with its distal attachment on the dorsum of the hand in the second stage of the series of surgeries, allowed to mature and then reattached to a remote receptor site, say the face in the third stage. The procedure of reconnecting of blood supply to the free end of the pedicle is repeated and the tube is left to mature in each stage of pedicle transfer. After the tube has matured, having established viable blood supply from its receptor site, it is cut open along its length and the full thickness skin with soft tissue is spread out over exposed bony areas of the face, to cover the wound and reconstruct the area. However, before the reconstruction the receptor site must be devoid of any infection and all scar tissue must be removed through excision. Once the reconstruction has been done, the part is enclosed in a custom made pressure garment, with or without silicone pressure pads, to help prevent edema, allow molding of the grafted soft tissue to the desired shape and prevent further scarring. This helps the graft to "take" satisfactorily.

Postoperative Rehabilitation of Burn

Every burn patient should be supplied with compressive garments such as gloves, mask, splints and conformers custom made by the occupational therapist, as soon as the wound has stabilized, before undergoing early reconstructive surgery. This helps prevent hypertrophy of scar and minimize contractures. Reconstructive operations are performed to restore functional and psychological needs. In children early reconstruction is often necessary to prevent development and growth impairment. The role of the family in the process of reintegration to normal life is crucial.*

Plan of Postoperative Rehabilitation

The postoperative rehabilitation is started on the day of surgery with corrective positioning. The goal is to prevent edema and contractures. It is often necessary to maintain the desired position by splinting. If the patient is in good condition active exercises and ambulation is performed.

The majority of patients are operated for the first time on the third or fourth day after burning. Surgeons try to remove most of the burned tissue in the first attempt. The postoperative period up to five days is very unfavorable for rehabilitation, and isometric exercises only are recommended in order to preserve the grafted areas. On the seventh day hydrotherapy is started by immersion in warm water and the take of grafts is evaluated. If most of the wounds are healed immersion hydrotherapy is continued every day; if there are open wounds of large necrotic areas shower spray is used every day to facilitate exercises and to prepare the patient for the next operation.

Early Problems in the Postoperative Convalescent Phase

Healed and grafted areas are sensitive and fragile. New skin may often break and blisters develop.

Patients are shown and taught how to clean, lubricate and massage the new skin. The possibility of scar formation and hypertrophic reactions should be explained to the patient or the family and the necessity for continuous pressure on these areas stressed. Splinting is necessary especially during the night—remember the position of comfort is always the position of contracture.

---

*Adapted form an article of Brcit A. University Medical Center, Ljubljana, Yugoslavia; Annals of the MBC -vol. 2 -n' 2 -June 1989.

Splints, conformers, masks, gloves and other compressive garments are produced during treatment in the burn unit. It is not necessary to have expensive materials and equipment. Plaster splints are very simple to produce. Elastic fabric for pressure garments is commercially available. With an ordinary sewing machine excellent gloves and masks can be produced by the occupational therapist in the Unit.

Especially for children, the school teacher and play therapist are very important during hospitalization to keep their minds busy and active. It is necessary to teach children how to use compressive garments or splints, which they very often dislike.

Short hospitalization time is very important and it follows a simple rule: hospitalization time should be equal to the percentage of burned area (e.g. 30 percent burn requires 30 days' hospitalization time).

The role of the surgeon at this stage is to recognize contractures which may hinder rehabilitation and to perform early release. This is especially important in the hands. Of no less importance are esthetical disfigurements of the face, which must be corrected for cosmetic and psychological reasons.

PHASE 4

Rehabilitation of the Burn Patient

Rehabilitation Goals and Planning[3]

Early surgery of the burn wound, especially primary tangential excision of the dead tissue creates favorable conditions for effective early healing and thus for rehabilitation. A rehabilitation team must be organized to follow the burn patient through acute care from admission, during hospitalization till discharge. The members of this team are surgeon, nurse, physiotherapists, occupational-therapist, psychologist, dietitian and orthotist. For major burns, follow-up treatment in the Rehabilitation Centre follows discharge from acute care.

Burn rehabilitation is undeniably difficult and time-consuming, but outlining short-term and long-term treatment goals and modalities is worthwhile. These goals and daily schedules ideally are posted where the patient and family can review them easily, thereby reinforcing the expectation that the goals be met. Treatment goals and strategies vary, depending on the patient's injury, stage of treatment, age, and comorbidities. Goals range from minimizing loss of range of motion (ROM) in the critically-ill patient to establishing a work hardening program in recovered patients.

- In critically-ill patients, goals are to limit loss of ROM, reduce edema, and prevent predictable contractures through positioning and splinting. This process generally involves twice-a-day therapy sessions, which take advantage of planned anesthetics to allow more aggressive joint ROM exercises.

- In patients who have recovered from critical illness but still are hospitalized, treatment is much more time-consuming, as well as physically and emotionally demanding of the patient and therapist.

Points to Ponder

- Appropriate therapist time must be budgeted.
- Realistic therapeutic goals and plan of care should be devised by the treatment team, which should include the patient and family.
- Before discharge from hospital, appropriate functional goals for the patient should be to achieve the ability to stand, ambulate, feed, and toilet.
- Regular meetings to discuss progress and a posted daily schedule are essential for motivation of the patient.

Principles of Physiotherapy in Care of Burn Patients

As a primary caregiver a physiotherapist is expected to present with the burn team in the ER. The job of the therapist begins immediately after burn and is carried over the entire period of the recovery till final rehabilitation of the patient is achieved.

Physiotherapy primarily involves:

- Positioning
- Splinting
- Assisting in pain and wound management
- Selective mobilization of body segments.

Positioning

The positioning of the burn patient is vital in bringing about the best functional outcomes in postoperative rehabilitation. It should begin immediately after the surgery and carried out until the scars from the last operative procedure are matured and all contractile forces cease to exist. Positioning should be designed for the specific individual's needs and be closely monitored and altered as the patient's medical status changes. It should not compromise mobility and function as these will greatly affect the final functional outcome. The statement that "the position of comfort is the position most likely to lead into contractures" is not only applicable to every burn patient but also to all who has sustained serious injury.

Points to Ponder

Positioning must always be done in a way that it:

- Reduces edema
- Maintains joint alignment
- Maintains soft tissues optimally elongated
- Prevents contracture formation
- Maintains ROM

- Promotes wound healing
- Relieves pressure
- Protects joints, exposed tendons and new grafts/flaps.

While selecting a position the therapist must always consider:

- TBSA affected by the burn
- Depth of the burn
- Associated injuries
- Exposed tendons/joints
- Patient's postoperative status.

Complications resulting from prolonged or improper positioning include:

- Pressure ulcers
- Nerve lesions
- Decreased ROM
- Joint malalignment.

General Guideline to Optimum Positioning for Different Body Segments[3]

Head—appropriate position: Head should be in 30° elevation.

In head and face burn, massive edema may greatly distort the face, but that this will disappear in a short time. Edema is usually at its maximum in the first 12 to 24 hours after the burn, when the patient must be watched carefully, because respiratory obstruction may occur suddenly. Head end of a regular hospital bed can be elevated with two 12 inches tall wooden blocks placed under the head end legs of the bed. In a three section hospital bed, the head end may be elevated to 30 degrees and foot section may be raised at the knee by 15 degrees, placing the patient in a fowler's position.

Special considerations: Foot board must be provided at the foot end of the bed to prevent sliding down the bed when head elevated.

Neck—appropriate position: Neck should be in midline with 10–15° of extension.

Neck flexion contractures, very common in neck burns, can lead to major cosmetic deformities, ventilatory difficulties, problems with salivation, vocalization and in extreme cases dislocation of the mandible. The therapist must use a Roll behind the neck to keep the neck in extension, held in place by a chin strap if needed. One should never use a pillow for positioning the neck or the head of a burn patient. Neck contractures make for difficult intubation in case of an emergency.

Special considerations: Intubated patients must be positioned with neck in neutral or in slight extension for maintaining good airway clearance.

Shoulder—appropriate position: Shoulder should be positioned in 90° abduction with 15–20° horizontal adduction and slight external rotation.

Shoulder joints usually become fixed in adduction and internal rotation, particularly if the medial aspect of the arm, the shoulder girdle and axilla has been burnt. Such contracture are extremely difficult to release manually once they have developed, hence every effort should be made to prevent them.

Special considerations: The therapist should monitor radial pulse and reposition the arm frequently to avoid compression of the brachial plexus which may lead to a neuropathy. Look frequently for sensory abnormalities such as tingling and numbness and/or motor weakness or deficits.

Elbow—appropriate position: Elbow in 30° flexion with the forearm in mid supination is the optimum position from the functional point of view.

Although flexion is the functional position, contractures develop more frequently in this position. The affected joint must be mobilized as early and as much as possible.

Special considerations: Avoid locking the elbow in either full extension or flexion.

Wrist and hand—appropriate position: Ideal position is, wrist in 0–30° extension, MCP joints in 70–90° flexion, and IP joints in full extension. The thumb should be positioned in a combination of palmar and radial abduction maintaining the first web space in a stretched position. The thick skin on the palms of a patient's hands usually protects them, so most burns occur on the back of the hand (dorsum). The hand swells, and as the edema organizes the hand stiffens. One can minimize this edema by raising the burnt hand, hanging it from a drip pole.

Severely burnt hands are not suited to the exposure treatment because the crust cracks when a patient uses his fingers; nor are they well suited to the occlusive method because he cannot exercise his hand inside a big bulky dressing. The plastic bag method is usually best. This keeps his fingers moist and mobile, and makes even a severe burn almost completely painless. Even if both his hands are burnt he can still do many things for himself. An antiseptic in the bag is desirable but not essential. Recognizing the depth of a burn is difficult in the hand, but is important, because small deep burns may be best treated by immediate excision and grafting.

Special considerations: A dropped wrist not only leads to functional limitations, but can also cause compression to the median and ulnar nerves and disturb the venous return resulting in edema. Exposed tendons and joints should be positioned in a static cock up splint at all times without exceptions (Fig. 6.16). During dressing changes of the hand with exposed structures the splint may be briefly removed while the affected structures are manually supported. The splint should be reapplied immediately after the dressing is completed.

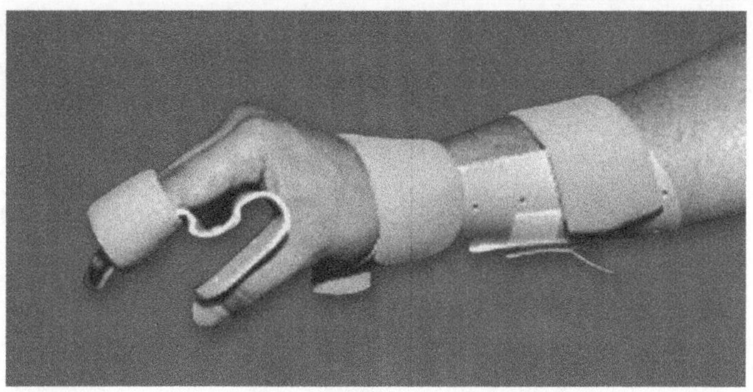

Fig. 6.16: Static cock up splint

Dynamic (lively) splints are ideal when a patient's hand starts to recover, so change his fixed splint for one which allows him to move his fingers, but still holds his hand in the best position when it is resting. The easiest way to make a dynamic splint is to make, a plaster cock-up splint, and to fix a piece of thick wire to it. Attach rubber bands to the wire and pass these round his proximal phalanges to allow him to exercise his fingers (Fig. 6. 17).

When grafting a burnt hand is needed, one must graft early, or the patient will lose the function in his hand unnecessarily. The common deformities that can follow are seen in B, C, D and E, that can usually develop in a badly burnt hand but can be prevented by: Splinting a patient's burnt hand in the position of safety as in A, in Figure 6.18. Start physiotherapy as early as is practical and since there is no universal splint for a burnt hand, one must consider each patient's needs separately.

Hip joints—appropriate position: Neutral flexion-extension and rotation, 10–15° hip abduction and knee extension.

The hip joints tend to develop contracture in flexion and adduction.

The combination of hip flexion and abduction tightness can lead to hip dislocation.

Special considerations: In patients with no ventilatory problems the prone position facilitates hip as well as knee extension.

Knee joints—appropriate position: Full knee extension.

The knee joints tend to develop contracture in flexion. One should however avoid locking the knee in full extension and mobilize the joint as early and frequently as possible to gain and maintain flexion range.

Special considerations: Avoid elevation of the legs with knees unsupported because it might cause undue stretching of the posterior structures of the knee joint and may lead to laxity of the cruciates.

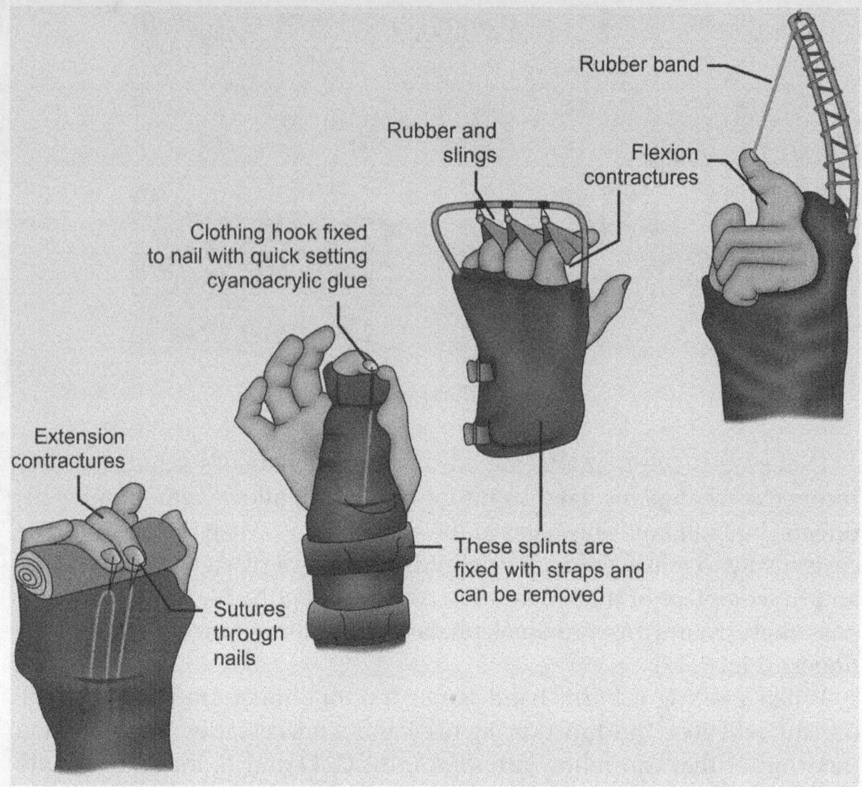

Fig. 6.17: Dynamic hand splint

Foot and ankle—appropriate position: The ankle joint should be positioned in neutral with the help of a foot board or a L splint. This position should be maintained while the patient is lying in the prone or supine position.

One must place soft cushion under the calf and the heel while the patient is supine. Hard surfaces encourage venous stasis in the calf, leading to DVT and can cause heel pressure ulcers.

Special considerations: Plantar flexion and inversion lead to the equinovarus deformity. Hence at every opportunity the neutral alignment of the ankle and foot must be ensured. Ankle-foot pumping must also be done actively or passively at two hourly intervals to prevent DVT.

Basic Principles of Splinting in Burn (Also See Annexure 6.1)

Introduction: Splints are vital in burn rehabilitation as they are utilized throughout the patient's recovery in obtaining appropriate positioning of the entire body. No matter how the therapist approaches splinting materials, designs, application schedules the goal is to bring about the best functional outcome at the completion of rehabilitation. The therapist must

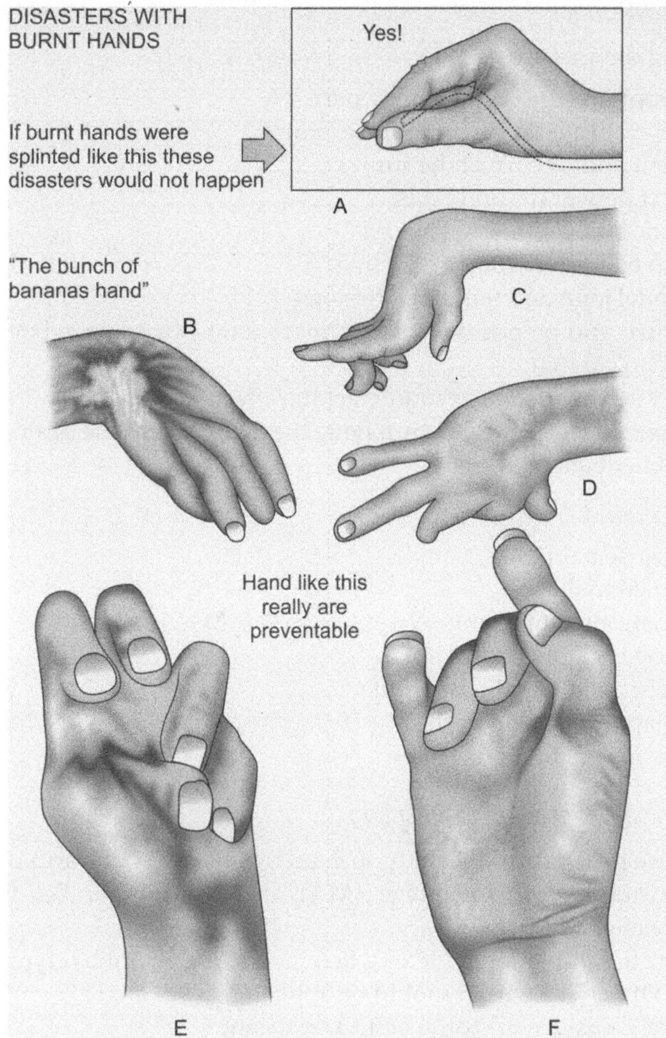

Fig. 6.18: A—correct method of splinting a burnt hand; B, C, D, E, F—common deformities that may develop in a badly burnt hand

be aware of the anatomy and kinesiology of the body part to be splinted prior to fabricating a splint or an orthotic device.

Splinting Definitions

Static splint: Static or passive splints indicate that the affected joint or joints are to be immobilized or be movement restricted.

Dynamic splint: A dynamic splint is one that achieves its effects by movement and force. "It is a form of manipulation". It may use forces generated by the patient's own muscles or externally imposed forces using rubber bands or springs.

Points to Ponder

Splinting devices are used to:

- Appropriately position a body part
- Support, protect and immobilize joints
- Prevent and/or correct deformity
- Protect new grafts and flaps
- Maintain and/or increase ROM
- Aid in edema and pain reduction
- Remodel joint and tendon adhesions
- Stabilize and/or position one or more joints enabling other joints to function correctly
- Assist weak muscles to counteract the effects of gravity
- Strengthen weak muscles by having the patients exercise against springs or rubber bands.

Splints should:

- Not cause pain
- Be functional
- Cosmetically appealing
- Be easy to apply and remove
- Be light weight and low profile
- Be of appropriate materials
- Allow for ventilation.

Mechanical Principles of Splinting

- Reduce pressure on the body surface: by increasing the area of contact.
- Gain mechanical advantage (MA) and control parallel forces by increasing the MA.
- Use optimal rotational forces when mobilizing a joint by dynamic traction. Dynamic traction should be applied at a 90° angle.
- *Torque:* Consider the torque effect on a joint.
- Stabilize proximal normal joints to correctly mobilize distal affected joints.
- Consider the effects of reciprocal parallel forces when designing splints and placing straps.
- Increase splint strength by contouring the material's surfaces.
- Eliminate friction and splint migration with proper padding.

Role of Physiotherapy in Pain and Wound Management in Burn Injury

Burn injuries and its treatments are a tremendous pain management challenge. It is often the case of too little too late as regards to painkillers in burn pain , because the degree of tissue damage in severe burns can initiate physiologic changes in nociceptive pathways, that often place the patient at risk for undertreatment. The use of established analgesic guidelines that address both background and procedural pain and associated anxiety can provide effective pain relief. The key to successful treatment is the continuous and accurate assessment of the patient's pain and the response to therapy. Medications, especially opioids, and its mode of administration, usually injected, should be regularly evaluated and adjusted to achieve maximum effect with minimal adverse side effects. Nurse's role is perhaps the most important in the primary evaluation of burn pain and its successful treatment. The therapist has a secondary role in management of burn pain. The therapist must be familiar with the schedule of painkillers for a particular patient and time the therapy sessions after about ½ hour of the painkiller injections. This way the patient will have minimum discomfort while performing various therapeutic exercises and handling by the therapist.

Dressing changes are also horror sessions of pain and bleeding for the patient. This can be significantly minimized by hydrotherapy.*

Hydrotherapy in Burn—A Viable Treatment Option

Introduction

The benefits of hydrotherapy as an adjuvant to the treatment of burns are universally recognized. Hydrotherapy in burn management involves both immersion in a tub or showers in running warm water of the burnt body part to help in the healing process. Commonly hydrotherapy starts on day 3–5 postburn, when patients have overcome initial shock and their general condition has stabilized. Though the actual hydrotherapy is done under the supervision of the physiotherapist, in most cases nurses are present and physicians available on call. Sterilized stainless steel tubs of varying sizes are used depending upon the area to be submerged. Water used is usually ordinary (tap) water, though sterilized water may also be used in some cases.

The advantages of hydrotherapy are:

- Improvement of the burn wound, i.e. separation of the soiled dressing, Escher and other tissue debris from the wound surface, cleaning of the wound and drainage of pus with minimum of bleeding and damage to fragile new skin
- Facilitation of physical therapy and mobilization with the helps of buoyancy
- Well-being, pain relief and comfort of the patient due to the soothing effect of flowing warm water on the raw area.

---

*Adapted from Montogomery RK; Critical Care Nursing Clinics North America. 2004 Mar;16(1):39-49.

Material

The whole body immersion tub, also known as Hubbard's Tank is made of stainless steel with dimensions: L 1.80 m × D 0.8 m × W 1.0 m and contains 80 liters of water. It has inlets with valves for filling preheated fresh tap water/sterilized, outlets with drain valves for removing dirty water, tangential air jet pumps for circulation of the water and thermostats to maintain optimum water temperature. The setup must have a mobile hoist consisting of two rotating electromechanical arms, with slings, a stretcher with sterilized vinyl cover and a transfer trolley, for transferring the patient from the bed to the tub with minimal handling. Arrangements must be made for heating the room as well as for preheating and sterilization of the water through ultraviolet radiation. The tub must be cleaned and sterilized with disinfectant solution after every session, and culture specimens from the tub, trolley, hoist straps and other parts are obtained periodically to detect infective agents.

Smaller areas like the hands or feet may be submerged in smaller tubs or whirlpool bath, following the aseptic precautions detailed above.

Showers are carried out for in an ordinary porcelain tub using tap water through a hand held telephone shower in a bathroom which is routinely cleaned and sterilized with disinfectant solutions.

Procedure

The tub is filled with water, the patient, after checking vital signs, is lifted the help of the hoist from the transfer trolley and gently placed in the tub. The debridement is started only after the patient has soaked in the warm water for at least 10 minutes. In a water temperature of about 35°C the patient feels comfortable and can relax. The dressing is allowed to separate from the wound surface by the flowing water and then wound is scrubbed with wet sterile gauze and betadine lotion. Loose necrotic debris is gently removed and pus evacuated. The whole procedure takes about 20–30 minutes to complete. When eschar incision or other procedures are performed, bleeding could be considerable. This procedure must be performed in the Operation Theater by the surgeon immediately after hydrotherapy session. Submerging in water softens the eschar and makes for easy separation from the wound surface.

When the general condition of the burned patient allows it or when the burns involve only the upper part of the body, we prefer shower therapy using water and betadine scrub, but the procedure lasts less than bath therapy (10 min versus 20 min). The temperature of the water depends on the patient's feeling of comfort, ranging from 24 to 34°C.

Bath therapy may be employed for a period of 10–20 days in the majority of cases for 10 to 30 minutes once daily or on every second day.

Analgesia may or may not be administered before hydrotherapy, since even gentle scrubbing of the wound surface can sometimes be quite painful. Patients are encouraged to perform movements under the guidance of the physiotherapist, and to actively participate in their bath, which is a source of satisfaction. Hair-washing, shaving of axilla and around orifices can be carried out at the same time.

Undesired side effects, such as pyrexia, chills and fatigue, have been universally observed, but are transient and of no clinical significance.

Role of the Physiotherapist in the Critically-ill Burn Patient

To attain the objective of optimal long-term function, rehabilitation efforts must begin at the outset of burn care. Physical and occupational therapists play essential roles in the acute treatment of all burn patients, even in the critically ill and during resuscitation of those with large injuries. The following are the three principal priorities for the burn therapist in the acute stage:

- Performing ROM
- Splinting and antideformity positioning
- Establishing a long-term relationship with the patient and family members to ensure compliance with therapy goals and to increase the patient's motivation for recovery.

  If a body part is left immobile for a long period of time, capsular contraction and shortening of tendon and muscle groups, which cross the joints, occur. This can be prevented by a program of passive ROM exercises, antideformity positioning, and splinting.
- Passive ROM exercise is best performed twice daily, with the therapist taking all joints through a full ROM. The therapist must be sensitive to the patient's pain, anxiety, wound status, extremity perfusion, and security of the patient's airway and various drips and drains.
- These procedures should be performed in coordination with the ICU staff. Attention to the security of endotracheal tubes, nasogastric tubes, and arterial and central venous catheters is paramount, as unexpected loss of these devices can contribute to damage or even death of the patient.
- Although these procedures are important, they cannot be accomplished effectively or humanly if they cause excessive pain and anxiety. Performing ROM often can be timed to coincide with dressing changes and wound cleansing, thereby minimizing the need for medication.
- Proper antideformity positioning minimizes shortening of tendons, collateral ligaments, and joint capsules and reduces edema.

  Although splints are used less frequently, there are several predictable contractures that occur in patients with burns that can be prevented by a proper ROM exercises, positioning, and splinting. These contractures generally develop in the flexed position of comfort, except in the hands.

- Flexion deformities of the neck can be minimized with thermoplastic neck splints, conformers, and split mattresses. In critically-ill patients, positioning the neck in slight extension is often all that can be done. Do not allow the ventilator tubing to pull the head so that a contracture develops; without proper care, a rotary contracture can develop, generally with the patient turned toward the ventilator.

Points to Ponder

- Contractures are especially likely to develop if wounds are not closed early. The speed at which contractures can develop is astonishing, if prevention strategies are not part of routine care.
- Axillary adduction contractures can be prevented by positioning the shoulders widely abducted with axillary splints, padded hanging troughs of thermoplastic material, or a variety of sling support devices mounted to the bed.
- Elbow flexion contractures are minimized by statically splinting the elbow in extension. Elbow extension splints can be removed to give flexion exercises to help retain a full ROM.
- Flexion contractures of the hips and knees are particularly common but can be prevented by careful positioning and with passive ROM exercises. Prevention of such contractures is important even in infants, as these contractures can interfere with subsequent ambulation. Prone positioning, although poorly tolerated by some, can assist in minimizing hip flexion contractures; knee immobilizers can minimize knee flexion contractures.
- The equinovarus deformity of the ankle and foot, in which the ankle is plantar flexed and the foot is in an inverted position, is a serious problem that can occur even if the ankles are not burned. This contracture can be prevented with static splinting of the ankles in the neutral position with a molded thermoplastic AFO and performing passive ROM exercises twice daily. Splints designed for this purpose can cause pressure injury over the metatarsal heads or calcaneum if improperly designed. These pressure injuries can be prevented by using padding to distribute pressure evenly across the metatarsal heads and by extending the footplate of the splint beyond the heel and cutting out the area around the calcaneum.
- Inspect all splints at least twice daily for evidence of poor fit or pressure injury, since improper fitment of splints can cause further injury to the skin.
- Another important aspect of antideformity positioning is placing affected extremities just above the level of the heart, which reduces edema.
- The therapist should provide regular updates to the patient and other team members about problems and progress as they develop.

Role of the Physiotherapist in the Recovering Burn Patient

As critical illness abates and wounds progressively close, the roles of the physical and occupational therapists, as well as, the demands on the patient expand and become more difficult. Patients become more aware of what has happened to them, and they can become fearful of the therapist and the potentially painful and uncomfortable therapy procedures.

The principal components of burn therapy that characterize the recovering period include the following:

- Continued passive ROM exercises
- Increasing active ROM and strengthening exercises
- Minimizing edema aggressively through massage, mechanical and electrotherapeutic compression techniques
- ADL training
- Initial scar management
- Preparing for work or play or school.

Long-term favorable outcome requires hardwork during this period, but it is important for the therapist not to push too hard. An early program of passive ROM greatly facilitates successful retention of normal ROM during this period. Intraoperative ROM exercises under anesthesia also can be useful; in coordination with the operating room team. Difficult passive ROM can be performed between induction of anesthesia and preparation of the surgical site. Other maneuvers that can be used to increase the patient's tolerance for passive ROM include the following:

- Timing of the ROM session with medication for dressing changes
- Administration of opiates or benzodiazepines ½ hour before the exercise session
- Gentle conversation and encouragement
- An unhurried approach to therapy sessions.

Burned and grafted extremities commonly have lingering edema that can contribute to joint stiffness. Reducing this edema facilitates rehabilitation efforts.

- The use of custom-fitted elastic garments this early after injury is expensive, as they frequently need to be downsized as the edema resolves; however, simply wrapping the fingers with self-adherent elastic helps reduce digital edema. Tubular elastic dressings, elastic wrap dressings, pneumatic compression splints, elevation, and retrograde effleurage massage also help reduce extremity edema.
- Local silicone pressure pads may be used to minimize evolving hypertrophic scars.

As final wound closure nears and hospital discharge approaches, the focus of rehabilitation efforts becomes practical. Performance of ADL tasks and the impending return to play/school/work become the most important considerations.

- Resisted ROM, isometric exercises, active strengthening, and gait training are important objectives.
- When treating children, it is important to use developmentally appropriate play to facilitate rehabilitation goals. For example, children with serious hand burns should be engaged in such play activities that require the use of their hands at a motor level that is consistent with their motor development. This prevents frustration and fear of failure in children.

For many burn patients, the first 18 months after discharge are more difficult than the acute stay. The principal rehabilitation goals at this time include the following:

- Progressive ROM and strengthening
- Evaluation of evolving problem areas
- Specific postoperative therapy after reconstructive operations
- Scar management.

Ideally, the same therapist who worked with the patient during the acute stage hospitalization should continue through the outpatient treatment. Not only does this continuity reassure the patient but also helps the therapist to monitor burn recovery more accurately. If, for reasons of distance or managed care, it is not possible to maintain this relationship, regular contact with the primary care therapist during review clinic visits back at the burn unit can achieve this goal indirectly. Unfortunately, it is not uncommon for ROM and strength to be lost during the first months after discharge. This is particularly true if there is inadequate outpatient rehabilitation, most commonly due to inexperienced therapist. The burn unit team should monitor the quality of outpatient rehabilitation services during review clinic visits at the burn unit. If the patient is losing substantial ROM and strength due to inadequate therapy, readmission for focused rehabilitation is appropriate.

Points to Ponder

- The realities of distance, transportation, and managed care often cause patients to work with inexperienced therapists. Therapists should visit the burn unit prior to the patient's discharge, discuss treatment approach, videotape therapy sessions with the patient's written permission, and maintain frequent telephone contact with the primary care therapist. Family education and involvement with rehabilitation plans may facilitate early identification of evolving problems and rectify rehabilitation efforts.
- Burn therapists play a central role in planning and performing reconstructive procedures in the months and years after acute discharge. They help to identify need for operations, plan sequencing of operations, and educate patients and families about preoperative care.

Planning appropriate postoperative rehabilitation activities helps patients optimize surgical outcome.

Areas of Concerns for Burns of the Upper and Lower Extremities

Upper Extremity

High-quality acute burn care minimizes early upper extremity reconstructive needs, but problems regularly occur. Perhaps the most common upper extremity deformities are dorsal hand and web space contractures.

- Dorsal hand contractures are prevented ideally by attention to proper positioning before surgery and postsurgically. If the initial excision of dead tissue was performed tangentially rather than at the level of the fascia, i.e. if there is some remnant dorsal subcutaneous fat, the release is likely to slide and accept a large piece of skin graft. Such release usually results in a resistance-free complete ROM of the metacarpophalangeal joints.
- Although web space contractures are common deformities that require surgical correction, they can be minimized by early surgery, followed by compressive gloves supplemented with web space conformers. In the normal web space, the leading edge of the palmar aspect of the web is distal to the dorsal aspect. In the typical dorsal web space contracture, this pattern is reversed. The syndactyly or webbed digit is usually a dorsal deformity. When severe, i.e. limiting digital abduction, such deformity should be corrected. The typically normal leading palmar edge of the web space must not be compromised.

Very deep burns of the elbow are notorious for producing restriction of ROM even with best possible care. Normal elbow ROM is required for performance of ADL such as feeding and toileting.

Limited elbow extension occurs commonly due to flexion contracture that responds to simple release; however, heterotopic ossification, i.e. when abnormal bone forms in the soft tissues around the triceps tendon and interferes with elbow motion, also may contribute (Fig. 6.19). An X-ray can be done to exclude it.

Restricted elbow extension may resolve spontaneously over the course of years, but it should be treated surgically if it interferes significantly with recovery. A careful dissection is required. The abnormal bone is removed so that the elbow joint is not blocked; it is important to visualize and protect the ulnar nerve during this surgery.

Axillary contracture is not uncommon and can interfere with important upper extremity functions such as feeding. Axillary release should encompass the entire rotational axis of the shoulder to facilitate complete ROM and the gap is closed with sheet skin graft. Postoperatively, abduction splints should maximize the ROM without creating traction or pressure on the brachial plexus or vessels.

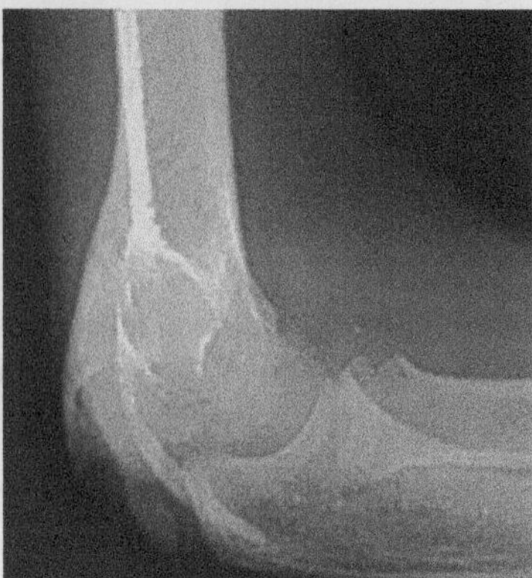

Fig. 6.19: Heterotopic bone formation

Lower Extremity

Patients who have been supine for long periods often tolerate immediate upright positioning poorly. Before starting assisted standing, such patients benefit from tilt table training and graduated sitting on bed to overcome orthostatic hypotension. Lower extremity edema, which can hinder recovery, is prevented best by using gentle elastic wraps prior to placing the patient in an upright position.

The most common lower extremity deformities that require correction in patients who have sustained burns are:

1. Dorsal foot extension contractures,
2. Popliteal flexion contractures, and
3. Hip flexion contractures.

The latter two are particularly common in infants and very young children as they spend long periods of time with the hips and knees flexed and are particularly difficult to splint and give passive ROM exercises.

- A deep dorsal foot burn may result in a contracture of the metatarsophalangeal joints, so that the toes are brought off the ground, causing the patient to have an abnormal gait. When the abnormal gait is severe enough to interfere with ambulation, corrective surgery becomes necessary. An incisional release of the scar over the dorsum of the foot accepts a large piece of split thickness skin graft, particularly if the initial operation was performed in a layered fashion so that viable subcutaneous fat remains.
- Flexion contractures of the popliteal fossa also interfere with ambulation. Correction generally requires incisional release and grafting, followed by focused postoperative physiotherapy to maintain knee extension. Avoiding injury to the relatively superficial underlying neurovascular structures of the popliteal fossa is important.
- Flexion contractures at the hips are common in infants and very young children who spend little time with the hips in extension. The contracted

position of comfort is with the hip in flexion. This deformity interferes with ambulation and should be addressed early in recovery. Avoid injury to the femoral vessels and nerve, as the overlying contracted tissue may distort the normal anatomy.

Management of Scar

Hypertrophic scarring is a difficult problem for burn patients and scar management is an essential aspect of outpatient burn therapy. Perhaps the most virulent hypertrophic scarring is seen in deep dermal burns that heal spontaneously in three or more weeks; this seems especially true in areas of highly elastic skin, e.g. the lower face, submental triangle (below the lower jaw), anterior chest and neck. The wound hyperemia seen universally following burn wound healing should begin to resolve within about nine weeks after epithelialization. In wounds destined to become hypertrophic, increased neovascularization occurs with increasing rather than decreasing erythema after nine weeks, visible in the burnt hand (Fig. 6.20).

Available tools to modify the progression of hypertrophic scar formation are limited in number and effectiveness. These tools include scar massage, compression garments, topical silicone, steroid injections, and surgery. In some contractures over major joints, serial casting may be useful.

Regular and effective scar massage can be effective in limited areas of scarring, and it is convenient since it can be performed by family members. Ideally, this technique is performed several times each day. Lanolin-based moisturizers lotion such as Nivea or Vaselin, which minimize drying of recently healed burns and skin grafts, are applied. Evolving hypertrophic areas then are massaged in a firm and slow manner (Fig. 6.21).

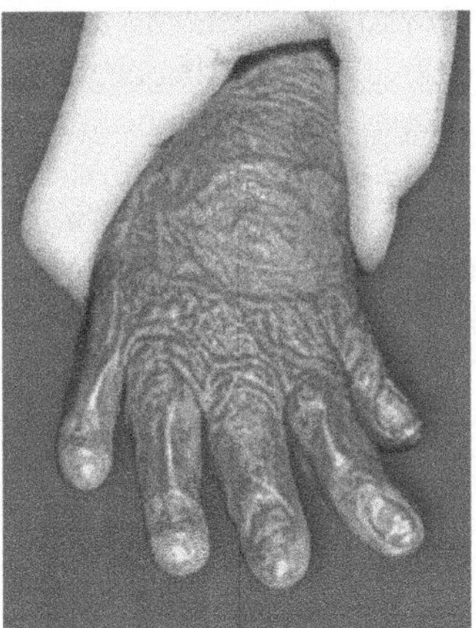

Fig. 6.20: The physiology of hypertrophic scarring is not fully understood. Perhaps the most virulent hypertrophic scarring is seen in deep dermal burns that heal spontaneously over the course of 3 or more weeks, particularly in highly elastic skin, e.g. the lower face, submental triangle, anterior neck, chest, etc.

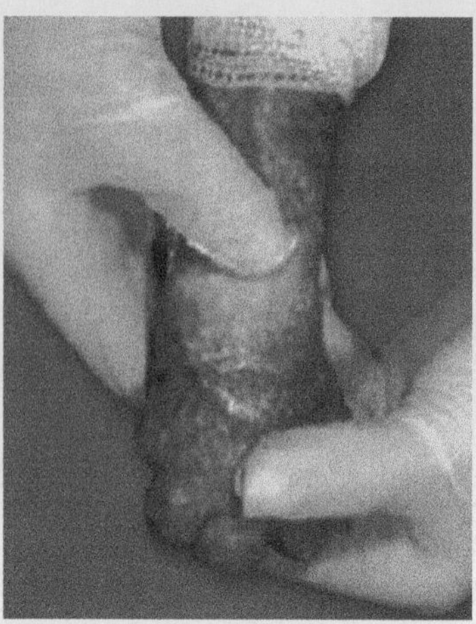

Fig. 6.21: Scar massage optimally is performed several times each day. Use firm, slow pressure on evolving hypertrophic areas after applying lanolin-based bland skin creams/ lotions such as Nivea

Despite the controversy over its use, compression garments seem to improve control of broad areas of hypertrophic scarring, particularly in young children in whom the scarring process seems to be more severe. Compression garments should be worn 23 hours a day until wound erythema begins to abate, usually about 12–18 months after injury. In growing and young children, frequent refitting and replacement of compression garments are required. Garment fit must be verified after manufacture, as a poorly fitting garment is less effective and can be uncomfortable.

Local silicone pressure pads, applied to the healed wound as a sheet, are effective when applied to small areas of a troublesome hypertrophic scar. Have the silicone in place 24 hours a day is ideal, except during bathing. Some children develop a rash beneath the topical silicone, but this rash quickly resolves with removal of the silicone; in these patients, 12-hour or every-other-day application seems to help. Silicone sheets can be placed beneath compression garments or can be held in place by one of several elastic devices. Firm pressure is not required for the silicone to be effective.

For only localized and very symptomatic areas of early hypertrophic scars, especially if they are in highly cosmetic locations or associated with severe itching (pruritus), direct steroid injections or hydrocortisone phonophoresis can be useful.

Points to Ponder

- Limit the total dose of steroid so that systemic effects do not occur.
- These injections or ultrasound applications are painful, as they require high pressure to infiltrate the dense hypertrophic scars and in children sedation usually is required.
- Only localized and very symptomatic areas are treated in this fashion.

Extreme Pruritus or Itching is a Frequent Part of Burn Wound Healing

- Pruritus typically begins shortly after the wound has healed, peaks in intensity 4–6 months after injury, and then gradually subsides in most patients. It can be especially troubling at night.
- In most patients, it is adequately treated with massage, moisturizers, and oral antihistamines at night. Alternative approaches are available, although none work reliably for everyone.
- In patients particularly troubled by pruritus, a sequential therapeutic trial of each of the following local medication often identifies one particularly helpful method: application of topical creams containing vitamin E, topical antihistamine creams, topical cold compresses, frequent application of moisturizing creams, or colloidal baths.
- Localized highly pruritic scars often respond to a steroid injection.
- In rare cases, pruritus becomes so intense that excoriations develop.
- These wounds can become infected with *Staphylococcus aureus*, which further increases the pruritus.
- To allow healing of excoriated areas, some patients require admission for wound care and antibiotics to control the pruritus and infection. Surgical excision or incision and skin grafting are useful maneuvers when other scar management tools are ineffective.

REFERENCES

1. Bass CB. Burns. In: Manual of patient care in plastic surgery. Little Brown, Boston, 1982.
2. Gordon DM. Nursing care of the burned child. In: Artz Moncrief J, Pruit B. (Eds.) Burns: A team approach. WB Saunders, Philadelphia, 1979.
3. Kemble HJV, Lamb BE. Practical burns management. Hodder and Stoughton, London, 1987.

ANNEXURE 6.1

SPLINTING GUIDE FOR BURN THE WHOLE BODY

Face

- ***Silicone thermoplastic splinting for scar management*** combines the mold ability of thermoplastic splinting materials with a therapeutic surface of silicone sheeting. One can use standard negative and positive molds forming techniques to shape the material over a plaster mold, trim as desired, and attach straps as needed. And since silicone sheeting works without pressure, one can achieve effective scar management of

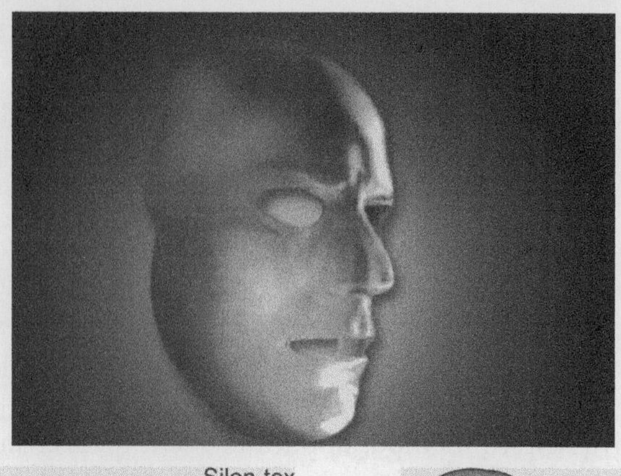

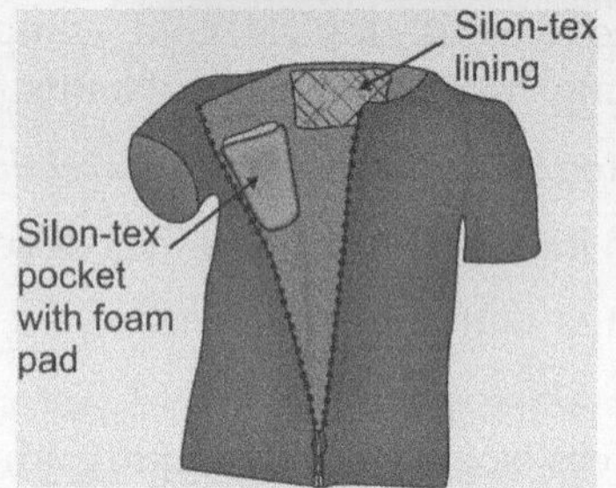

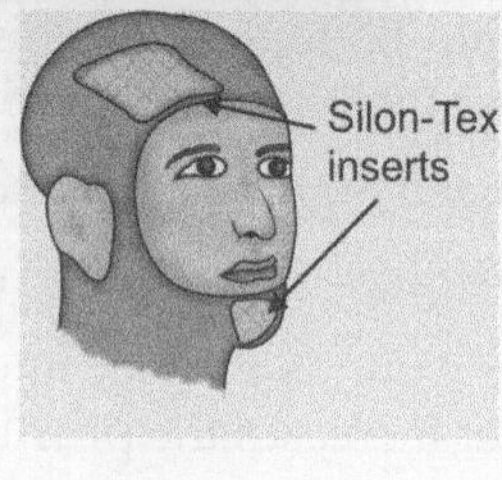

soft areas of the face... closer to the eyes, the nostrils, and lips and is cosmetically appealing.

- ***Silicone elastomer face mask/body suit*** prevents and corrects scar hypertrophy, negative and positive molds required to customize a face mask for an individual patient.

Neck

- ***Soft neck collar***:
  The soft foam cervical collar is a neck support that offers soft comfortable support while helping to reduce head and cervical vertebrae movement.

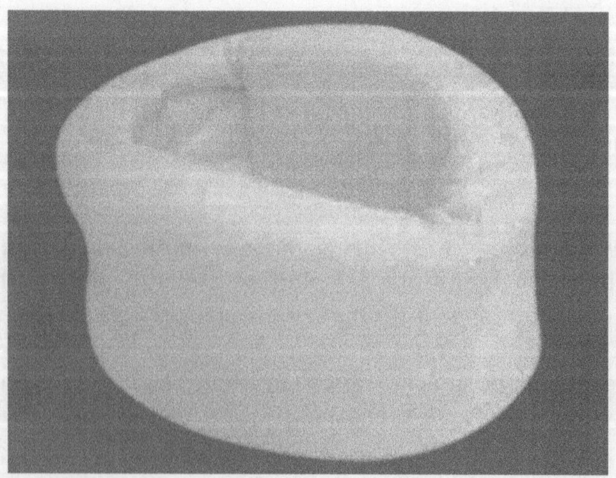

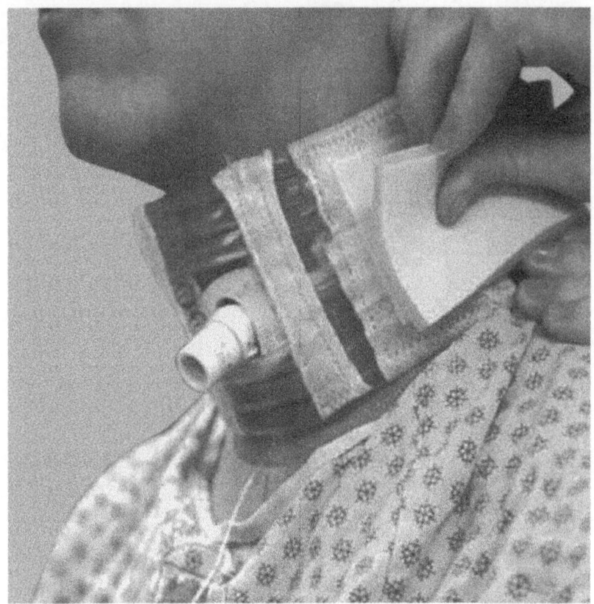

- ***Anterior neck conformer with tracheostomy aperture***
  Critically-ill patients with burns often require long-term ventilator support with tracheostomy placement. When these patients also have neck burns the therapist must go beyond the typical approaches to neck splinting.

Tracheostomy tube is a limiting factor in early positioning and application of pressure devices. However, it is a fact that early neck positioning is critical for patient with neck burn. Hence, a neck positioning device that is sturdy enough to benefit the patient while also being easily accessible for respiratory treatments and airway care and in case of emergencies is essential.

Axilla/Shoulder

- ***Axillary pads***

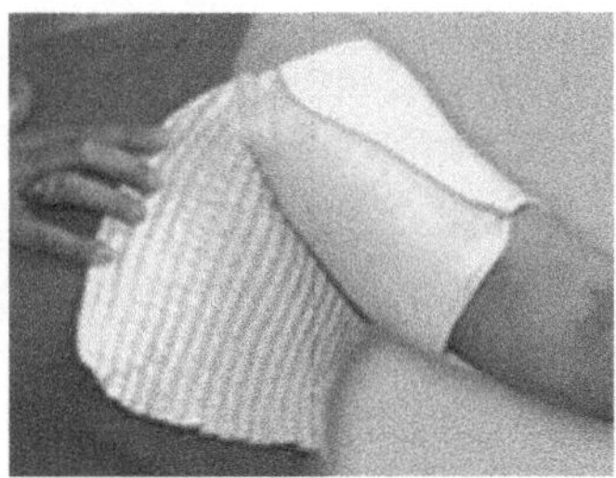

- ***Airplane splints***
  Special considerations for shoulder girdle—avoid over stretch on the brachial plexus.

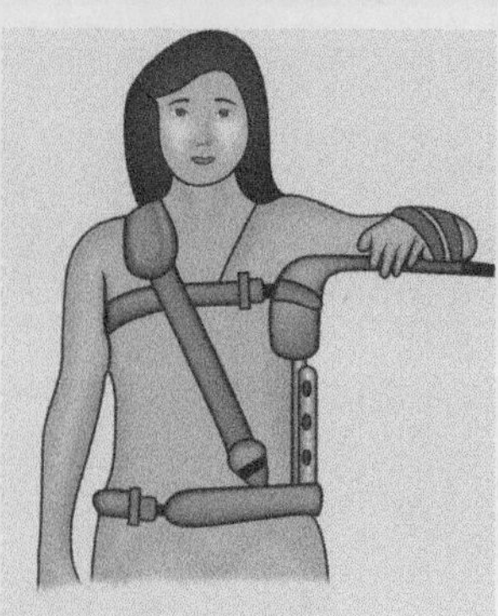

Elbow

Static elbow splint—anterior elbow conformer slab.

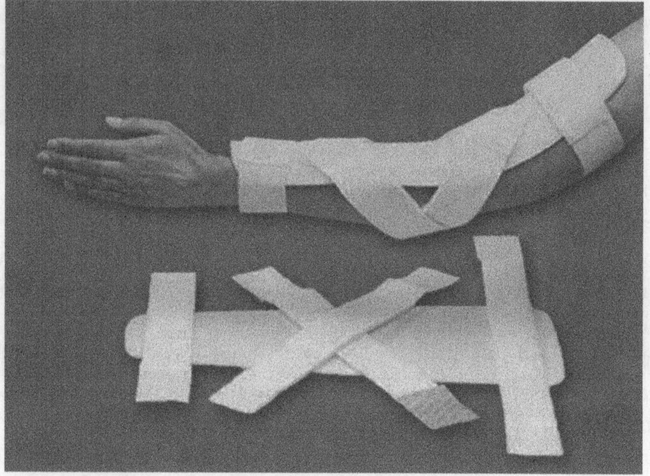

Dynamic elbow splint—flexion or extension.

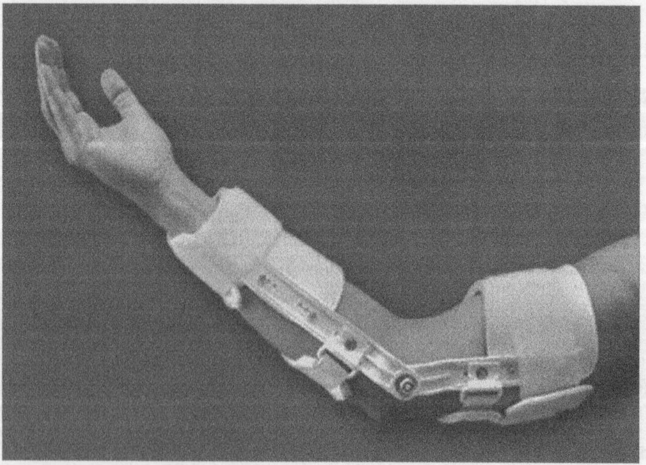

Wrist

Static splints

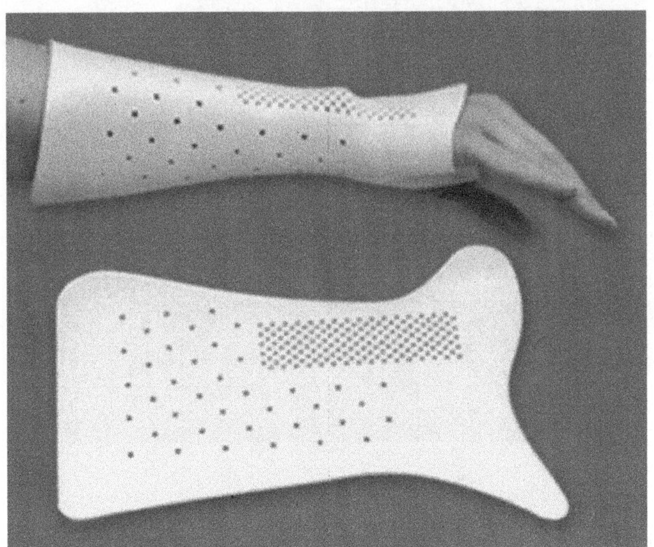

Volar/dorsal thermoplastic wrist cock-up splint

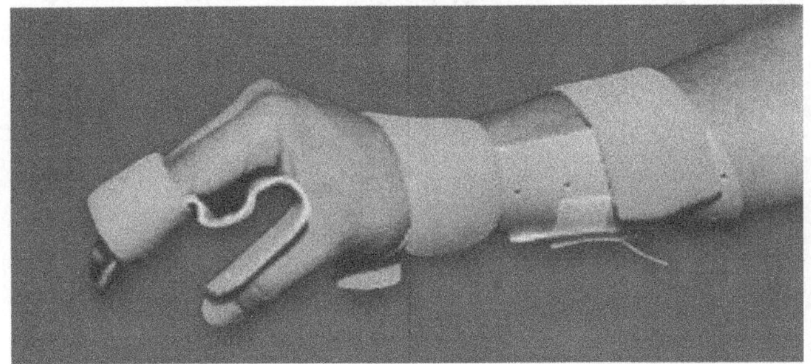

Palmar wrist splint with a thumb component

Dynamic Splints

Wrist radial/ulnar deviation splint

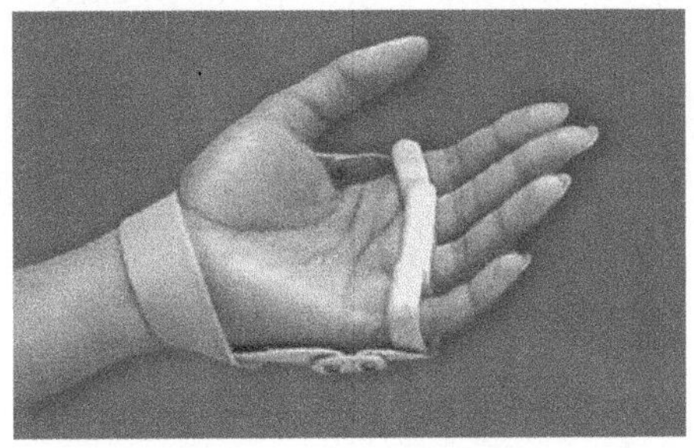

Wrist flexion/extension/deviation

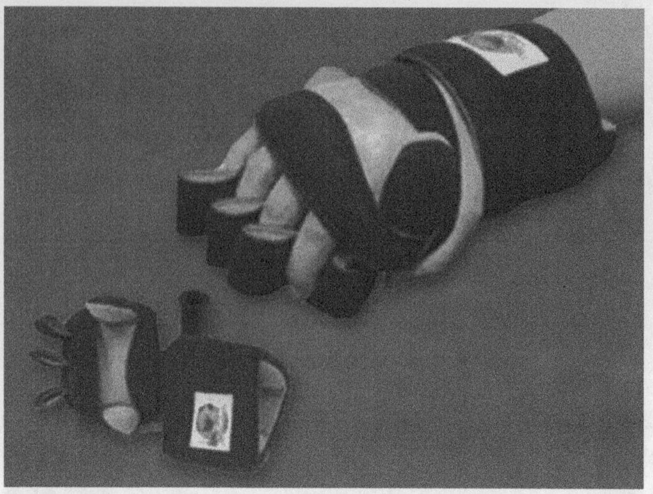

Hand

Pressure gloves for the hand with built in digital spacer—to be worn for 1–2 years.

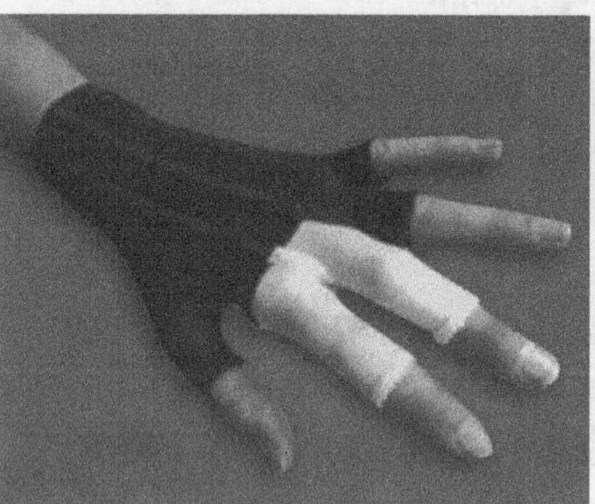

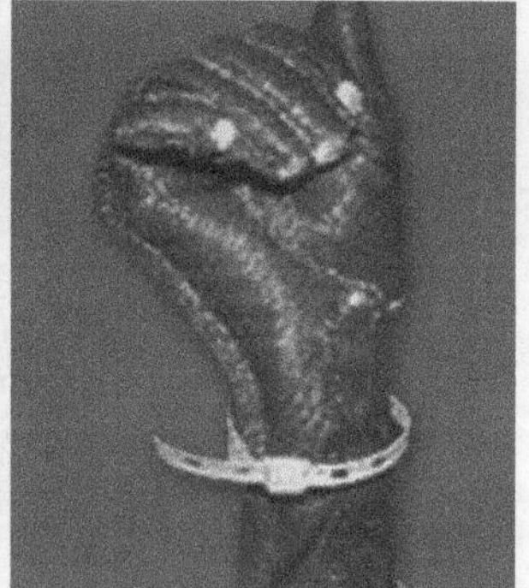

Ideal splinting position for burnt hand: Proper functional positioning for splinting of serious hand burns is the metacarpophalangeal joints are kept at 80–90° of flexion, the interphalangeal joints in extension, the wrist is at 35–45° of extension, and the first web space is open.

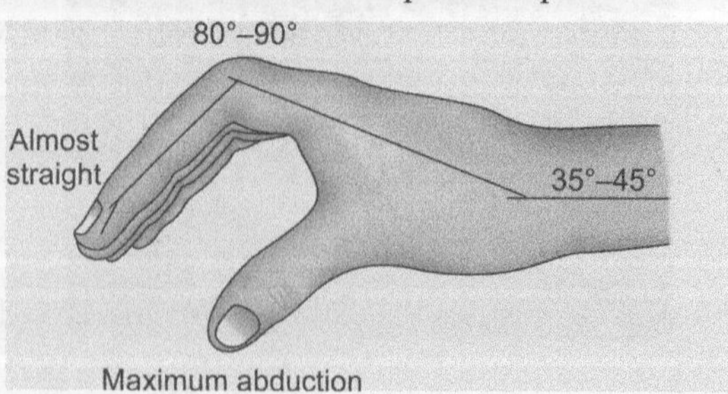

Types of Hand Splints

Functional hand position confirmer splint with wrist and forearm support.

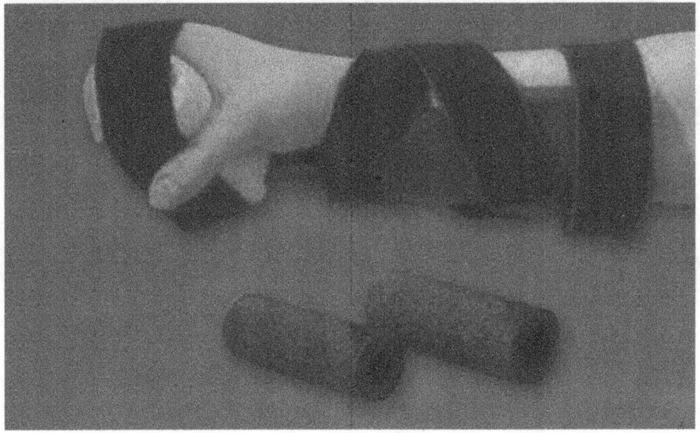

Resting pan cake splint with stabilizer straps for thumb in near opposition.

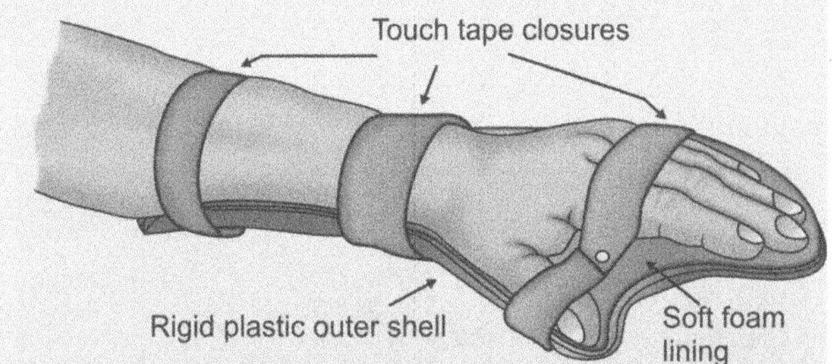

Functional hand position confirmer splint with thumb web spacer (c-bar).

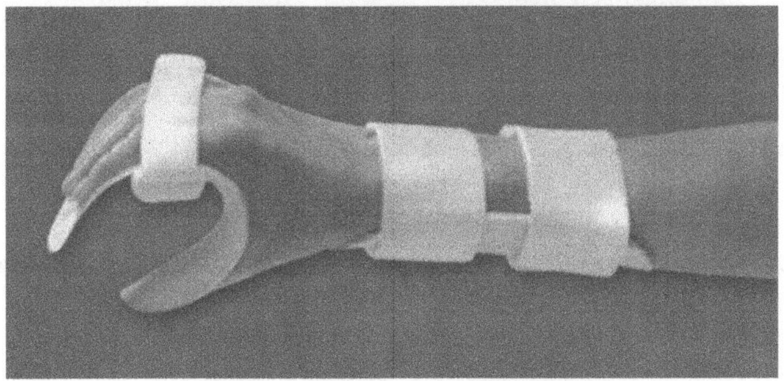

Digital gutter splint—single digit volar splint, clamp type and multiple digit kit.

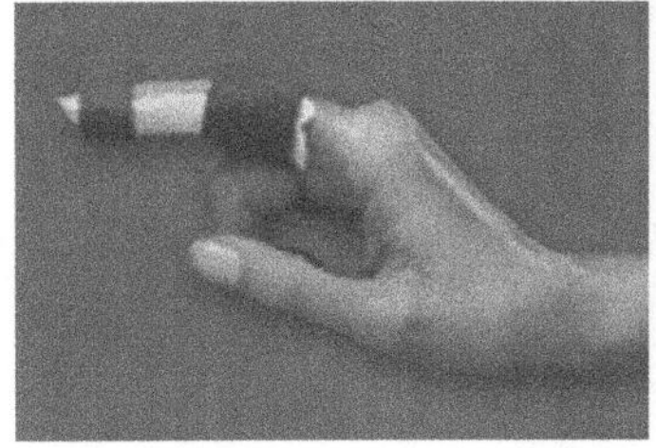
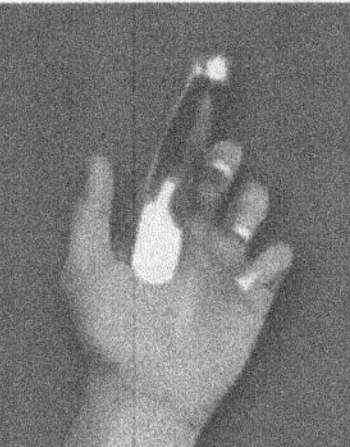
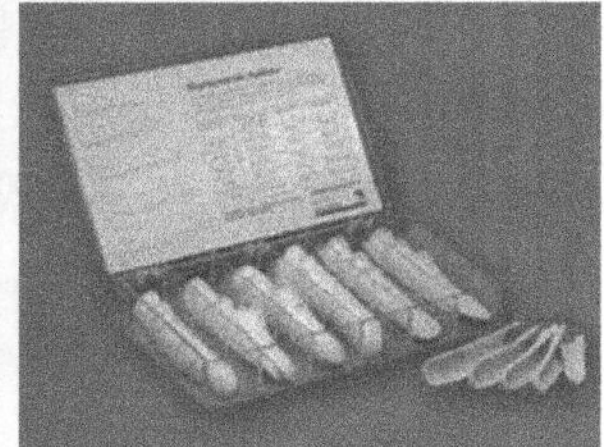

Advanced model

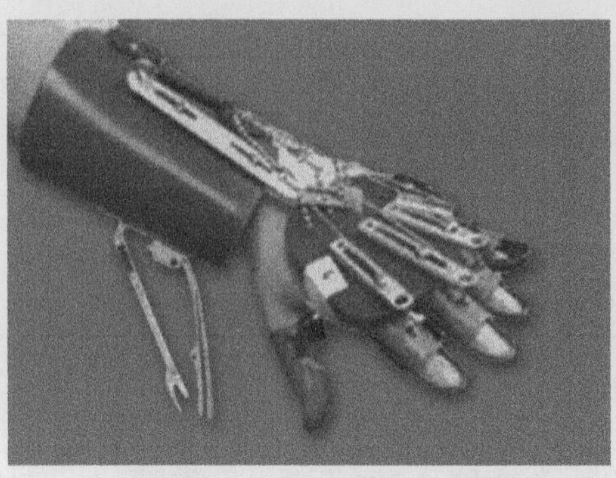

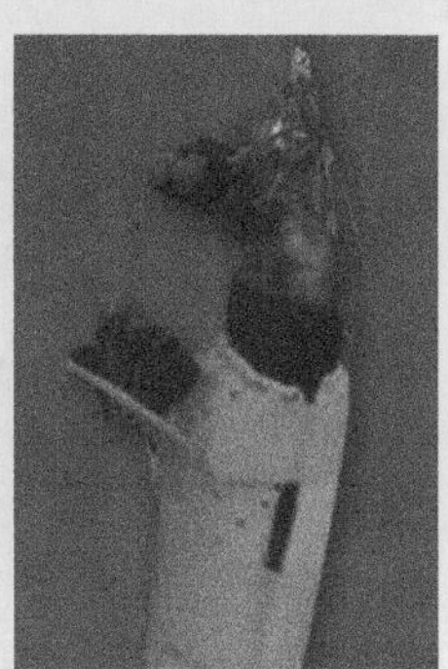

Dynamic wrist and hand splints—provides MCP/IP joint flexion/extension splints, thumb outrigger, knuckle benders and spring loaded flexion/extension.

Special considerations for finger joints—try to maintain angle of pull at 90°.

Hip

3-point extension hip/knee splint—prevents hip knee contracture.

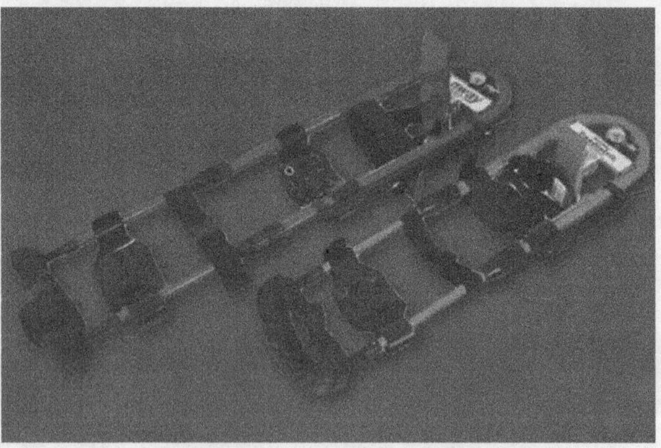

Knee

Static posterior knee conformer splint with pneumatic compression.

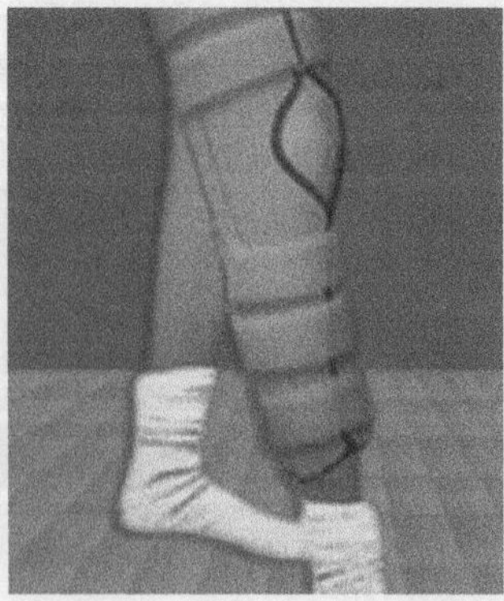

Ankle/Foot

Compression burn garment for leg.

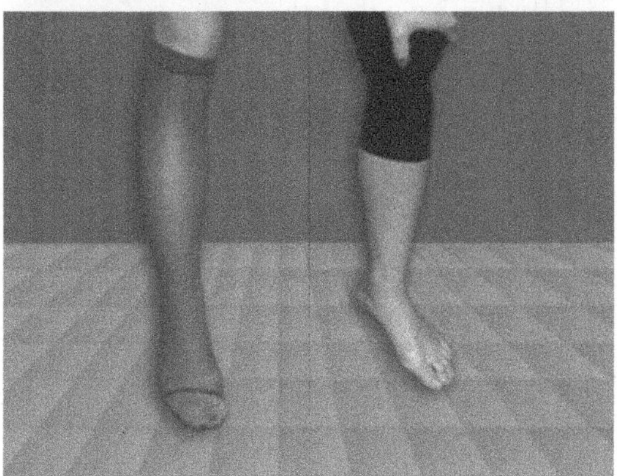

Static pneumatic AFO—A pneumatic splint that provides comfort, compression and security through circumferential compression and immobilization. Rocker Bottom Sole assists in gait, transferring weight from heel to toe while walking. Contoured spatula stirrups anatomically conforms to and immobilizes lower leg and ankle comfortably.

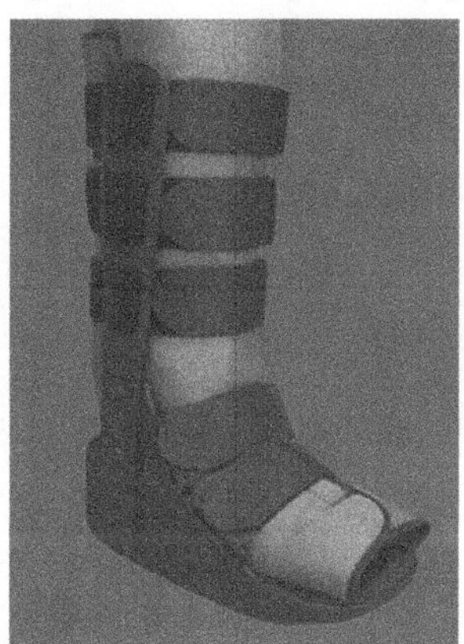

Static molded AFO shoe inserts

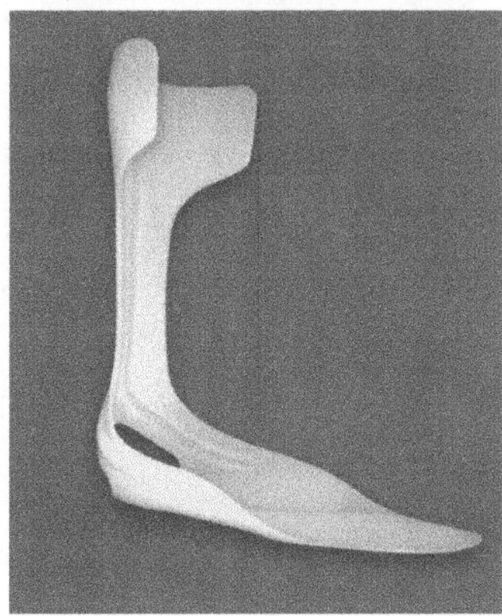

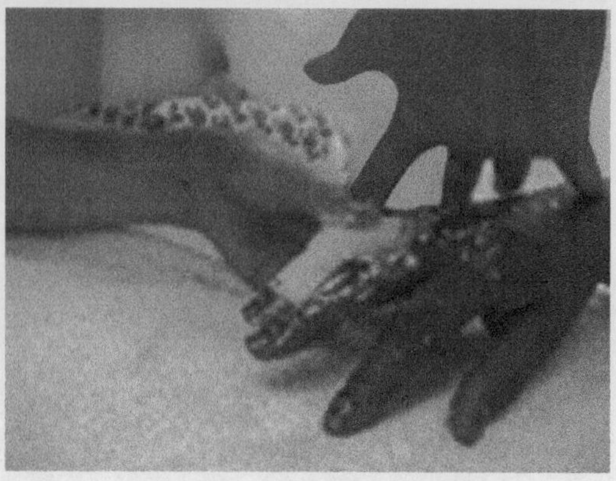

Serial Plastering

Serial plastering of fingers with flexion contracture

- Provides a prolong sustained stretch
- A fast, relatively inexpensive method of correcting burn scar contractures
- Flexion contractures of over 30° respond well to casting
- Provides circumferential evenly distributed pressure
- It offers a successful alternative to dynamic splinting when patient compliance is an issue, i.e. in pediatric cases.

ANNEXURE 6.2

TYPES OF GRAFT

Accordion graft: A full-thickness skin graft in which slits have been made so that it may be stretched to cover a larger area.

Arteriovenous graft: An arteriovenous fistula consisting of a venous autograft or xenograft or a synthetic tube grafted onto the artery and vein.

Avascular graft: A graft of tissue in which not even transient vascularization is achieved.

Blair-Brown graft: A split-skin graft of intermediate thickness.

Bone graft: A piece of bone used to take the place of a removed bone or bony defect.

Cable graft: A nerve graft made up of several sections of nerve in the manner of a cable.

Coronary artery bypass graft (CABG) see under bypass surgery of the heart.

Delayed graft: A skin graft sutured back into its bed and subsequently shifted to a new recipient site.

Dermal graft: Skin from which epidermis and subcutaneous fat have been removed; used instead of fascia in various plastic procedures.

Fascia graft: One taken from the fascia lata or the lumbar fascia.

Fascicular graft: A nerve graft in which bundles of nerve fibers are approximated and sutured separately.

Full-thickness graft: A skin graft consisting of the full thickness of the skin, with little or none of the subcutaneous tissue.

Heterodermic graft: A skin graft taken from a donor of another species.

Krause-Wolfe graft: Full thickness graft.

Lamellar graft: Replacement of the superficial layers of an opaque cornea by a thin layer of clear cornea from a donor eye.

Nerve graft: Replacement of an area of defective nerve with a segment from a sound one.

Omental grafts: Free or attached segments of omentum used to cover suture lines following gastrointestinal or colonic surgery.

Pedicle graft: A tube soft tissue with intact skin cover raised on the abdomen and transferred surgically to remote areas in stages.

Penetrating graft: A full-thickness corneal transplant.

Periosteal graft: A piece of periosteum to cover a denuded bone.

Pinch graft: A piece of skin graft about 14 inch in diameter, obtained by elevating the skin with a needle and slicing it off with a knife.

Sieve graft: A skin graft from which tiny circular islands of skin are removed so that a larger denuded area can be covered, the sieve-like portion being placed over one area, and the individual islands over surrounding or other denuded areas.

Split-skin graft: A skin graft consisting of only superficial portion of the skin thickness.

Thick-split skin graft: A skin graft cut in pieces, often including about two-thirds of the full thickness of the skin.

White graft: A graft devoid of blood supply.

(*Courtesy:* Dorland's Medical Dictionary for Health Consumers. © 2007 by Saunders, an imprint of Elsevier, Inc. All rights reserved).

Chapter

Physiotherapy in Women's Health—Obstetrics and Gynecology

INTRODUCTION

The woman's body is wonderfully complex and delicate. However, multiple roles as the mother, daughter, wife, homemaker, wage earner can be physically demanding and mentally taxing for women. A woman might share some common health risks with men, but because of their special reproductive role, they are also at risk of some distinctly female disorders.

Women's health broadly refers to health issues specific to human female anatomy and physiology. Disorders in women often relate to female reproductive organs, breasts and to conditions caused by abnormal secretion of female hormones.

Study of the normal female reproductive function such as menstruation, contraception, pregnancy and childbirth is collectively known as Obstetrics, whereas, various diseases of the female reproductive organs, including cancer of the uterus and ovary, are dealt with by the clinical specialty of Gynecology.

Beyond this, women's health also relates to significant biological differences between men and women in rates of susceptibility, symptoms and response to treatment in many major areas of health, such as heart disease, malnutrition and bone health.

Current knowledge emphasizes that regular physical activity may hold the key to prevent many of the disorders related to woman's health. It only takes a little more than 10 minutes of physical activity a day to start seeing and feeling the improvements, and to live longer, healthy life. Physical activity in the form of supervised exercises under the guidance of a specialist physio is invaluable in pregnancy, after childbirth and in postoperative states of gynecological surgeries. Therapeutic modalities like massage, exercises, deep heat, LASER, electromagnetic fields and ultrasonic energy have wide applications in preventing and assisting the recovery in various obstetrics complications and gynecological disorders. The following chapter focuses on several common obstetric complications and gynecological disorders that may be treated successfully by using physical modalities is a complementary measure to medical and surgical treatment. The following chapter deals with some common gynecological disorders normally encountered by physiotherapists in their clinical practice.

PELVIC INFLAMMATORY DISEASES (PID)

Pelvic inflammatory diseases (PID) are commonly caused by infection of the woman's reproductive organs. Infection spreads upward from the vagina to the cervix on to the uterus, fallopian tubes, ovaries and surrounding structures (Fig 7.1).

Some of these conditions are also referred to as:

- *Cervicitis:* Inflammation of the cervix
- *Salpingitis:* Inflammation of the fallopian tubes
- *Endometritis:* Inflammation present in the inner lining of the uterus
- *Peritonitis:* Inflammation of the peritoneum, the membrane that lines the abdominal cavity and covers most of the abdominal organs.

Causes

All of these conditions may be considered as individual diseases but most clinicians group them together as variations of PID, especially if they are caused by infection of either *Chlamydia trachomatis* or *Neisseria gonorrhoeae.* Although PID can occur at any age, sexually active adolescent females and women younger than 35 years are most suceptible to PID.

Pelvic inflammatory diseases (PID) can cause a wide variety of symptoms. Some women can be very ill and have severe pain and fever, while others may have no symptoms at all. Thus, PID is not always easy to diagnose and it is important for women between 15–35 to be screened by a specilist regularly, even if they do not have any risk factors or manifest symptoms of PID.

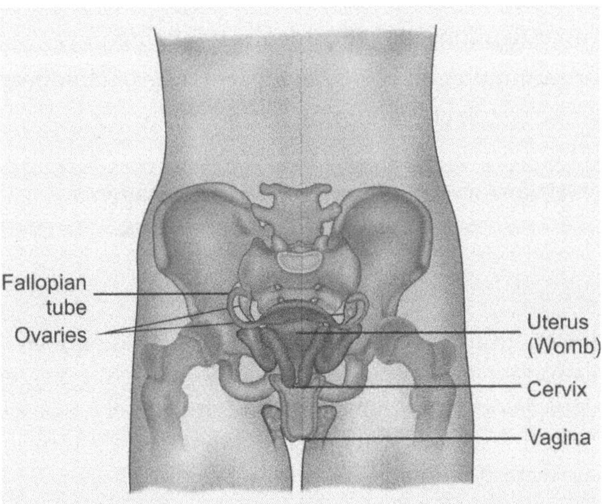

Fig. 7.1: Organs commonly affected by PID

Symptoms of Pelvic Inflammatory Disease

If a woman has PID, she may have any or all of these symptoms:

- Abdominal pain—especially lower abdominal pain or tenderness
- Low back pain
- Abnormal menstrual bleeding
- Unusually heavy vaginal discharges with/without foul odor
- Painful urination
- Painful sexual intercourse.

Pelvic inflammatory diseases (PID) symptoms may be worse at the end of a menstrual cycle and during several days thereafter.

Given the long-term complications PID can cause, such as infertility and ectopic pregnancy, it is recommended that females seek immediate medical attention if they have any of the above symptoms.

Exams and Tests

A health care practitioner usually can diagnose PID by taking the individual's medical history, doing a physical exam, and ordering appropriate tests.

Physical exam findings in PID often include the following:

- Persistent fever—a temperature greater than 101°F (38.3°C)
- Abnormal vaginal discharge
- Lower abdominal and sacral tenderness
- Tenderness when the cervix is moved during a bimanual or speculum exam
- Tenderness in uterus and ovaries.

Laboratory investigations may include the following:

- A urine or serum pregnancy test if the female is of childbearing age
- Urine routine test to check for pus cells
- TC, DC, ESR
- Cervical PAP smear cultures to detect infective agents
- HIV test.

IMAGING

A pelvic ultrasonogram can be an important tool in diagnosing complications such as tubo-ovarian abscesses, ovarian torsion, cysts, endometrial thickening and ectopic pregnancy. Although unlikely to occur in pregnancy, PID is the most commonly missed diagnosis in ectopic pregnancies and can occur during the first 12 weeks of pregnancy.

EXPLORATORY LAPAROSCOPIC SURGERY

A gynecologist can insert a metal probe with a camera and a light source attached to the tip, through small surgical incisions in and around the lower abdomen to view the reproductive organs and evaluate whether inflammation or adhesion is present. The abdomen is distended by pumping in air so that closely packed visceral organs can be separated from one another for visual inspection. If the surgeon feels the defects are small enough for surgical correction it is done through the laparoscope, using microsurgical instruments, in the same sitting. Alternatively the surgeon may use surgical hard LASER to burn adhesions and patches of endometrial tissue growing outside the uterus. Such surgeries are minimally invasive, cause minimal complications and require very short hospital stay (Fig. 7.2).

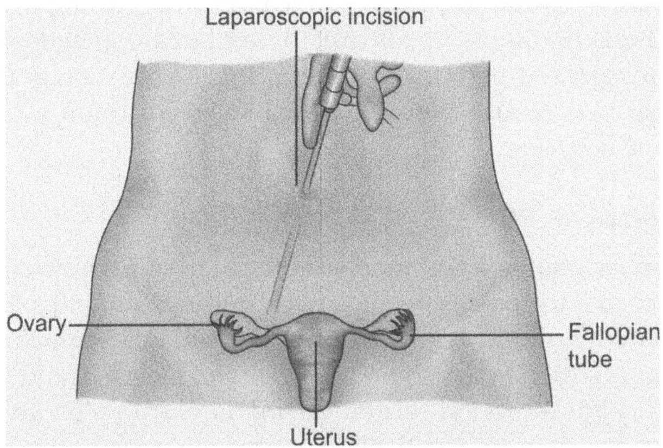

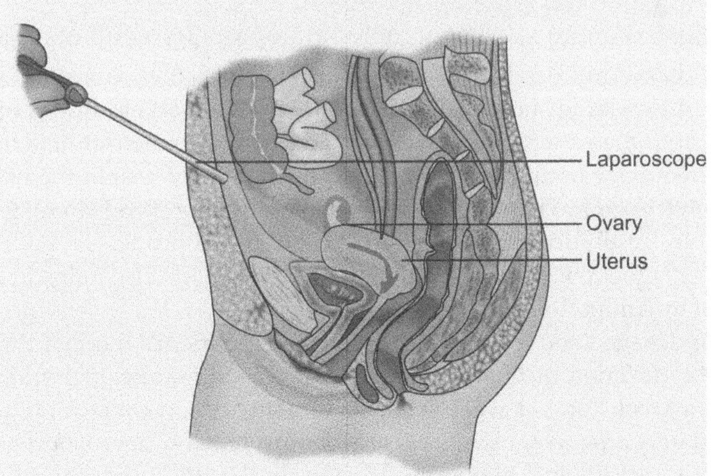

Fig. 7.2: Laparoscopic surgery of the pelvis—used for visual confirmation of a disorder such as adhesion, tumor and for microsurgical or LASER ablation of the diseased tissue

MEDICAL TREATMENT OF PELVIC INFLAMMATORY DISEASE

An antibiotic therapy for PID should be started as soon as the diagnosis is made. Pain medication may be given if the patient needs them.

Because samples of the bacteria from the upper genital tract are difficult to obtain and because many different organisms may be responsible for PID, especially if it is not the person's first occurrence, the doctor will usually prescribe at least two antibiotics at the same time that are effective against a wide range of infectious bacteria. The duration of treatments varies according to the severity of the disease. Symptoms may resolve before the infection is fully cured and even if the person may feel much better, they should still finish taking all the antibiotics prescribed.

Surgery

Untreated PID can cause chronic pelvic pain and scarring in about some women. These conditions are difficult to treat but are sometimes improved with laparoscopic surgery for manual or LASER ablation of pelvic adhesions. Surgery may also be needed to remove or drain a tubo-ovarian abscess if present (Fig. 7.2).

Physiotherapy in PID

Chronic pelvic pain is a common complication of PID. Physiotherapy is recommended if the pain is persistant for at least six months duration and is severe enough to impact a woman's functioning. The pain may occur both during and/or apart from the menstrual period and are usually caused by pelvic adhesion related disorders. Such pain may refer from their point of origin to sacral plate, groin, inner or posterior aspect of thigh, usually along the dermatomes of S 1–3.

Chronic PID related low back pain may benefit from application of pelvic diathermy. Pelvic diathermy is applied with the contraplaner placement of two large short-wave diathermy (SWD) pad electrodes over the lower abdomen and under lower back, creating a condensor field to apply high frequency oscillating current, to generate deep heat in the tissues of the pelvic region. The deep heat helps in increasing blood circulation and promotes resolution of chronic inflammation and provides relief of pain. Electromagnetic field generated between SWD pads also helps in resolution of inflammation and tissue healing.

The dosage should be adjusted as per the patient's thermal threshold and the duration of treatment should be 15–30 minutes per sitting, 2–3 times a week for 3–4 weeks. The treatment should preferrably to start immidately after a menstrual cycle and must end 5–7 days before onset of the next cycle. Pelvic diathermy is contraindicated during the menstrual cycle. This is most suitable when the pain and tenderness is diffuse in nature.

Alternatively, long-wave diathermy (LWD) is very effective in managing focal tenderness of reproductive organs. This modality combines the localization of ultrasound therapy with deep thermal effect of SWD. The indifferent electrode is placed under the sacrum and the hand probe is moved in concentric circles ov er the tender area with minimum pressure but firm contact. Average dosage is level V and the duration of application is 10–15 minutes, 2–3 days a week, for 3–4 weeks.

In application of both SWD and LWD the therapist must be cautious regarding loss of thermal sensation, acute infection, presence of an IUD or frequent spotting in between periods. These are absolute contraindications for application of pelvic diathermy.

Transcutaneous electrical nerve stimulation (TENS), applied in burst mode, at maximum intensity tolerated by the patient, can be applied over the representative dermatomes showing referral of pain. The passive electrode is placed over the sacrum and the active electrode over the painful dermatome. A number of channels may be used to cover the entire area of referral. The duration of treatment can be 20–30 minutes in a sitting. However, the duration can be as high as eight hours if the patient can be provided with a small portable TENS unit and trained to use it as a personal pain managing device. The primary advantage of TENS is that one can use this device even during menstruation and in presence of IUD or infection and that the treatment can be continued by the patient at home or during work.

Prevention

Therapists play an important role in counseling the patient of PID. The following steps may be taken to avoid or to keep PID from becoming worse:

- Practice safe sex, use condoms. Use only water-based lubricants with condoms.
- IUD—recently inserted intrauterine devices (IUDs) increases the risk of getting PID. Screening by a specilist must be done every three months.
- Have one sexual partner to reduce the chance of infections.
- General cleanliness—douches are not recommended; the vagina cleans itself naturally. Regular showers and baths are enough to keep the body clean. Wipe or wash from front to back after a bowel movement. This keeps bacteria away from entering the vagina.

PELVIC ADHESION RELATED DISORDERS (PARD)

Pelvic adhesions are scar tissue which forms between visceral organs and their surrounding tissues. In women, endometriosis can cause local inflammation, leading to adhesions. Adhesions may also form as a result of endometrial tissue bleeding into the visceral membrane causing

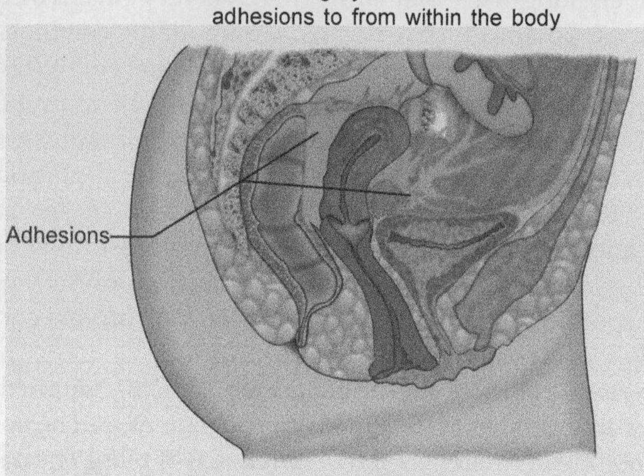

Fig. 7.3: Pelvic adhesions

inflammation, and as this "heal", scar tissue forms. Adhesions may also form as a result of infection.

In the female pelvis, adhesions may cause a number of problems including infertility, painful intercourse and chronic pelvic pain. Adhesions involving the bowel can cause bowel obstruction or blockage. They are also the main cause of intestinal or urinary tract obstruction and can be one of the major factors in female infertility due to obstruction of fallopian tubes (Fig. 7.3).

Visceral organs are most sensitive to stretching and distension, causing pain. Adhesions are believed to cause pelvic pain by tethering organs and tissues and causing traction on nerves. It is, however, important to understand, that not all adhesions cause pain, they may simply interfere with the normal function of the gut, bladder, bowel, ovary and fallopian tube.

Management of Pelvic Adhesions

It is now accepted that surgical excision of adhesions provides relief from pain. The problem is that such excision involves surgical trauma and the adhesions almost always recur. Surgeons are therefore reluctant to perform surgical excision and prefer LASER ablation of adhesions through laparoscopy (Fig. 7.2).

Other nonsurgical treatments include trigger point injections, drug treatments, physical therapies, and dietary changes.

Physiotherapy in PARD

Over the years, various therapeutic methods have been tested. The use of vibration, manipulation and low dose laser are well-established in the field of gynecological physiotherapy.

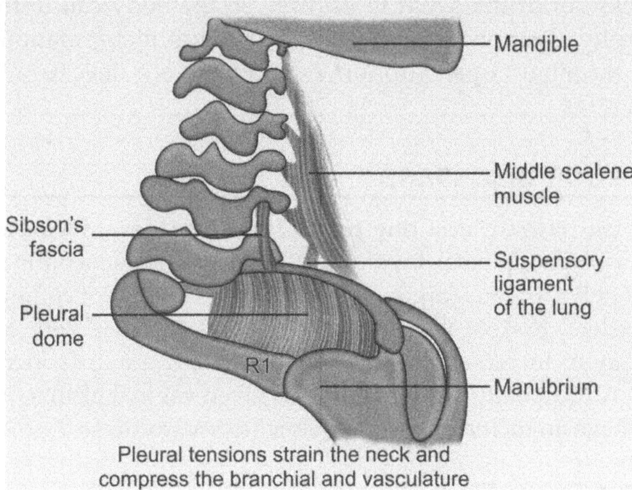

Fig. 7.6: Pleural dome suspension mechanism

structure contains highly variable proportions of collagen, elastin, smooth muscle fiber and striated muscle fiber. This variability has led to this same structure to be named a fascia, ligament or muscle in different texts. Contractures and adhesions of the pleura are common, almost considered a 'normal' feature of aging. Pleural restrictions are easily visible during surgery or dissection. We take more than 20,000 breaths per day. If there are pleural adhesions and contractures, these 20,000 aberrant breaths are a fine cause for repetitive strain injuries. Since the lungs are suspended from the cervical vertebrae, this puts a tremendous strain on the neck. The cervical paraspinal musculature becomes tight in its attempt to resist this pull (Fig. 7.6).[2]

Scalene muscles which are not only tight but also pulled down is a sign of strong pleural restrictions. Freeing the pleura often quickly relieves neck strain and improves head position. The brachial plexus passes adjacent to or through the middle scalene and pleural pull on the middle scalene routinely impinge on these nerves supplying the arm and hand. The blood vessels supplying the arm and hand passes as a bundle with the brachial nerves and are similarly compromised by pleural restrictions transferred to the scalene by the suspensor ligament of the lungs. History of respiratory illness is therefore a documented risk factor for thoracic inlet syndrome.[2]

Incorporating visceral manipulation into structural integration provides the keys to fuller and more efficient core/sleeve integration. The manipulative strategies used for visceral manipulation were originally developed by Osteopaths for use on fascia and ligaments. Now we physiotherapists can learn these efficient, low force methods in visceral manipulation classes and then apply them to other connective tissue as well. The assessment methods taught with visceral manipulation allow us to quickly prioritize what to do first, so the body can unfold easily and naturally. Caution: Do not attempt visceral manipulation without thorough training. Organ support membranes are delicate and highly reactive tissues.

PELVIC FLOOR DISORDERS

Most women have at least one pelvic floor disorder. Involuntary urine loss (urinary incontinence), involuntary fecal loss (fecal incontinence), and shifting of pelvic organs (organ prolapse) are examples of common pelvic floor disorders. Risk of pelvic floor disorders increase with advancing age in women. Increased weight was another factor that increases the incidence. Additionally, women that had given vaginal birth to more than one child have an increased risk of pelvic floor disorders.

How do the Pelvic Floor Muscles Work?

The thin pelvic floor muscles typically receive little attention during anatomy classes and in textbooks. Because dissection of these muscles is tedious, most students and clinicians tend to focus their attention on other obvious and physiologically active pelvic organs.

Two layers of muscles exist in the pelvic floor: the superficial urogenital diaphragm consisting of *bulbocavernosus, iliocavernosus,* and *transverses perinea muscles*; the *deep levator ani group* consisting of *pubococcygeus, iliococcygeus,* and *coccygeus muscles* (Fig. 7.7).

In quadrupeds, the levator ani group is the tail-wagging muscles. In bipedal mammals, however, the levator ani group provides support to pelvic and intra-abdominal organs against gravity in an upright posture. That's why humans and other apes do not have tails. The thin skeletal muscles of the levator ani group function much like the diaphragm in that both are under voluntary and involuntary control. Voluntary control of the muscles permits control of bladder and bowel function or insertional sex

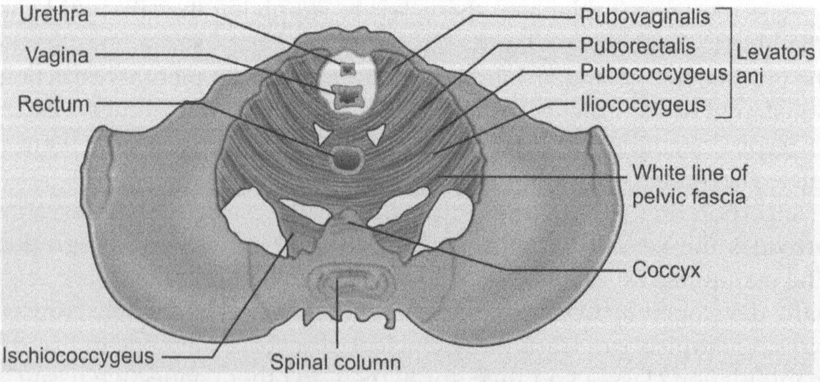

Fig. 7.7: The pelvic floor

at socially acceptable moments. On the other hand, involuntary—or automatic—activation of these muscles occurs when intra-abdominal pressure increases while standing, coughing, bouncing, etc. or in response to anxiety or stress. Weakness or damage to the muscles can occur due to nerve injury or rupture during vaginal delivery. Since these skeletal muscles are under voluntary control, conditioning regimens through Kegel's exercises, pelvic floor stimulation, etc. can strengthen weak muscles and restore function.

Urinary Incontinence

Words used to describe bladder control problems include the following:

- *Urgency:* The feeling of having to urinate very soon
- *Hesitancy:* When trying to urinate, difficulty getting a urine stream going
- *Frequency:* Feeling that you have to urinate often
- *Dysuria:* Pain with urination
- *Hematuria:* Visible blood in the urine, or pinkish urine
- *Nocturia:* Urination at night (having to wake up to urinate)
- *Dribbling:* Continuing to drip or dribble urine after finishing urination
- *Straining:* Having to strain or bear down on the external sphincter to urinate.

The exact number of people with incontinence is not known, but the total number of people affected may be far greater than current estimates. Though these numbers are staggering, about half of incontinent patients do not tell their physician or family members of their problem, because most of these individuals assume nothing can be done for incontinence or feel that leakage is a normal part of aging.

For millions, incontinence is not just a medical problem. It is a problem that also affects their emotional, psychological, and social well-being. Many people are afraid to participate in normal daily activities that might take them too far from a toilet. So it is particularly important to note that the great majority of incontinence causes can be treated successfully.

Pelvic Anatomy

The bladder stores urine. When you urinate, the bladder muscle contract to squeeze the urine out. Urine leaves the body through the urethra. The urethra is kept closed by the sphincter muscles squeezing like rubber bands. The pelvic floor muscles are part of this sphincter mechanism and help keep the urethra closed. Once the bladder becomes full, the brain is signaled that you need to get to a bathroom. When the toilet is reached, the brain signals the sphincter and pelvic floor muscles to relax, allowing urine to pass out through the urethra. The bladder tightens up, allowing the urine to flow out of it.

Normal Bladder Control

With normal bladder control one urinates only when one needs or want to. Good bladder control means that all parts of the system must work in sync. Urinary control relies on the finely coordinated activities of the smooth muscle tissue of the urethra and bladder, skeletal muscles of the pelvic floor, voluntary inhibition, and the autonomic nervous system. To control bladder function correctly following must occur in sequence (Fig. 7.8).

- The pelvic floor muscles must hold up the urethra and bladder
- The urethra must be open and shut by the sphincter muscles
- The bladder and pelvic floor muscles must be controlled by the nerves.

Urinary incontinence can result from anatomic, physiologic, or pathologic (disease) factors. Congenital and acquired disorders of muscle innervation (e.g., ALS, spina bifida, multiple sclerosis) may also cause inadequate urinary storage or control eventually.

Causes of acute or temporary incontinence are childbirth, limited mobility, side effect of medication, urinary tract infection or constipation.

Causes of chronic or longstanding incontinence are congenital defects, bladder muscle weakness, blocked urethra due to benign prostate hyperplasia in male, tumor, etc. brain or spinal cord injury, peripheral nerve disorders and most commonly pelvic floor muscle weakness.

Some common causes of incontinence are the following:

- *Smoking*: Known to irritate the bladder
- *Obesity:* Excess body fat can reduce muscle tone, including the pelvic floor muscles
- *Chronic constipation:* Straining at bowel can weaken the pelvic floor muscles
- *Diabetes:* Damage nerves and reduces sensation

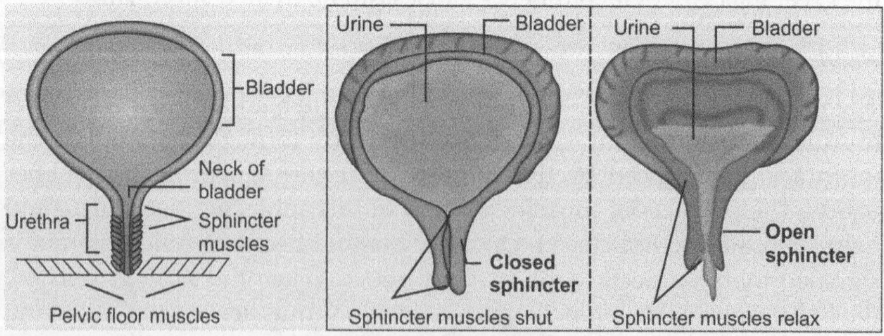

Fig. 7.8: Normal micturition

- *Spinal cord injury:* Signals between the bladder and the brain travel via the spinal cord. Damage to the cord can interrupt those signals, disrupting bladder function
- *Disability or impaired mobility:* People who have diseases such as arthritis, which make walking painful or slow, may have "accidents" before they can reach a toilet. Similarly, people who are permanently or temporarily confined to a bed or a wheelchair often have problems because of their inability to get to a toilet easily
- *Neurologic:* Conditions such as stroke, multiple sclerosis, muscular dystrophy, polio, Alzheimer disease or Parkinson disease can cause incontinence. The problem can be a direct result of a disrupted nervous system or an indirect result of having restricted movement
- *Pregnancy:* Pregnant women have problems controlling their bladder during pregnancy, which stops after delivery. Risk factors for postpartum incontinence include vaginal delivery, long second stage of labor, i.e. the time after the cervix is fully dilated, or after episiotomy—an incision to enlarge the vaginal opening during delivery, or exposure to oxytocin—a hormone that is given to start or speed up labor
- *Hysterectomy:* Women who have had a hysterectomy may have incontinence later in life.

Types of Urinary Incontinence

There are four types of urinary incontinence. A brief explanation of each follows:

Stress Incontinence

Stress incontinence is the most common type of leakage encountered. Stress incontinence is the loss of urine that occurs with any maneuver that increases intra-abdominal pressure, such as coughing, sneezing, lifting, laughing, during intercourse and changing position. This typically occurs in women that experience loss of support in the anterior vaginal wall leading to dropping of the bladder neck and urethra during increases in abdominal pressure. Most investigators feel that the descent of the bladder neck and urethra out of the normal intra-abdominal position into the pelvis prevents closure of these structures during times when pressure is exerted on the bladder body. Some feel that the change in the angle of the bladder neck and urethra are responsible for the leakage. Stress incontinence can occur in men as well, often seen following transurethral prostate surgery.

Urge Incontinence

Leakage that occurs when there is a sudden uncontrollable need to urinate is called urge incontinence. With urge incontinence, the bladder contracts and squeezes out urine involuntarily. Sometimes a large amount of urine is released. The bladder muscle in many of these patients is overactive and usually provides very little warning to the patient that urination is eminent. With urge incontinence it is often necessary to use a bathroom as frequently as every two hours, and bed-wetting is common. Urge incontinence often occurs in those people with spinal cord injuries, multiple sclerosis, strokes, or diseases of the spinal cord. Urge incontinence may occur in male patients with an obstructing prostate. Women with loss of tone to the vaginal wall, bladder and urethra also develop urge incontinence.

Overflow Incontinence

Overflow incontinence occurs when the bladder is inefficiently emptied, leaving large amounts of urine in the bladder. As the volume increases, the resistance provided by the bladder, neck and urethra may be overcome, and urine loss may occur. This type of incontinence is a constant dripping of urine. It's caused by an overfilled bladder. This pattern is common in diabetics, male patients with enlarged prostates, urethral structures and in some patients with spinal cord injuries. In some cases this may be caused by medications taken for other conditions.

Functional Incontinence

This type of incontinence occurs when one has normal urine control but have trouble getting to the bathroom in time. Functional incontinence is common in disabled or demented patients and is the most common type of incontinence in the nursing home setting. Patients with functional incontinence have normal orderly bladder activity but are unable to respond to this signal, due to immobility or impaired mental status. As a consequence, they become incontinent unless they are prompted to void on a schedule.

Diagnosis

Evaluation of the incontinent patient will focus on categorizing the type of incontinence being experienced. An urination diary should be used to note urination patterns recording the times one urinates and the amounts of urine one produces. With this understanding, specific therapy can be recommended that is individualized to each patient.

One needs to physically examine the patient for signs of medical conditions causing incontinence, such as tumors that block the urinary tract, stool impaction, and poor reflexes or sensations, which may be evidence of a nerve-related cause. The vaginal exam can reveal anatomic causes, such as a dropped bladder (cystocele), a prolapsed uterus or structural abnormalities in the urethra. A rectal exam is sometimes necessary to assess the sphincter tone and possible fecal backup.

Common tests to detect incontinence are:

- *Stress test:* One relaxes and then coughs vigorously as the one watches for loss of urine.
- *Urinalysis:* Urine is tested for evidence of infection, urinary stones, or other contributing causes.
- *Ultrasound:* Sound waves are used to "see" the kidneys, ureters, bladder, and urethra.
- *Post-void residual measurement:* This measures how well the patient is able to empty the bladder when or how much urine is left in the bladder after urinating. This is done for people whose symptoms suggest overflow incontinence. The measurement can be done in either of two ways, either with an ultrasound or a catheter.
- *Cystoscopy:* A thin tube with a tiny camera is inserted in the urethra and used to see the urethra and bladder. This is so the doctor can look for any abnormalities in the bladder and lower urinary tract.
- *Urodynamics:* Various techniques measure pressure in the bladder and the flow of urine. This testing involves inserting a small tube into the bladder and examining the bladder and urethral sphincter function.

Treatment

Treatment options are multiple and based on the type of incontinence:

1. *Stress incontinence* is urine loss during physical activity that increases abdominal pressure, e.g. coughing, sneezing, laughing. Treatment options include:
   - Nonsurgical treatments are electrical stimulation of pelvic floor muscles, biofeedback, pelvic floor muscle exercises
   - Injectable collagen
   - Medications
   - Surgical treatments (TVT slings).

   The primary aim of treatment in case of stress incontinence is strengthening of the pelvic floor muscles, which helps support the bladder neck and the urethra and prevents it from incomplete closure (Fig. 7.9).
2. *Urge incontinence,* also called detrusor instability, is urine loss with urgent need to void and involuntary bladder contraction. Treatment options include:
   - Nonsurgical treatments are electrical stimulation of pelvic floor muscles, biofeedback
   - Medications
   - Surgical treatments.
3. *Overflow incontinence* is constant dribbling of urine; bladder never completely empties. Treatment options include:
   - Medications
   - Intermittent self-catheterization
   - Surgery to relieve prostatic obstruction.

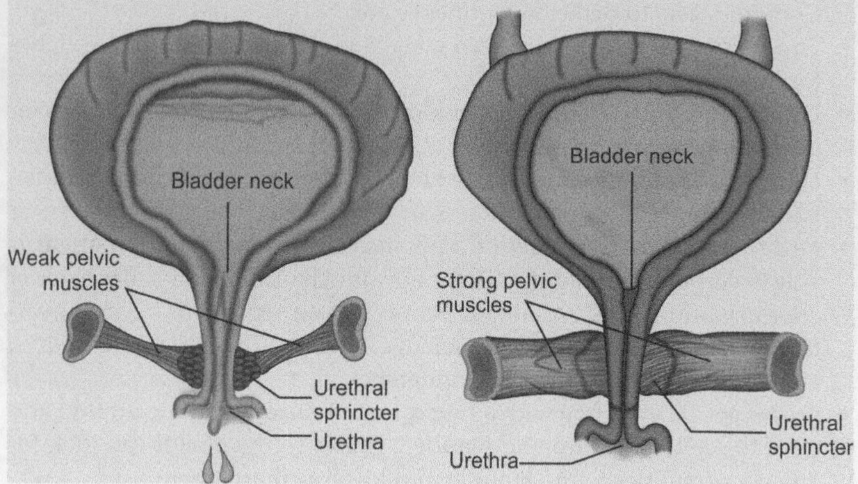

Fig. 7.9: Role of pelvic floor muscles in controlling stress incontinence

4. *Functional incontinence* is caused by inability of an individual to reach toilet in time due to either physical or mental impairment. Since very little can be done to address the root cause, under such circumstances there is only preventive action to be taken, such as using a diaper or condom catheter with urine bag.

Noninvasive Treatment Methods

Behavioral modifications are one of the first line treatment options for all incontinence and are the least invasive. These include:

- *Bladder training:* Teaches people to resist the urge to void and gradually expand the intervals between voiding.
- *Toileting assistance:* Uses routine or scheduled toileting, habit training schedules, and prompted voiding to empty the bladder regularly to prevent leaking.
- *Vaginal weight training:* Small weights are held within the vagina by tightening the vaginal muscles. Should be performed for 15 minutes, twice daily, for 4 to 6 weeks.
- *Biofeedback:* Used in conjunction with Kegel's exercises, biofeedback helps people gain awareness and control of their pelvic muscles.
- *Pelvic floor electrical stimulation:* Mild electrical pulses stimulate muscle contractions. Should be done in conjunction with biofeedback and Kegel's exercises (Fig 7.10).
- A pessary is a stiff ring that is inserted by a physio or nurse into the vagina, where it presses against the wall of the vagina and the nearby urethra. The pressure helps reposition the urethra, leading to less stress leakage. One should watch for possible vaginal and urinary tract infections if using pessaries.

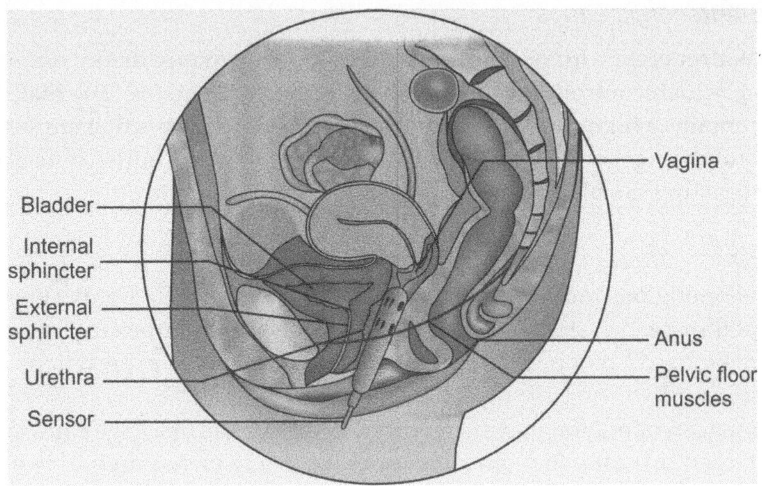

Fig. 7.10: Pelvic floor stimulation—bipolar vaginal sensors/electrodes are used to deliver suitably modulated surged currents or IFT to the sphincters and the pelvic floor muscles

Medical Therapy

Estrogens, given through either oral or vaginal route can increase the tone of urethral muscle by up-regulating the alpha-adrenergic receptors in the surrounding area, and they enhance alpha-adrenergic contractile response of pelvic floor muscles, which helps in urethral support.

Mucosal turgidity of periurethral tissue through proper nourishment enhances urethral mucosal stickiness. The result is an improved mucosal seal effect, which prevents intrinsic sphincter deficiency. Estrogen supplementation appears to be the most effective in postmenopausal women with mild-to-moderate incontinence. Both urge and stress incontinence may benefit from estrogen supplementation.

Anticholinergic Drugs

Anticholinergic drugs increase the amount of urine that the bladder can hold. These drugs also decrease the pressure associated with the urge to urinate, however, it is contraindicated in case of allergy to anticholinergics, poorly controlled narrow-angle glaucoma and bladder or bowel obstruction.

Tricyclic Antidepressants

Historically, these drugs were used to treat major depression; however, they have an additional use in treatment of bladder dysfunction. They facilitate urine storage by decreasing bladder contractility and increasing outlet resistance.

Alpha-Adrenergic Drugs

Alpha-adrenergic drugs mimic actions of the sympathetic nervous system, which controls various involuntary body functions. The bladder neck contains a high concentration of sympathetic receptors that are sensitive to alpha-agonists. Alpha-agonists increase bladder outlet resistance by contracting the bladder neck.

Surgery

Several operations for incontinence exist to treat specific anatomical problems of the organ system of micturition. The decision to use surgery must always be based on an accurate diagnosis and realistic expectations for the surgery.

In men, an operation may be required to relieve the blockage caused by an enlarged prostate. In women, an operation may be required to restore the support of the pelvic floor muscles or to reconstruct or compress the sphincter. Stress incontinence is the most common type of incontinence that is treated with surgery.

TVT (Tension-Free Vaginal Tape)

Tension-free vaginal tape (TVT), is a minimally invasive surgical procedure used to surgically to treat some women with stress urinary incontinence. The procedure can be performed under local or spinal anesthesia and takes only about 30–60 minutes to complete. After anesthesia takes effect, surgeon will insert a mesh tape through a small incision in the vagina. Then the surgeon "weaves" the tape beneath the urethra and pulls the tape up through two tiny punctures in the skin's surface just above the pubic bone or near the creases of the thighs. At the end of the procedure, the surgeon will "snip" the tape, just under the skin's surface, and close the two small incisions. Unlike other procedures, no sutures or anchors are necessary, except for small absorbable sutures to close the small vaginal incision.

The TVT stops urine leakage the way the body was designed to by supporting the urethra. Normally, the urethra is supported by the pelvic floor muscle to maintain a tight seal and prevent involuntary urine loss. In women with stress incontinence, the weakened pelvic floor muscle and connective tissue cannot support the urethra in its normal position. To correct this, a ribbon-like strip of mesh is inserted under the urethra to provide support whenever the patient stresses this area, such as during coughing, sneezing, or walking. This allows the urethra to remain appropriately closed, preventing involuntary urine loss. The unique elastic properties of the TVT prevent the mesh from affecting normal voiding (Source: HP Dietz et al. Mechanical properties of urogynecologic implant materials. International Urogynecology Journal. 0937-3462).

The recovery period following the procedure is short, and patients experience few complications and minimal scarring after surgery and the patient can go back to her routine in just a day or two. It is also clinically proven: 98 percent of women who participated in a study begun seven years ago are still dry, or experience significantly less leakage (Source: Nilsson et al. 7-Year Follow-up on the Tension-free Vaginal Tape (TVT) Procedure; International Urology, IUGA Abstract #116 (89): October 2003).

Although rare, complications associated with the treatment include injury to blood vessels, difficulty urinating, and bladder and bowel injury. Rarely, the tape may be slightly "tight" or "loose". If it is too tight, it may be more difficult to urinate or empty the bladder. If it is too loose there may still be some residual leakage.

Injection Therapy

Injecting material to increase the bulk around the urethra can improve the function of the urethral sphincter and compresses the urethra near the neck of the bladder.

Injectable agents can help women who are not candidates for surgery and have very weak urethral sphincter without urethral hypermobility. Injectable agents also may help men with intrinsic sphincter deficiency that has lasted longer than 1 year.

Injectable materials include collagen—naturally occurring protein found in skin, bone, and connective tissue, fat from the patient's body, and polytetrafluoroethylene (PTFE) or durasphere—both synthetic compounds.

Artificial Sphincter

An artificial urethral sphincter may help patients who are incontinent after surgery for prostate cancer or stress incontinence, trauma victims, and in patients with birth defects in the urinary tract.

The device has three components: A pump, a balloon reservoir, and a cuff that encircles and closes the urethra. All three components are filled with fluid, e.g. saline. The cuff is connected to the pump, which is surgically implanted in the scrotum in men or the labia in women. The pump is activated by squeezing or pressing a button. The fluid in the cuff empties into the reservoir, the urethra opens, and the bladder empties. Fluid from the reservoir returns to the cuff, which again closes the urethra. Possible complications include infection, tissue breakdown, and mechanical failure.

Sacral Nerve Stimulation

Sacral nerve internal stimulation therapy is a reversible treatment for people with urge incontinence caused by overactive bladders who do not respond to behavioral treatments or medication. It is an implanted neurostimulation system that sends mild electrical pulses to the sacral nerve,

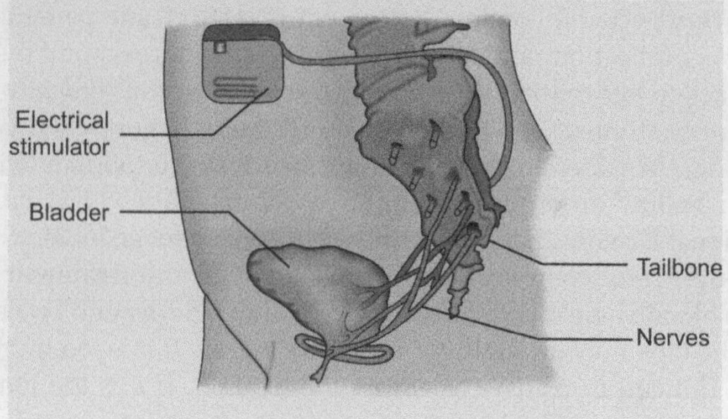

Fig. 7.11: Implanted sacral nerve stimulator

which influences bladder control muscles. Stimulation of this nerve may relieve the symptoms related to urge incontinence (Fig. 7.11).

Prior to doing implantation, the effectiveness of the therapy is tested on an outpatient basis with an external stimulator. For a period of three to five days, the patient records voiding patterns that occur with stimulation. The record is compared to recorded voiding patterns without stimulation. The comparison demonstrates whether the device effectively reduces symptoms. If the test is successful, the patient may choose to have the device implanted.

The procedure requires general anesthesia. A lead is placed near the sacral nerve and is passed under the skin to a neurostimulator, which is about the size of a cigarette lighter. The neurostimulator is placed under the skin in the upper buttock.

Adjustments of pulse duration, frequency and intensity can be made with a remote programming device that sends a radio signal through the skin to the neurostimulator. Another programming device is given to the patient to further adjust the level of stimulation, if necessary. The system can be turned off at any time.

Possible adverse effects of sacral nerve stimulator implant include the following:

- Change in bowel function
- Infection
- Lead movement
- Pain at implant sites
- Unpleasant stimulation or sensation.

Prevention of Incontinence—Tips for the Patients

- Avoid foods and drinks that may irritate the bladder. These include alcohol, caffeine, carbonated drinks, chocolate, citrus fruits, and acidic fruits and juices.

- Do not drink too much fluid. Six to eight cups a day is adequate, more if you are exercising, sweating a lot, or the weather is hot.
- Urinate regularly.
- Do not ignore the urge to urinate or to have a bowel movement.
- If you are overweight, try to get to a healthier weight.
- If necessary, wear absorbent pads to catch urine.
- Maintain proper hygiene. This will help you feel more confident and will prevent odors and skin irritation.
- Do Kegel's exercises: Exercising the muscles of your pelvic floor may benefit women with either stress or urge incontinence.

Pelvic Floor Myalgia

Like all skeletal muscles, pelvic floor muscles are prone to develop painful disorders such as myalgia. Such myalgia in a male may arise from prolonged periods of cycling or motorcycling and manifests as saddle soreness. In a women pelvic floor myalgia may arise from vulvar vestibular inflammation, painful penetrative sex or even chronic constipation. Painful intercourse due to vaginismus can be common manifestation of pelvic floor myalgia. Physical therapy is the recommended treatment for pelvic floor myalgia though the challenge is finding a physical therapist with the necessary experience and sensitivity to treat these patients. However, in recent years, more and more physical therapists have become trained and gained expertise in managing pelvic floor complaints by treating incontinent patients.

The same techniques used in incontinence, to evaluate and strengthen pelvic floor muscles using biofeedback techniques, are also useful in treating hypertonus and vaginismus. Because vulvar vestibulitis often coexists with vaginismus, most research efforts have evaluated these conditions together. In one prospective study, 22 of 28 subjects with vulvar vestibulitis, who were followed for 6 months, responded well to physical therapy and EMG biofeedback.[1] In a randomized trial of treatment options for vulvar vestibulitis, another researcher saw pain significantly diminish among women treated with physical therapy.[3,4]

Vaginal dilators are an alternative approach, particularly when access to a skilled physical therapist is limited. Made of silicone or plastic and available in a variety of sizes, the vaginal dilators enable a woman to gain confidence, knowledge, and awareness of her vagina and pelvic floor muscles in the privacy of her own home (Fig. 7.12).

The goal of vaginal dilator therapy is strictly clinical; to discover what triggers the pelvic floor muscles to go into spasm and to develop strategies to keep the pelvic floor relaxed and soft. With increased knowledge about her body's response, the woman becomes able to gently introduce dilators of progressively larger sizes into the vagina. With this knowledge and confidence, the insertion of dilators becomes comfortable and routine,

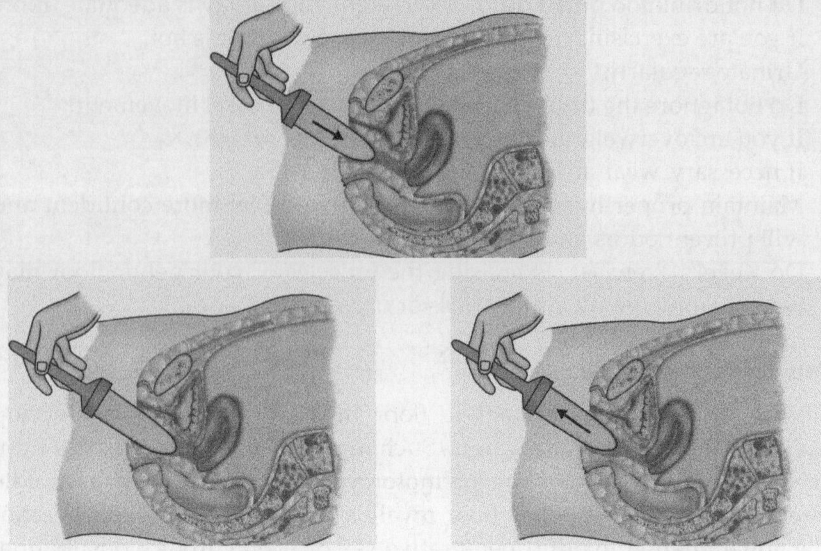

Fig. 7.12: Vaginal dilation—techniques of use; in supine position with hip knee flexed—slowly insert dilator into the vagina as far as it will go

and that skill is then transferred to her sexual activities. When vaginal dilators are combined with psychosexual counseling, success rates exceed 97 percent.[4] Silicone vaginal dilators are designed for home use in treating levator ani myalgia. This alternative approach is particularly useful in regions with limited access to a skilled physical therapist.

Move the dilator from side to side for approximately five minutes and then remove the dilator.

Points to Ponder: Tips to Patients on Using Vaginal Dilators

- Use the dilator 2–3 times a week.
- Examine the dilator before each use to be sure that it is smooth.
- Starting with the smallest size dilator, attach the handle to the dilator and apply some gel to the fatter rounded end of the dilator or to the entrance of the vagina. Lie on your back in bed with your knees bent and slightly apart.
- Insert the rounded end of the dilator into the vagina gently and as deeply as you can without discomfort, moving the dilator from side to side for five minutes (Fig 7.12). Do not use force inserting the dilator.
- After use clean dilator with hot soapy water, rinsing it well.
- If you are able to take the present size easily, then next time try using the next size dilator and progress up the sizes.
- Do not be alarmed if there is slight bleeding or spotting following dilator it is normal.

Future

A novel approach to managing pelvic floor myalgia involves local infiltration of botulinum toxin type A (BOTOX) to selectively reduce muscle tension.[5,6] Although the preliminary data from small case series are encouraging, long-term effects and the possibility that overtreatment could cause pelvic organ prolapse or incontinence should limit the use of BOTOX for pelvic floor myalgia to clinical trials.

HYSTERECTOMY

Hysterectomy is surgical removal of the uterus, resulting in inability to become pregnant. This surgery may be done for a variety of reasons including, but not restricted to, chronic pelvic inflammatory disease, uterine fibroids and cancer (Fig. 7.13). A hysterectomy may be done through a transverse or lower abdominal median or a vaginal incision.

The uterus may be completely removed, partially removed, or may be removed with the tubes and ovaries. A partial hysterectomy is removal of just the upper portion of the uterus, leaving the cervix and the base of the uterus are left intact. A total hysterectomy is removal of the entire uterus and the cervix. A radical hysterectomy is the removal of the uterus, both fallopian tubes, both ovaries, and the upper part of the vagina (Fig. 7.14).

The average hospital stay is from five to seven days. Complete recovery may require two weeks to two months. Recovery from a vaginal hysterectomy is faster than from a abdominal hysterectomy. If the bladder was involved, then a catheter may remain in place for three to four days to help the bladder pass urine. Moving about as soon as possible will help to avoid blood clots in the legs. Walking to the bathroom as soon as possible is recommended. Normal diet is encouraged as soon as possible after bowel function returns. Avoid lifting heavy objects for a few weeks following surgery. Sexual activities should be avoided for six to eight weeks after a hysterectomy. Most patients recover completely from hysterectomy. Removal of the ovaries causes immediate menopause and hormone replacement therapy (estrogen) may be recommended.

Cesarean Delivery—An Overview

If a woman is unable to deliver vaginally, the fetus is delivered surgically by performing a cesarean delivery. Cesarean delivery (also called a cesarean section or C-section) is the surgical delivery of a baby by an incision through the mother's abdomen and uterus. This procedure is performed when it is determined to be a safer method than a vaginal delivery for the mother, baby, or both (Fig. 7.15).

In a cesarean delivery, an incision is made through the lower abdominal wall and into the uterus. The incision may be vertical or transverse.

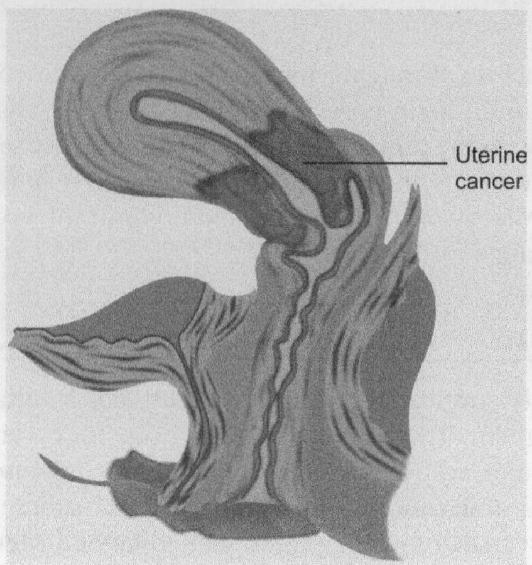

Fig. 7.13: Primary indication for hysterectomy—uterine cancer

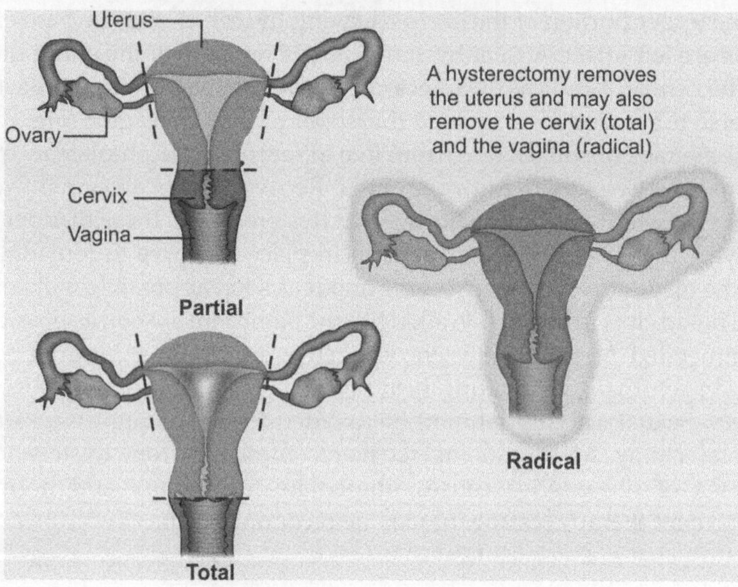

Fig. 7.14: Types of hysterectomy

However, the type of incision is determined by conditions of the mother and the fetus.

A transverse incision extends across the pubic hairline, whereas, a vertical incision extends from the navel to the pubic hairline. A transverse uterine incision is used most often, because it heals well and there is less bleeding. Transverse uterine incisions also increase the chance for vaginal birth in a future pregnancy.

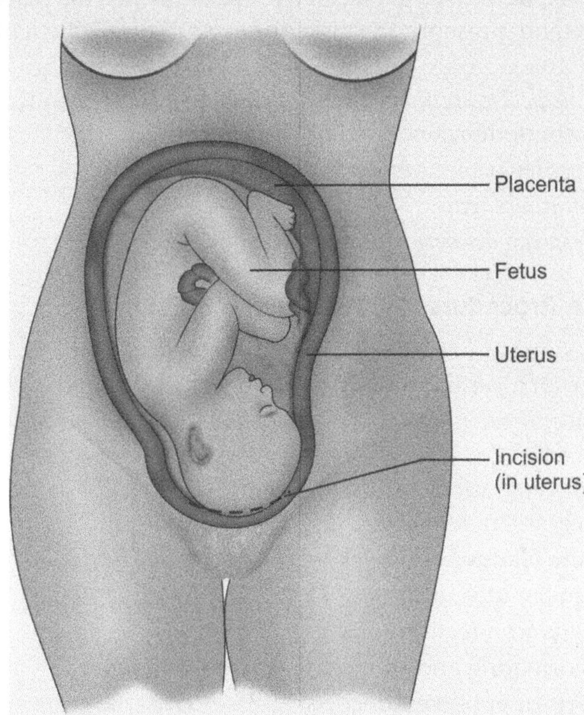

Fig. 7.15: Cesarean section

Reasons for the Procedure

Some cesarean deliveries are planned and scheduled accordingly, while others may be performed as a result of complications that occur during labor.

There are several conditions which may make a cesarean delivery more likely. These include, but are not limited to, the following:

- *Fetal distress indicated by abnormal fetal heart rate:* The fetal heart rate during labor is a good indicator of how well the fetus is handling the contractions of labor. The heart rate is usually monitored electronically during labor, with the normal range varying between 120 to 160 beats per minute. If the fetal heart rate indicates a problem, immediate action can be taken, such as giving the mother oxygen, increasing fluids, and changing the mother's position. A cesarean delivery may be necessary.
- *Abnormal position of the fetus during birth:* The normal position for the fetus during birth is head-down, facing the mother's back. However, sometimes a fetus is not in the right position, making delivery more difficult through the birth canal.
- *Sluggish labor* that fails to progress normally.
- *Baby is too large* to be delivered vaginally.

- *Placental complications,* e.g. placenta previa, in which the placenta blocks the cervix and presents the risk of becoming detached prematurely from the fetus.
- *Maternal medical conditions* such as diabetes, high blood pressure, or human immunodeficiency virus (HIV) infection.
- *Active herpes lesions* in the mother's vagina or cervix.
- *Twins or multiples fetus.*
- *Previous cesarean delivery.*

Risks of the Procedure

As with any surgical procedure, complications may occur. Some possible complications of a cesarean delivery may include, but are not limited to, the following:

- Bleeding
- Abnormal separation of the placenta, especially in women with previous cesarean delivery
- Injury to the bladder or bowel
- Infection in the uterus
- Surgical wound infection
- Difficulty urinating and/or urinary tract infection
- Delayed return of bowel function
- Blood clots.

After cesarean a woman may or may not be able to have a vaginal birth with a future pregnancy. This depends on the type of uterine incision used for the cesarean birth and because the scar may not be strong enough to hold together during labor contractions.

The Procedure

A cesarean delivery is usually performed in an operating room under strict aseptic conditions. In most cases, the patient will be awake for a cesarean delivery because most cesarean deliveries today are performed with a regional anesthesia such as an epidural or spinal. Only in rare situations will a mother require general anesthesia for this type of birth. With spinal/epidural anesthesia, the patient will have no feeling from waist down, and will be awake and able to hear and see the baby as soon as he/ she is born.

Generally, a cesarean delivery follows this process:

1. Patient is undressed completely and dressed in a hospital gown and positioned on an operating or examination table in Lithotomy position.
2. A urinary catheter may be inserted before coming to the operating room and an intravenous (IV) line may be started in the patient's arm or hand.

3. For safety reasons, straps will be placed over the legs to secure the patient position on the table.
4. Hair around the surgical site over the abdomen is shaved and the skin cleansed with an antiseptic solution and draped with sterile sheet. A drape is also be placed above the chest to screen the surgical site from the patient.
5. The anesthesiologist will continuously monitor the heart rate, blood pressure, breathing, and blood oxygen level during the procedure.
6. Once the anesthesia has taken effect, an abdominal skin incision is made above the pubic bone, either in transverse or vertical line and an electrocautery machine is used to seal off bleeding blood vessles. Deeper incisions is made through the lower abdominal muscles until the uterine wall is reached. A final incision is then made on the wall of the uterus. This incision may be either transverse or vertical. The amniotic sac is opened, and the baby is delivered through the opening and the umbilical cord is cut and the placenta removed. The uterus is then be examined for any tears or remaining pieces of placenta. Catgut self-absorbing sutures are used to close the incision in the uterine wall and the uterus repositioned in the pelvic cavity. The muscle and other tissue are closed in layers with self-absorbing sutures and the skin incision is closed with silk sutures or surgical staples. A sterile bandage/dressing is then applied over the surgical wound.
7. Medication to help the uterus contract and expel the placenta, whole blood to compensate for the blood loss during surgery, dextrose/Ringer lactate/normal saline to compensate for electrolyte and nutrition and antibiotics to prevent secondary infection is given through IV.

Postoperative Care

In the Hospital

The patient will be taken to the recovery room for observation immediately after surgery. Nurses will monitor blood pressure, breathing, pulse, bleeding, and the firmness of the uterus at frequent intervals.

Usually, the baby can be brought to the mother while she is in the recovery room. In some cases, babies born by cesarean will first need to be monitored in the nursery for a short time. Breastfeeding can begin in the recovery area, just as with a vaginal delivery.

After about one to two hours in the recovery area, the patient will be moved to her room/ward for the rest of the hospital stay. As the anesthesia wears off, she may receive pain medication as needed, through an infusion pump connected to intravenous line. In some cases, pain medication may be given through the epidural catheter until it is removed.

In addition to the soreness of the abdomen, the patient may also have abdominal cramps due to intestinal gas as the peristalsis begins working again after surgery. She should be encouraged to get out of bed. Moving around and walking are helpful in relieving gas pains. She may also feel some uterine contractions called after-pains for a few days. The uterus continues to contract and get smaller over several weeks.

The urinary catheter will be removed usually by the next day after surgery. Antibiotics may be given through IV while in the hospital and tablets to continue at home.

At Home

The patient will need to wear a sanitary pad for bleeding. It is normal to have vaginal bleeding for several days after birth, followed by a discharge that changes from dark red/brown to a lighter color over several weeks.

One should not douche, use tampons, or have intercourse until the time recommended by the physician and may also have other activity restrictions, including no strenuous activity, driving, or heavy lifting. A follow-up visit with physician will be needed usually two to three weeks after the procedure and physician should be informed if the patient has any of the following:

- Heavy bleeding
- Foul-smelling drainage from vagina
- Fever and/or chills
- Severe abdominal pain
- Increased pain, redness, swelling, or bleeding or other drainage from the incision site
- Leg pain.

Day 1

To reduce the effects of a general anesthetic, one should practice the following exercises hourly throughout the day.

Deep Breathing Exercises

Adequate pain relief is essential because deep breathing could be uncomfortable. Practice the breathing exercises sitting up in bed, supported by pillows, or out in a chair.

Take a deep breath in through the nose, hold for two seconds and then sigh the air out of the mouth. Repeat four times and then try to 'huff' the air out (Fig. 7.16).

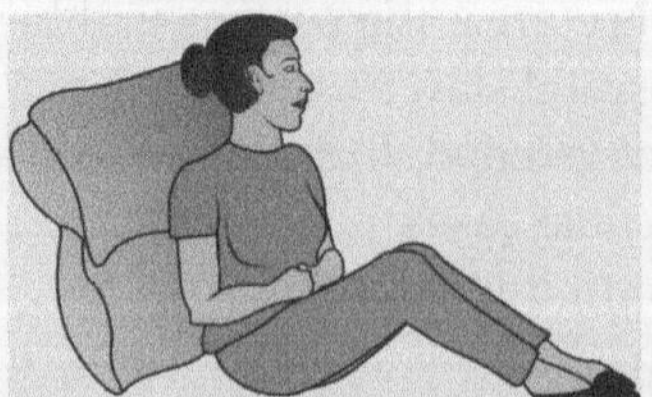

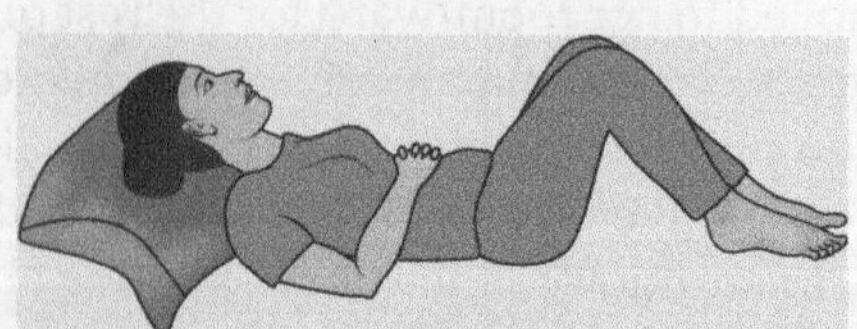

Fig. 7.16: Breathing exercises in supported sitting and supine lying

Huffing

Take a deep breath in, and then breathe out quickly and forcefully blowing through the mouth. This will help loosen any secretions sticking to the walls of the airway.

Coughing

One should be able to cough strongly and effectively to clear any excess secretions. Patients worry about sutures giving way and this may reduce the effectively of the cough. They may find it more comfortable to cough in the same position as for deep breathing exercises. Support the abdominal incision by holding a small towel or pillow firmly over the abdomen. If the operation is through the vaginal route, place a small cushion between the legs.

Circulatory Exercises

These are designed to improve circulation in legs whilst lying in bed or sitting in a chair exercise every hour.

Ankles

Bend and stretch the ankles up and down firmly and quickly. Repeat 10 times (Fig. 7.17).

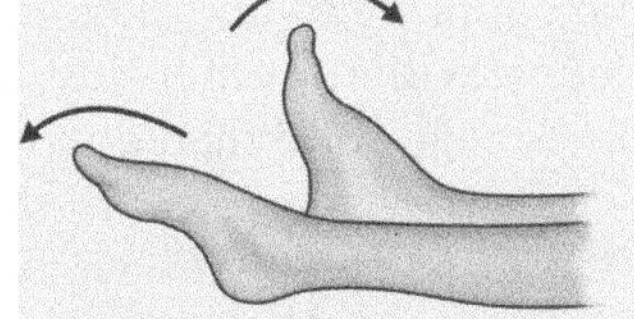

Fig. 7.17: Ankle and foot exercise

Knees

Tighten thighs by pushing the backs of your knees down against the bed contracting the quadriceps and G. Max isometrically. Repeat five times.

Day 2 Onwards

Start all exercises in supine lying with the head on a pillow, knees bent and a shoulder-width apart, feet flat on the bed.

Abdominal Exercise

Gently place hands on lower abdomen. Breathe in through the nose and on expiration feel the abdominal muscles tighten, try to hold for a count of three and then relax. Breathe in and out normally. Practice this exercise three times a day till able to hold for 10 seconds and can repeat 10 times (Fig. 7.18 top).

Pelvic Tilting

Place hands in the hollow of the back. Tighten abdominal muscles and try to flatten the lower back onto the hands and tilt the bottom. Breathe normally. Hold for three seconds and release gently. Try to progress this exercise by tightening abdominal muscles and also pulling up the pelvic floor before continuing as above (Fig. 7.18 Left).

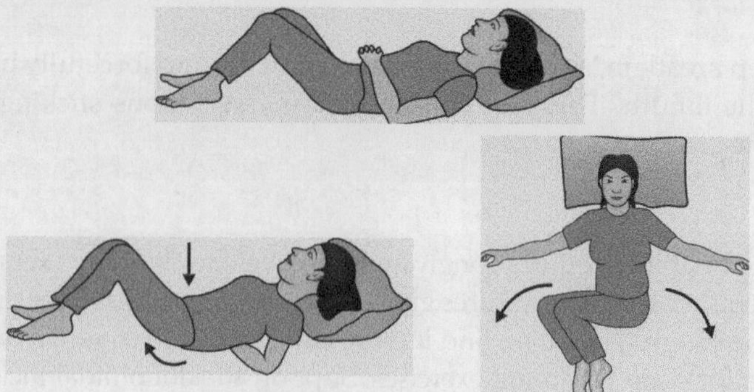

Fig. 7.18: Top—isometric abdominal exercises; Left—pelvic tilting; Right—knee rolling

Knee Rolling

Tighten abdominal muscles and gently lower both knees to one side rotating the spine as far as is comfortable. Bring them back to the middle and relax. Repeat to the other side (Fig. 7.18 Right).

Knee Bends

Tighten your tummy muscles (Exercise 1). Keep your back flat on the bed and bend one hip and knee up as far as is comfortable. Try to hold up to the count of 10 and then replace the leg, so the foot is back on the bed. Repeat with the other side. Repeat each of these exercises four times, three times a day, and then do more as you feel able.

To Get Out of Bed

Bend both knees and roll onto your side by moving your shoulders and knees together. Push up by pressing your upper hand down onto the bed while you lower your feet to the floor. Sit on the edge of the bed and then stand by pushing up with your legs and hands.

Posture and Back Care

It is very important to be aware of one's posture and to take special care for about six weeks after surgery. A good posture will help prevent backache.

Precautions while sitting—Sit upright in a back supportive chair, with both feet flat on the floor. Do not slouch. It helps to place a small cushion or rolled towel in the small of the back to give lumbar support.

Precautions while standing or walking—Avoid supporting the abdomen with hands and slouching forwards. Stand upright with shoulders back, and bottom and tummy tucked in.

Precautions while lifting—Do not lift heavy objects. Try to pull up the pelvic floor, tighten abdominal muscles and breathe out as you lift. Remember to bend your knees and keep your back straight. Hold larger objects close to your body.

Advice on Discharge

Continue with exercises taught by the therapist for at least six weeks. Take a daily rest on bed for about an hour after lunch. Walking is a very valuable exercise. Try to walk for about 20 minutes at least once a day. Hills and stairs are quite safe, but build-up speed and distance gradually. One should not expect to return to full-time work until after six weeks. One should refrain from sexual intercourse for about six weeks.

Do's and Don'ts of Household Activities

Do's

Independent personal hygiene; light housework, such as dusting, ironing, washing and drying dishes; preparing light meals.

Don'ts

Heavy lifting; shaking a heavy bed sheet; cooking a large meal using the oven; heavy housework.

Take things slowly. Be very careful for the first six weeks after the operation. Gradually build-up activity over the next six weeks until able to resume normal lifestyle.

Exercise during Pregnancy

Correct posture and appropriate exercises are important tools to prepare a woman's body for the demanding task of carrying the fetus, labor, birth, postnatal recovery and the strenuous mothering tasks after the baby is born.

Posture

The spine is probably one of the most ignored and least appreciated parts of the body. The vertebrae does far more that just keep our bodies in a vertical position—its many functions include supporting the internal organs, providing protection for the spinal cord and acting as an attachment for ligaments and muscles for the girdles and extremities. Therefore it is not surprising that when one experiences backache, the effects can be felt in almost any part of the body.

The ways in which women stand, sit and lie is very important in pregnancy, because there is now extra strain being placed on the joints, ligaments and muscles, firstly through the added weight of the growing fetus and secondly because of hormones produced during pregnancy soften ligaments in and around the lower back and pelvis in preparation for the birth. Many of the discomforts associated with pregnancy can be avoided or relieved through correct posture, so one must remember the following golden rules and prevent suffering.

Standing

As the pregnancy progresses, the weight of the uterus automatically tends to pull the abdomen forward and down, the woman standing in a 'hunched-up' position and placing unnecessary strain on the lumbar spine, thus resulting in backache. To correct this one should relax the shoulders and retract them slightly to obtain the correct pelvic tilt by pulling the buttocks inward thus raising the front of the pelvis and distribute body weight evenly on both feet, to prevent the pelvis from 'drooping' to one side.

Sitting

When sitting, one should check that the back is well-supported either by own muscles or by the firmness of the chair. A pregnant lady may find it more comfortable and easier to rise from a hard straight-backed chair. This does forces one to concentrate on posture and will also prevent the uterus from placing pressure on alimentary canal and stomach which could result in gastric reflux or heartburn.

Points to Ponder

- If the chair one is using at work does not offer enough support, ask for a more comfortable one or take a few firm cushions along to provide extra padding
- Wherever possible, try sitting in the reverse position, with arms resting on the back of the chair
- Place a box or a stack of books under the feet to keep them slightly raised and prevent from constantly leaning forward
- If the job requires one to sit for long periods, one should remember to get up and move around more than in nonpregnant state
- Sitting on a firm surface with legs crossed, may also be a comfortable position, which will also allow the pelvic muscles to stretch in preparation for labor.

Kneeling

Kneeling on all fours reduces the pressure of the uterus off the back, and many expectant women find kneeling positions comfortable both during pregnancy and labor. Support upper body with arms or try leaning onto the seat of a chair, or in full kneeling place a cushion between the buttocks and heels to avoid pressure.

Bending

When bending down never attempt to try and retrieve something of the floor with straightened legs. Always use the hips and knees when bending over, keeping the back straight and the buttocks over the feet. Also one should ensure that all work surfaces are of the correct height, so there is no need to place added strain on the back by bending over.

Lifting

It is generally safer to leave the lifting of heavy objects to others, as during pregnancy there is a greater possibility of causing damage to the already stressed muscles and joints. However, if the mother to be has a toddler to care for or are required to lift fairly heavy objects, she must remember to bend her knees, and hold the object as close to her body as possible.

Lying Down

In the later stages of pregnancy women may find it more comfortable to prop themselves up with extra pillows that can support their neck and upper half of the body. This is also particularly helpful if they are suffering from heartburn or feel breathless. A pregnant woman may also experience dizziness later in pregnancy due to her circulation being hampered by her sleeping position. If this occurs, she should try bending her knees and keeping her head and shoulders well-raised with the support of extra pillows.

Many women suffer with insomnia during pregnancy and this is somewhat worsened by the discomfort of enlarging abdomen. They may try lying in the 'recovery' position, i.e. high side lying on one side of the body, being supported by few pillows, to catch up on that much needed sleep.

Exercises during and after Pregnancy

Regular exercise can improve blood circulation, help heart work more efficiently and can help control weight in pregnant women. It helps the patient to relax and feel better. The general benefits of regular exercises include:

- Psychological and social benefits, bringing a sense of well-being
- Reduction in aches and pains of pregnancy, e.g. backache, cramp
- Increased circulation minimizes varicose veins and swelling
- Improved stamina, giving you more energy to cope with the growing demands of pregnancy
- Improved posture and body awareness
- More controlled weight gain
- Reduction in the minor ailments of pregnancy such as stiffness, tension, constipation and insomnia
- Aids postnatal recovery
- Improves ability to cope with labor and childbirth.

Appropriate Exercise

- *Gentle swimming*—swimming is a wonderful activity during pregnancy as not only does it relieve bodily strain, it also tones many of the muscle groups with minimal effort.

  If previously an active swimmer, front crawl or back stroke in later stages of pregnancy is recommended.
- *Aquanatal,* a form of water aerobics specifically for pregnancy.
- *Walking*—a simple brisk walk first thing in the morning will work well in expectant mothers, particularly in the later months of pregnancy when other exercises become progressively difficult.
- *Antenatal group exercises* offer great support to the expectant mom, by helping her tune into her body and developing a few lasting friendships. Many of these classes help prepare the women for active labor as well as providing gentle exercise specifically to the pelvic floor during pregnancy under close supervision of an experienced physiotherapist.

It is not advisable to start any new activity during pregnancy apart from those mentioned above.

Dedicated Antenatal Exercises—Group/Individual

Warming-up Exercises

- Stand up straight, feet slightly apart, and weight evenly distributed on each foot. Bend forward from the waist downwards as if trying to touch the toes, and then slowly bring the body back up to upright position. Repeat five times.
- Remain in the standing position, remembering to concentrate on correct posture. Place hands on the hips, and rotate the head, neck and spine from the waist to the left, and back again, and then to the right and back again. Pausing briefly while facing forward. Repeat five times.
- Remaining in the standing position, let arms rest loosely by the sides, while still keeping the back straight. Bend laterally from the waist down to one side, then the other, letting the hands follow the trace of the leg while bending sideways on both sides alternately. Repeat five times.

Stretching Exercises

- Adopt a squatting position with a forward hand hold. Keeping the back as straight as possible and gently spread knees outwards with your elbows. Repeat a few times.
- Kneel sitting on a firm surface with knees far apart. Relax the upper body, resting hands on front of the thighs, and then gently glide forward, sliding hands along the floor until you feel the stretch in buttocks and groin. Remain in that position for at least one minute, breathing deeply. Slowly release the stretch by following the same pattern backwards until achieving the starting position.

Ankle and Foot Exercises

- Sit on the floor with long sitting with hands palm-down behind for support. Point toes down towards the floor, hold for a few seconds, and then extend them upwards. Relax the foot completely, and repeat. This exercise is particularly helpful for those suffering with calf-cramping. Repeat five times.
- Remain in the same position, placing a firm pillow or rolled-up blanket under the calf of one leg, so that the ankle hangs loosely. Now roll the foot round in each direction, always coming up in the middle, out and then round, five times in each direction, then repeat with the other foot.

Arm and Shoulder Exercises

- Stand up straight, weight evenly distributed, and feet slightly apart. Lift both shoulder, bringing it as close to the ear as possible, but without drooping or poking the head forward. Roll the shoulder girdles alternately or together in a complete circle one way five times and repeat in the opposite direction.
- Remain in the same position, with arms firmly by the sides. Raise one arm straight up above the head, and gently swing it down and around, attempting to complete a circle motion, repeating in the opposite direction. Repeat five times in each direction with each arm.

Abdominal Exercises

- Lie on a firm surface with the head and neck supported with a pillow. Keep knees bent and slightly apart, and arms relaxed by the sides. Contract stomach muscles while breathing out, and hold for a count of five, then relax completely while breathing in, keeping the neck and shoulders totally relaxed. Repeat five times.
- Remaining in the same position, flex the hip knees alternately, keeping neck and shoulders on the floor and totally relaxed. Repeat five times.

Back Exercises

- Prone kneel on all fours, with knees slightly apart. Drop the head down and hunch the back towards the ceiling while breathing out, hold for a count of four. Then gently release, dropping the spine downwards while breathing in and raising the head upwards at the same time. Repeat five times.
- Remain prone kneeling, and bring one knee inwards towards the dropped head. Gently kick it out towards the rear, raising the head. Repeat five times with each leg.

Pelvic Exercises

Obtaining the correct pelvic tilt during pregnancy will go a long way in helping the body to adapt to it's changing shape, improve over-all circulation, hopefully relieve some of the pregnancy discomforts and strengthen abdominal and pelvic floor muscles in preparation for labor and those first few strenuous weeks of motherhood.

Pelvic Tilt

Sit on the edge of a hard chair with knees apart. Gently hollow the back, noticing how the pelvis tilts downwards. Now round the lower back, tightening the abdominal muscles. This exercise may also be done in standing position.

Pelvic Floor

Supine lying with head and neck supported by a pillow, hip knee flexed and arms relaxed at sides. Tense the muscles around the vagina, urethra and rectum (as if to stop the flow of urine). Hold for a count of three, and then relax completely. On doing this exercise correctly, you will notice how the knees pull slightly inwards and buttock muscles become tense. This exercise can be practiced almost anywhere without anyone noticing as it does not necessarily require a lying position.

Reasons for Toning the Pelvic Floor Muscles

- Minimizing the effects of stress incontinence in the later stages of pregnancy.
- Giving added support to enlarging uterus and growing baby, thus offering more in the way of comfort during pregnancy.
- Well-toned pelvic floor muscles, also aid in preventing a prolapsed uterus following the birth.
- Increases sexual pleasure for both partners'.

The Golden Rules of Exercise during Pregnancy

- Do not begin a new strenuous exercise activity—stick to what you are familiar with and enjoy.
- Begin slowly, gradually building up a pattern—Rome was not built in a day.
- If you are already part of an aerobics class, ask for the instructor's advice on simple yet effective exercises.
- Stop if it hurts.
- All exercise should be followed with a few minutes of deep breathing and total relaxation.

Relaxation

'Relaxation' in a sense is totally different from 'resting'—one may be resting, either sitting or lying, but that does not mean that the body is totally relaxed. Pregnancy is a wonderful time to become in-tuned with the body's needs, and learning total relaxation techniques will go a long way in ensuring a healthy body and mind, now and forever.

Are you Tense?—A Short Self-assessment

- Do you find it difficult to unwind in the evenings?
- Do you have to make a conscious effort to relax the shoulders?
- Are you frequently irritable and impatient?
- Do you need to resort to alcohol or tobacco to calm your nerves?
- Are headaches a part of your everyday life?
- Have your sleep pattern altered?
- Have your memory and concentration deteriorated?

Many people will answer 'yes' to most, if not all of these questions, and on recognizing these signs of stress, total relaxation techniques will help live a better life.

Preparation

- Sit in a comfortable position on a chair keeping legs crossed and stretched out in front or long sitting on the floor, with the back, neck and head being supported. Take time to find a position that offers you maximum comfort, one where constant adjustment won't be necessary.
- Rest hands on the thighs, or support them with pillows on each side of the trunk.
- Close your eyes, and relax neck and shoulders completely.
- Breathe in and out slowly through the mouth, feeling each breath, and notice how the body relaxes on exhaling. Practice this, until the breathing has settled into a relaxed pattern.

Muscle Relaxation

- Begin by concentrating on each facial muscle. Tense each area of the face and then relax it completely, letting the jaw hang loosely. It is very important that you work on one area at a time, moving from the forehead down towards the chin, leaving each section in a relaxed state.
- Now retract and elevate the shoulders, back and neck, then release completely.
- Move over to the abdominal area, and on inhaling, tighten abdominal muscles. Slowly breathe out, relaxing the abdominal muscles and lower back—always remembering to keep the shoulders well-relaxed.
- Tighten the buttock and pelvic floor muscles and then relax them completely on exhalation—feeling the body sinking further and further back into the chair.
- Tense the thigh and calf muscles on inhalation, and let the tension flow out on exhaling.
- Flex your feet on inhaling, and relax them on the exhaling.

Mind Control

This is probably the more difficult of the two to achieve, as once the body is totally relaxed, the mind seems to wander, and could, depending on your thoughts recreate all the tension that you have just managed to relieve. When practicing relaxation techniques, it is vital that you set time aside for 'yourself' should be unhurried and not just done in-between other pressing duties. If possible, practice the relaxation sessions in a dimly-lit room, where there is unlikely to be any disturbances. Try calming the mind, by visualizing a pleasant location. Imagine that you are sitting on a rock, overlooking the ocean, alone with nature and can hear the splashing sounds of the waves. Once you have managed to obtain the feeling of total relaxation, sit or lie back and enjoy the serenity within yourself, noting how the body feels in this state, so that you will be able to recognize any signs of future tension. The blood pressure may have been lowered during this exercise, so it is wise that while getting up, do it slowly, moving each part of the body to promote blood circulation, thus preventing dizziness. Relaxation comes more easily to some that to others, but in time it will grow in any one allowing one to become fully aware of the body and mind.

The precautions for the pregnant exercises are:

- Do not raise the body temperature needlessly, since the body temperature will already be slightly raised and the heart rate will naturally fluctuate.
- Avoid over-stretching or over-loading the pelvic joints, especially the hips, as the hormone Relaxin helps to relax the connective tissue around pelvic joints making them more vulnerable to stretch or stress injury.
- Avoid isometric contractions as they decrease circulation and increase blood pressure.
- Avoid supine lying after 16 weeks as this may cause dizziness or nausea and may reduce blood flow to the fetus.
- Stretches should be performed for no longer than 10 seconds, as longer stretching may make the joints less stable and more vulnerable to injury. As pregnancy continues into weeks 15–27 weeks, avoid any sudden changes in direction, any high impact exercises, or any sudden increases in exercise intensity.
- Exercises over the head can still be performed, but avoid weight training exercises above the head.
- Do squats and lunges to tone legs, but avoid inner/outer thigh resistance training (Abduction/adduction exercises) during pregnancy. Stop and seek medical advice in case of following symptoms:
- Spotting blood.
- Experiencing any deep pelvic/abdominal pain.
- Experiencing general pain/discomfort.
- Experiencing general pain/discomfort especially in the pelvic region.

Postnatal Exercise

Postnatal exercises can commence on completion of a satisfactory postnatal checkup generally after six weeks of delivery. In case of cesarean section, the delay will be a minimum of eight weeks or up to 12 weeks in emergency cesarean or if the recovery has been slower than usual, before commencing any sort of exercise. The only exercises advisable prior to six or eight weeks postdelivery are exercises such as walking, pelvic tilts and pelvic floor exercises in supine position.

It is essential to start off gently and increase the intensity level of the exercise very gradually. Emphasis must be put on pelvic floor exercises, back care and postural work. Avoid heavy lifting exercises initially and always bend the knees to pick up the baby, which will prevent straining the back. Activities such as brisk walking, aqua exercise or swimming are excellent activities to start exercising again because of the reduced risk of injuries to joints and pelvic floor muscles. Exercises that work the stomach muscles should be very gentle to begin with and must be performed carefully and correctly.

It is important to build-up fitness level gently and in a controlled manner due to the hormone relaxin still being present in the body for up to five months, particularly if breastfeeding the hormone will remain in the system for longer.

REFERENCES

Visceral Manipulation

1. Barral JP, Mercier P. Visceral manipulation. Eastland Press, 1988.
2. Burch JP. Interdisciplinary structural integration: Finding the balance. Massage and Bodywork, April/May 2001;22-31.

Pelvic Floor Disorders

1. Glazer HI, Rodke G, Swencionis C, et al. Treatment of vulvar vestibulitis syndrome with electromyographic biofeedback of pelvic floor musculature. J Reprod Med 1995;40:283-90.
2. Bergeron S, Bouchard C, Fortier M, et al. The surgical treatment of vulvar vestibulitis syndrome: A follow-up study. J Sex Marital Ther 1997;23:317-25.
3. Abramov L, Wolman I, David MP. Vaginismus: An important factor in the evaluation and management of vulvar vestibulitis syndrome. Gynecol Obstet Invest 1994;38:194-7.
4. Schnyder U, Schnyder-Luthi C, Ballinari P, et al. Therapy for vaginismus: In vivo versus in vitro desensitization. Can J Psychiatr 1998;43:941-4.
5. Jarvis SK, Abbott JA, Lenart MB, et al. Pilot study of botulinum toxin type A in the treatment of chronic pelvic pain associated with spasm of the levator ani muscles. Aust N Z J Obstet Gynaecol 2004;44:46-50.
6. Thomson AJ, Jarvis SK, Lenart M, et al. The use of botulinum toxin type A (BOTOX) as treatment for intractable chronic pelvic pain associated with spasm of the levator ani muscles. BJOG 2005;112:247-9.

Postnatal Exercise

Postnatal exercises can commence on completion of a satisfactory postnatal check up, generally after six weeks of delivery. In case of caesarean section, the delivery will be a minimum of eight weeks or up to 12 weeks in [illegible] if the recovery has been slow [illegible] eight weeks postpartum [illegible] exercises such as walking, pelvic tilts and pelvic floor exercises [illegible].

It is sensible to start off gently and progressively increase the level of the exercises very gradually. Emphasis must be put on pelvic floor exercises, back care and posture work. Avoid high impact exercises initially and always bend the knees to pick up the baby which will protect the back. Activities such as brisk walking, aqua aerobics and swimming are excellent activities to start exercising again because of the reduced risk of injuries to joints and pelvic floor muscles. Exercises that work the stomach muscles should be very gentle to begin with and must be [illegible] carefully and gradually.

[illegible]

REFERENCES

Visceral Manipulation

[illegible]

Pelvic Floor Disorders

[illegible]

Index

Page numbers followed by *f* refer to figure and *t* refer to table

E

F

G

H

I

T

U

V

W

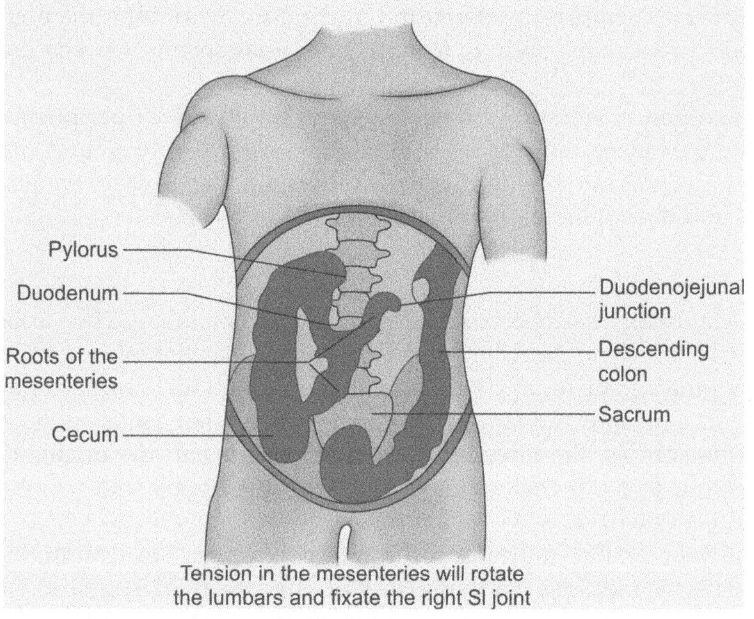

Fig. 7.5: Roots of the mesenteries showing relative positioning of visceral organs within the support matrix

Tension in the mesenteries, and particularly tension in the roots of the mesenteries, will rotate the lumbar spine and fixate the right sacroiliac joint. It is a routine demonstration in visceral manipulation classes to first assess lumbar and sacral position and mobility, and then free the mesenteries. Post-treatment testing of the lumbar and sacroiliac joints shows that a very few minutes of light visceral manipulation makes profound change in lumbosacral position and mobility.[2]

Thorax

The lungs are surrounded by two layers of pleural membranes. The pleura are essentially fascial sheets associated with organs. The inner or visceral pleura form the surface of the lungs. The outer or parietal pleura form the inner surface of the chest cavity.

Between the two layers is a small amount of serous fluid. This lubricant and the space it occupies are maintained at slight negative pressure. This negative pressure means the two pleural surfaces cannot move away from each other and just like two sheets of wet glass, they can slide on each other but cannot be pulled apart.

The top of the parietal pleura forms a dome 2–3 cm above the first rib. The apex of this dome is suspended in part from the bottom side of the middle scalene muscle by the suspensor ligament of the lung. In addition, Sibson's structure attaches the pleural apex to the anterior surface of the transverse process of C_7, sometimes C_6, and occasionally also C_5. Sibson's of support. Therapists, as structural integrators, work with the organ of support to assist the body to form a better relationship between gravity and body.

The organ of support also contains a vast network of peripheral and autonomic innervations. Much of what therapists do as structural integrators is a conversation with this nervous system, particularly the gamma loops and the autonomic nervous system.

Core

A crucial bodily balance exists between surface and core. The surface of the body is easy to describe but the nature and location of core has been an ongoing debate for all of structural integration's half century of development. Currently, advanced Rolfing instructor Jan Sultan and others describe core as 'the visceral space', not referring to the organs themselves, but to the membranous container of the organs and its inherent pressure system.

The membranes supporting the internal organs have multiple and extensive connections with the rest of the organ of support. French Osteopath Jean-Pierre Barral has demonstrated that manipulation of the visceral support system has profound and lasting effects on the organization of the rest of the body. The visceral support membranes have rich autonomic innervations: the number of neurons in the visceral support system exceeds the number of neurons in the spinal cord and brainstem. The several nerve plexus of the visceral support system are literally another brain, named the Enteric brain, and function as a crucial entry point for our conversation with the nervous system. Here are two examples of how the visceral support system affects structure, one in the abdomen and one in the thorax.[1]

Abdomen

The 25 feet of the small intestine are supported by a membrane called the mesentery. If the small intestines are removed with the mesentery attached, and the small intestine is stretched out in a line, the mesentery appears as a 6-inch long curtain hanging from one edge of the intestine. In the body, the edge of the mesentery not attached to the intestine is collected and attached along a 6-inch long line running from the duodenojejunal junction in the upper left quadrant of the abdomen, to the ileocecal valve in the lower right quadrant. Between these two end points the mesenteries attach to the back wall of the abdomen crossing the lumbar spine at a diagonal and also crosses the superior portion of the right sacroiliac joint attaching to both sacrum and ilium. The diagonal line of attachment of the mesenteries to the back wall of the abdomen is called the Roots of the Mesenteries (Fig. 7.5).

Vibration

Use of vibratory massage, applied to the viscera of the lower abdominal region, using electromechanical vibrating platforms, vibrating belts or hand held vibrators can give substantial relief to cramping pain caused by PARD.

Mechanical vibration at variable frequency and amplitude can be safely applied to pelvic adhesions through soles of the feet in standing position or through buttocks in sitting position using a vibrating platform. Vibrating platform exercises also provide significant additional health benefits for women such as increased venous return and vascular tone; improved core and lower extremity muscle tone and power; better postural tone and stability.

Mechanical vibrations may also be applied in the form of rhythmic oscillatory motion through the long axis of the spinal column with the patient in supine position. Such oscillatory motion can induce visceral motion, causing release of protective spasm and stretching of adhesions in the visceral mesenteries (Fig. 7.5). Oscillatory motion in supine position may induce postural hypotension and therefore may be applied with caution in patients with disorders of heart and blood pressure. After the session the patient must be asked to rest for at least five minutes in supine position before being allowed to get up.

Skilled therapists may also use hand held vibrator with large pad (10–15 cm diameter) attachment, to apply localized vibration through the abdominal wall. The degree of pressure applied to the abdominal conditions wall has to be very carefully controlled so as not to cause discomfort to the patient.

The selection of the mode, duration and frequency of vibration as well as selecting suitable patient position is done by the therapist based on patient feedback, since each patient of PARD is unique and may vary widely in their response to vibration. The therapist also has to be careful to avoid vibration therapy in immediate postoperative cases, menstruating patients or patients with active inflammation of the pelvis, indicated by tenderness and raised temperature of the lower abdominal area, in presence of painful micturition or colitis and in presence of IUD.

VISCERAL MANIPULATION

Elisabeth Dicke of Germany developed tissue manipulation technique for the viscera in 1929, which was found to be effective in relieving symptoms chronic pelvic pain syndrome due to PARD. The conditions that benefited from this nonsurgical approach include vulvodynia, vulvar-vestibulitis, dyspareunia (painful intercourse), vaginismus, interstitial cystitis and chronic pelvic pain. This technique however was never accepted by mainstream practitioners, who preffered medicine and electrotherapy for treatment of pelvic pain.

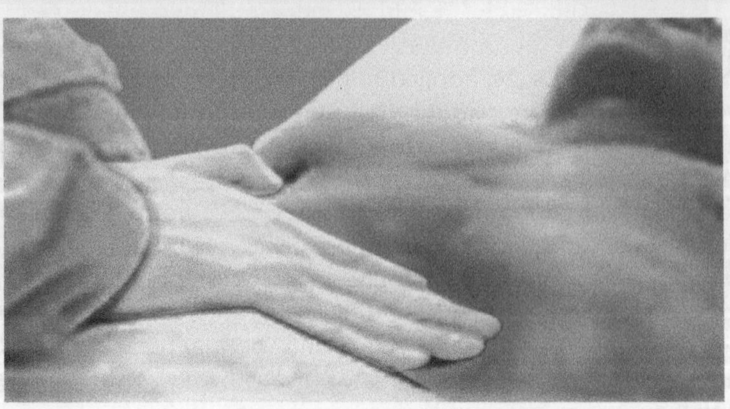

Fig. 7.4: Visceral manipulation

In recent times however, with growing public distrust towards drug based treatment, osteopathic visceral manipulation, alongside physiotherapy, has generated widespread professional interest in treatment of pelvic pain.

Jean Pierre-Barral, a french osteopathic physician, developed the art of visceral manipulation. Visceral manipulation is a gentle hands-on therapy that works with the body's visceral system, such as the heart, liver, intestines and other internal organs. The therapist lightly places their hands in very specific locations on the client's body and manually works to encourage the normal mobility and tone of the viscera and their surrounding structures, releasing restrictions and thus helping the organs to move and glide freely and encouraging the organ to a more balanced position (Fig. 7.4). This gentle therapy can help to improve the function of any organ or organ system within the viscera and improve the health of the body in general.[1]

Visceral manipulation is believed by its practitioners to be beneficial for the following disorders: Bloating, constipation, GERD, chronic pelvic pain, bladder incontinence, pelvic pain, headaches, migraines, anxiety and depression.[1]

Principles of Visceral Manipulation

Osteopathic principles of visceral manipulation are based on structural integration which emphasizes the interaction of the human body with earth's gravity. The following describes how structural integration and visceral manipulation work with each other.

Fascial Continuity

The human body is held together and given its shape by connective tissue. Developing early in fetal growth, all of the connective tissue in the human body is continuous. About 20 percent of the weight of the human body is connective tissue. Collectively this connective tissue matrix is the organ